New and Emerging Diseases

Editors

SUE CHEN
NICOLE R. WYRE

VETERINARY CLINICS OF NORTH AMERICA: EXOTIC ANIMAL PRACTICE

www.vetexotic.theclinics.com

Consulting Editor
AGNES E. RUPLEY

May 2013 • Volume 16 • Number 2

ELSEVIER

1600 John F. Kennedy Boulevard • Suite 1800 • Philadelphia, Pennsylvania, 19103-2899
http://www.vetexotic.theclinics.com

VETERINARY CLINICS OF NORTH AMERICA: EXOTIC ANIMAL PRACTICE Volume 16, Number 2
May 2013 ISSN 1094-9194, ISBN-13: 978-1-4557-7348-0

Editor: John Vassallo; j.vassallo@elsevier.com
Development Editor: Teia Stone

Veterinary Clinics of North America: Exotic Animal Practice (ISSN 1094-9194) is published in January, May, and September by Elsevier, Inc., 360 Park Avenue South, New York, NY 10010-1710. Subscription prices are $243.00 per year for US individuals, $389.00 per year for US institutions, $124.00 per year for US students and residents, $289.00 per year for Canadian individuals, $457.00 per year for Canadian institutions, $326.00 per year for international individuals, $457.00 per year for international institutions and $159.00 per year for Canadian and foreign students/residents. To receive student/resident rate, orders must be accompanied by name of affiliated institution, date of term, and the *signature* of program/residency coordinator on institution letterhead. Orders will be billed at individual rate until proof of status is received. Foreign air speed delivery is included in all *Clinics* subscription prices. All prices are subject to change without notice. **POSTMASTER:** Send address changes to *Veterinary Clinics of North America: Exotic Animal Practice*, Elsevier Health Sciences Division, Subscription Customer Service, 3251 Riverport Lane, Maryland Heights, MO 63043. **Customer Service: Telephone: 1-800-654-2452** (U.S. and Canada); **1-314-447-8871** (outside U.S. and Canada). Fax: 1-314-447-8029. E-mail:**journalscustomerservice-usa@elsevier.com** (for print support); **journalsonlinesupport-usa@elsevier.com** (for online support).

Reprints. For copies of 100 or more of articles in this publication, please contact the Commercial Reprints Department, Elsevier Inc., 360 Park Avenue South, New York, New York 10010-1710. Tel.: (212)-633-3813; Fax: (212)-633-1935; E-mail: reprints@elsevier.com.

Veterinary Clinics of North America: Exotic Animal Practice is covered in *MEDLINE/PubMed (Index Medicus).*

Printed and bound by CPI Group (UK) Ltd, Croydon, CR0 4YY
Transferred to digital print 2013

Contributors

CONSULTING EDITOR

AGNES E. RUPLEY, DVM
Diplomate, American Board of Veterinary Practitioners–Avian Practice; Director and Chief Veterinarian, All Pets Medical & Laser Surgical Center, College Station, Texas

EDITORS

SUE CHEN, DVM
Diplomate, American Board of Veterinary Practitioners–Avian Practice; Associate Veterinarian, Gulf Coast Avian and Exotics, Gulf Coast Veterinary Specialists, Houston, Texas

NICOLE R. WYRE, DVM
Diplomate, American Board of Veterinary Practitioners–Avian Practice; Service Head, Exotic Companion Animal Medicine and Surgery Section, Department of Clinical Studies, Matthew J. Ryan Veterinary Hospital, University of Pennsylvania, Philadelphia, Pennsylvania

AUTHORS

JOÃO BRANDÃO, LMV
School of Veterinary Medicine, Louisiana State University, Baton Rouge, Louisiana

SUE CHEN, DVM
Diplomate, American Board of Veterinary Practitioners–Avian Practice; Associate Veterinarian, Gulf Coast Avian and Exotics, Gulf Coast Veterinary Specialists, Houston, Texas

JULIE DECUBELLIS, DVM, MS
Clinical Instructor, Department of Zoological Companion Animal Medicine, Cummings School of Veterinary Medicine, Tufts University, North Grafton, Massachusetts

THOMAS M. DONNELLY, BVSc
Diploma in Veterinary Pathology; Diplomate, American College of Laboratory Animal Medicine; Diplomate, American Board of Veterinary Practitioners–Exotic Companion Mammals; The Kenneth S. Warren Institute, Ossining, New York

PAUL M. GIBBONS, DVM, MS
Diplomate, American Board of Veterinary Practitioners–Reptile and Amphibian Practice; Turtle Conservancy Behler Chelonian Center, Ojai, California

JENNIFER GRAHAM, DVM
Diplomate, American Board of Veterinary Practitioners–Avian Practice and Exotic Companion Mammal Practice; Diplomate, American College of Zoological Medicine; Assistant Professor, Department of Zoological Companion Animal Medicine, Cummings School of Veterinary Medicine, Tufts University, North Grafton, Massachusetts; Affiliate Assistant Professor, Department of Comparative Medicine, University of Washington School of Medicine, Seattle, Washington

SHARMAN M. HOPPES, DVM
Diplomate, American Board of Veterinary Practitioners–Avian Practice; Clinical Associate Professor, Department of Small Animal Clinical Sciences, College of Veterinary Medicine and Biomedical Sciences, Texas A&M University, College Station, Texas

PETER J. KERR, BVSc, PhD
CSIRO Entomology, Canberra, ACT, Australia

ERIC KLAPHAKE, DVM
Diplomate, American Board of Veterinary Practitioners–Avian Practice; Diplomate, American College of Zoological Medicine; Diplomate, American Board of Veterinary Practitioners–Reptile and Amphibian Practice; Veterinarian, Cheyenne Mountain Zoo, Colorado Springs, Colorado

LA'TOYA V. LATNEY, DVM
Lecturer and Attending Clinician, Exotic Companion Animal Medicine and Surgery Section, Department of Clinical Studies, Matthew J. Ryan Veterinary Hospital, University of Pennsylvania, Philadelphia, Pennsylvania

CHRISTOPH MANS, med vet
Clinical Instructor in Zoological Medicine, Department of Medical Sciences, Special Species Health Service, School of Veterinary Medicine, University of Wisconsin, Madison, Wisconsin

JÖRG MAYER, DVM, MSc
Diplomate, American Board of Veterinary Practitioners–Exotic Companion Mammals Practice; Diplomate, European College of Zoological Medicine Small Mammal; Associate Professor, College of Veterinary Medicine, University of Georgia, Athens, Georgia

COLIN McDERMOTT, VMD
Relief Veterinarian, National Aquarium in Baltimore, Baltimore, Maryland; Exotic Companion Animal Medicine and Surgery Section, Department of Clinical Studies, Matthew J. Ryan Veterinary Hospital, University of Pennsylvania, Philadelphia, Pennsylvania

DENNIS MICHELS, VMD
Intern, Gulf Coast Avian and Exotics, Gulf Coast Veterinary Specialists, Houston, Texas

GLENN H. OLSEN, DVM, MS, PhD
Veterinary Medical Officer, USGS Patuxent Wildlife Research Center, Laurel Maryland

BRIAN PALMEIRO, VMD
Diplomate, American College of Veterinary Dermatology; Lehigh Valley Veterinary Dermatology and Fish Hospital, Pet Fish Doctor, Allentown, Pennsylvania

SUSAN J. PELLO, VMD, MS
Small and Exotic Animal Veterinarian, Animal and Bird Health Care Center, Cherry Hill, New Jersey; Consulting Veterinarian, Hawk Mountain Sanctuary, Kempton, Pennsylvania

H.L. SHIVAPRASAD, BVSc, MS, PhD
Diplomate, American College of Poultry Veterinarians; Professor, Avian Pathology, California Animal Health and Food Safety Laboratory System - Tulare Branch, University of California, Tulare, California

ZACHARY J. STEFFES, DVM
Pet Hospital of Peñasquitas, San Diego, California

IAN TIZARD, BVMs, BSc, PhD
Diplomate, American College of Veterinary Microbiologists; Professor, Department of Veterinary Pathobiology, College of Veterinary Medicine and Biomedical Sciences, Texas A&M University, College Station, Texas

CLAIRE VERGNEAU-GROSSET, DVM
Companion Avian and Exotic Animal Medicine, University of California, Davis, California

JAMES WELLEHAN, DVM, MS, PhD
Diplomate, American College of Zoological Medicine; Diplomate, American College of Veterinary Microbiologists; Assistant Professor, Zoological Medicine Service, College of Veterinary Medicine, University of Florida, Gainesville, Florida

NICOLE R. WYRE, DVM
Diplomate, American Board of Veterinary Practitioners–Avian Practice; Service Head, Exotic Companion Animal Medicine and Surgery Section, Department of Clinical Studies, Matthew J. Ryan Veterinary Hospital, University of Pennsylvania, Philadelphia, Pennsylvania

Contents

rhabdovirus, arenavirus, and paramyxovirus epidemiology, divergence, and host fidelity are presented. A new emerging bacterial disease of *Uromastyx* species, *Devriesea agamarum*, is reviewed. *Chrysosporium ophiodiicola*–associated mortality in North American snakes is discussed. *Cryptosporidium* and pentastomid infections in squamates are highlighted among emerging parasitic infections.

Avian bornavirus (ABV) has been shown the cause of proventricular dilatation disease (PDD) in psittacines. Many healthy birds are infected with ABV, and the development of PDD in such cases is unpredictable. As a result, the detection of ABV in a sick bird is not confirmation that it is suffering from PDD. Treatment studies are in their infancy. ABV is not restricted to psittacines. It has been found to cause PDD-like disease in canaries. It is also present at a high prevalence in North American geese, swans, and ducks. It is not believed that these waterfowl genotypes can cause disease in psittacines.

Of the many important avian wildlife diseases, aspergillosis, West Nile virus, avipoxvirus, Wellfleet Bay virus, avian influenza, and inclusion body disease of cranes are covered in this article. Wellfleet Bay virus, first identified in 2010, is considered an emerging disease. Avian influenza and West Nile virus have recently been in the public eye because of their zoonotic potential and links to wildlife. Several diseases labeled as reemerging are included because of recent outbreaks or, more importantly, recent research in areas such as genomics, which shed light on the mechanisms whereby these adaptable, persistent pathogens continue to spread and thrive.

Chinchillas have been successfully maintained in captivity for almost a century. They have only recently been recognized as excellent, long-lived, and robust pets. Most of the literature on diseases of chinchillas comes from farmed chinchillas, whereas reports of pet chinchilla diseases continue to be sparse. This review aims to provide information on current, poorly reported disorders of pet chinchillas, such as penile problems, urolithiasis, periodontal disease, otitis media, cardiac disease, pseudomonadal infections, and giardiasis. This review is intended to serve as a complement to current veterinary literature while providing valuable and clinically relevant information for veterinarians treating chinchillas.

Abnormal conditions of the thyroid and parathyroid in the guinea pig appear in the English-language scientific literature on an emerging basis. Although true descriptions of abnormal thyroid and parathyroid anatomy or morphology are not new findings, the clinical condition of abnormal thyroid or parathyroid function seems to be a more common observation by clinicians in recent years. This article is an overview of general clinical conditions and adequate diagnosis, and offers treatment options.

This article reviews diagnosis and management of gastrointestinal diseases in guinea pigs and rabbits. The review includes established causes of gastrointestinal disease in these species. The authors highlight syndromes that may be considered emerging or less-recognized causes of gastrointestinal stasis, including gastric dilation and volvulus in guinea pigs and lead toxicity, colonic entrapment, and liver torsion in rabbits. Practitioners should recommend initial diagnostics, including radiographs and blood work on guinea pigs and rabbits presenting with nonspecific signs of gastrointestinal stasis, to better determine possible cause and make the best treatment recommendations.

Viral diseases of rabbits have been used historically to study oncogenesis (e.g. rabbit fibroma virus, cottontail rabbit papillomavirus) and biologically to control feral rabbit populations (e.g. myxoma virus). However, clinicians seeing pet rabbits in North America infrequently encounter viral diseases although myxomatosis may be seen occasionally. The situation is different in Europe and Australia, where myxomatosis and rabbit hemorrhagic disease are endemic. Advances in epidemiology and virology have led to detection of other lapine viruses that are now recognized as agents of emerging infectious diseases. Rabbit caliciviruses, related to rabbit hemorrhagic disease, are generally avirulent, but lethal variants are being identified in Europe and North America. Enteric viruses including lapine rotavirus, rabbit enteric coronavirus and rabbit astrovirus are being acknowledged as contributors to the multifactorial enteritis complex of juvenile rabbits. Three avirulent leporid herpesviruses are found in domestic rabbits. A fourth highly pathogenic virus designated leporid herpesvirus 4 has been described in Canada and Alaska. This review considers viruses affecting rabbits by their clinical significance. Viruses of major and minor clinical significance are described, and viruses of laboratory significance are mentioned.

Since their introduction as pets several decades ago, ferrets have become an increasingly popular household pet. Great strides have been made in improving their diet and understanding common diseases (eg, insulinoma, hyperadrenocorticism, lymphoma) that affect them. With the frequency with which these conditions are seen, it sometimes is easy to forget that ferrets can be affected by other diseases. Some of these diseases, such as cryptococcosis, are known, but may be increasing in incidence and range, whereas others, such as hypothyroidism and pure red cell aplasia, may be underrecognized or underreported. This review highlights new and emerging diseases not already well reviewed in the literature.

x   *New and Emerging Diseases*

VETERINARY CLINICS OF NORTH AMERICA: EXOTIC ANIMAL PRACTICE

THE CLINICS ARE NOW AVAILABLE ONLINE!
Access your subscription at:
www.theclinics.com

Preface

New and Emerging Diseases

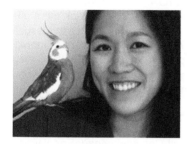
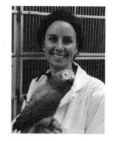

Sue Chen, DVM, Dipl. ABVP–Avian   Nicole R. Wyre, DVM, Dipl. ABVP–Avian
Editors

The term "emerging diseases" is generally used to describe infectious diseases that are appearing in a population for the first time, or that may have existed previously, but are rapidly increasing in incidence or changing in geographic range. As pathogens mutate, gain resistance to medications, or jump into new hosts, infectious diseases such as cryptococcosis in ferrets, are showing a re-emergence in different countries. Pathogenic organisms such as *Batrachochytridium dendobaditis* and Ranavirus are contributing to significant global population declines in amphibians, while others, such as avian influenza and West Nile virus, have zoonotic potential. We have taken the liberty to also include new noninfectious diseases in this issue as some conditions have only been recently described in those particular species. One example is pure red cell aplasia in ferrets. Additionally, we may not know if a condition has an infectious cause or we are still in the process of characterizing that infectious agent, as is the case for avian bornavirus and proventricular dilatation disease. The goal of this issue was to review the latest published information about new diseases in various exotics species, especially for those diseases not already well described. We also wanted to include updates on emerging diseases that may have been already described, but have novel diagnostic tests or innovative treatment protocols, such as many of the viral diseases of squamates.

Some of these diseases may not actually be "new," but may have been simply underrecognized or underreported. Interestingly, diseases such as hyperthyroidism in guinea pigs or inclusion body disease of cranes may have been long recognized in certain regions of the world, but may not have been seen elsewhere until now. Another example, Koi herpesvirus started off in one country but is now a global concern. Some diseases may have been previously experimentally induced, such as otitis media in laboratory chinchillas, but increasing numbers of natural infections are now being identified in our pet populations. By utilizing techniques used by researchers in the laboratory setting, we can now sample and treat middle ear infections in our pet chinchillas more effectively. Other diseases, such as gastric dilation

Vet Clin Exot Anim 16 (2013) xi–xii
http://dx.doi.org/10.1016/j.cvex.2013.02.005

and volvulus in guinea pigs and liver lobe torsions in rabbits, have been reported sporadically over the last several decades on necropsy, but only recently with improved diagnostic imaging and laboratory tests are we able to recognize the conditions early enough to successfully treat these patients.

The contributing authors are your colleagues that have come from a variety of backgrounds and represent an international group of individuals. We thank them all for their "blood, sweat, and tears" in reviewing the latest literature to produce this issue of *Veterinary Clinics of North America: Exotic Animal Practice*. We also want to thank John Vassallo for his guidance and assistance in putting this issue together. We certainly have learned a great deal in preparing this edition and we hope that you also glean some pearls of wisdom during your reading.

Sue Chen, DVM, Dipl. ABVP–Avian
Gulf Coast Avian and Exotics
Gulf Coast Veterinary Specialists
1111 West Loop South, Suite 110
Houston, TX 77027, USA

Nicole R. Wyre, DVM, Dipl. ABVP–Avian
Exotic Companion Animal Medicine and Surgery
Matthew J Ryan Veterinary Hospital
University of Pennsylvania
3900 Delancey Street
Philadelphia, PA 19104-6010, USA

E-mail addresses:
drchen@gcvs.com (S. Chen)
wyre@vet.upenn.edu (N.R. Wyre)

Selected Emerging Infectious Diseases of Ornamental Fish

Colin McDermott, VMD[a,b,*], Brian Palmeiro, VMD, DACVD[c]

KEYWORDS

- Koi herpesvirus • Ranavirus • Megalocytivirus • *Francisella* • *Cryptobia iubilans*
- *Exophiala*

KEY POINTS

- Emerging infectious diseases of fish include various viral, bacterial, parasitic, and fungal diseases, including goldfish herpesvirus, koi herpesvirus, Ranavirus, Megalocytivirus, Betanodavirus, *Francisella*, *Cryptobia iubilans*, and *Exophiala*.
- Although many emerging diseases do not have proper treatments or cures, exceptional husbandry and biosecurity is recommended for the prevention of all infectious diseases.
- As molecular techniques and diagnostics improve, more emerging diseases will be discovered, expanding our understanding of important diseases in ornamental fish.

INTRODUCTION

An emerging disease is one that has appeared in a population for the first time or that may have existed previously but is rapidly increasing in incidence, geographic range, or identification. The following discussion focuses on important emerging infectious diseases that affect ornamental fish in the aquarium and aquaculture industries. The following diseases were selected based on their clinical significance in ornamental fish medicine. Several of these diseases are listed by the World Organization for Animal Health (OIE) (**Box 1**).

VIRAL DISEASES

Because of the changing nature of viral taxonomy and classification, all viruses are named and discussed using the current nomenclature from the International Committee on Taxonomy of Viruses (ICTV) at the time of writing (ICTV 2011 Master

[a] National Aquarium in Baltimore, Pier 3, 501 East Pratt Street, Baltimore, MD 21202, USA; [b] Exotic Companion Animal Medicine and Surgery Section, Department of Clinical Studies, Matthew J Ryan Veterinary Hospital, University of Pennsylvania, 3900 Delancey Street, Philadelphia, PA 19104, USA; [c] Lehigh Valley Veterinary Dermatology and Fish Hospital, Pet Fish Doctor (www.petfishdoctor.com), 4580 Crackersport Road, Allentown, PA 18104, USA
* Corresponding author.
E-mail address: Cmcd.vmd@gmail.com

Vet Clin Exot Anim 16 (2013) 261–282
http://dx.doi.org/10.1016/j.cvex.2013.01.006
1094-9194/13/$ – see front matter © 2013 Elsevier Inc. All rights reserved.

> **Box 1**
> **OIE listed diseases of fish 2013**
>
> Epizootic hematopoietic necrosis[a]
>
> Epizootic ulcerative syndrome
>
> Infection with *Gyrodactylus salaris*
>
> Infectious hematopoietic necrosis
>
> Infectious salmon anemia
>
> Koi herpesvirus[a]
>
> Red sea bream iridoviral disease[a]
>
> Spring viremia of carp
>
> Viral hemorrhagic septicemia
>
>   [a] Discussed in this article.

Species List Version 2). Novel and unassigned viruses are discussed as applicable. Major emerging viral diseases of ornamental fish can be separated into distinct families, including Alloherpesviridae, Iridoviridae, and Nodaviridae.

Alloherpesviruses

Herpesviruses are enveloped, doubled-stranded DNA viruses with an icosahedral capsid. Herpesviruses show strong host specificity but some have the ability to infect multiple species with varying clinical signs. The order Herpesvirales can be broken down into 3 distinct families based on the types of animals they infect: Herpesviridae that infect mammals, birds, and reptiles; Alloherpesviridae that infect fish and amphibians; and Malacoherpesviridae, which contains the single recognized herpesvirus of bivalve mollusks (Oyster herpesvirus).[1] The family Alloherpesviridae can be further divided into 2 clades, one consisting of viruses from cyprinid and anguillid hosts and one consisting of viruses that affect ictalurid, salmonid, acipenserid, and ranid hosts.[2]

Cyprinid herpesvirus 1 (CyHV-1 or Carp pox) typically results in self-limiting hyperplastic cutaneous lesions; a full description of the virus and clinical signs can be found elsewhere.[3,4] Cyprinid herpesvirus 2 (CyHV-2) and cyprinid herpesvirus 3 (CyHV-3) are important emerging diseases of major concern for the ornamental fish trade and are discussed in further detail later.

Cyprinid herpesvirus 2

CyHV-2 (goldfish herpesvirus or herpesviral hematopoietic necrosis virus) was first described as a herpesvirus from an outbreak of disease in goldfish (*Carassius auratus*) in the autumn of 1992 and the spring of 1993 in western Japan.[5] Since then, the virus has been isolated from goldfish collections worldwide, including a recirculating aquaculture system on a small goldfish farm in California[6] and in hobby and breeder ponds in Delaware and Ohio.[7] The virus has be found internationally in Taiwan, Australia, and southern England.[8–10]

Prevalence studies in the United States have shown viral detection by polymerase chain reaction (PCR) from goldfish production facilities in all areas of the country. In a sampling of apparently healthy 6-month-old goldfish from 18 commercial farms across 3 East Coast states, 14 farms (78%) were found to have detectable levels of

CyHV-2.[7] This disease has a worldwide distribution but can go undetected in latent carriers or undiagnosed because of the limited availability of confirmatory diagnostic tests.

Clinical signs Clinical signs of CyHV-2 infection are largely nonspecific, and infections may only be suspected because of high mortality rates in farmed goldfish. When present, common antemortem clinical signs include lethargy, anorexia, inappetence, and respiratory signs; but they are often lacking, and mortalities may be the first and only clinical sign of infection.[11] Goldfish of any age may be infected with higher mortalities in juvenile fish. Mortalities may be acute and widespread or chronic with low-grade mortalities persisting over subsequent years.[9,10] In most reported cases, the onset of clinical signs was correlated with the change to spring or autumn temperatures (15°C–25°C).[10]

Diagnosis The initial diagnosis of the disease can be made from gross necropsy and histopathology. Major postmortem lesions include pale gills, coelomic effusion, splenomegaly with white nodules, and swollen kidneys (**Fig. 1**). In some cases, gross necropsy findings more typical for koi herpesvirus (KHV) are seen (enophthalmos, gill necrosis, notched nose). Histologic examination of the anterior kidney generally shows varying levels of necrosis. Necrotic lesions of the exocrine pancreas, hematopoietic tissues, spleen, and intestinal mucosa can also be seen.[5,6,9] Intranuclear inclusion bodies typical of herpesvirus infections may be present (**Fig. 2**).

A definitive diagnosis of the disease requires viral isolation in cell culture or PCR testing. The virus is infrequently isolated in cell culture and does not commonly produce a cytopathic effect in most cell lines.[6,7] A quantitative PCR has been developed and used experimentally to detect infections with CyHV-2 without cross reacting to other cyprinid herpesviruses. This PCR test has been used to detect virus in both clinically affected and apparently healthy, latently infected fish using spleen and posterior kidney samples.[7] Viral loads in clinically affected fish were significantly higher than those of apparently healthy fish. In most cases of moribund fish analyzed by quantitative PCR, fish with clinical signs had viral densities more than 10^6 copies per microgram host DNA.[7]

Treatment/Prevention There is no known treatment of CyHV-2 infection. Because of the apparent worldwide prevalence of the virus, the best way to control the disease is through prevention of outbreaks. Good husbandry and quarantine protocols are recommended to reduce the chance of a viral outbreak. Quantitative PCR may be more

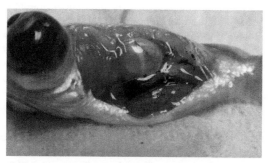

Fig. 1. Telescope goldfish (*Carassius auratus*) with goldfish herpesvirus infection. Note the pale gills. (*Courtesy of* Brian Palmeiro, VMD, DACVD, Allentown, PA.)

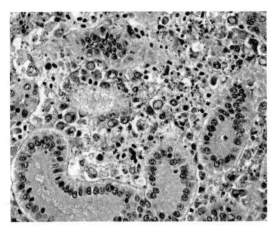

Fig. 2. Goldfish herpesvirus infection in the posterior kidney. Note the areas of necrosis and intranuclear inclusion bodies. (*Courtesy of* Thomas B. Waltzek, MS, DVM, PhD, Gainesville, FL.)

helpful than traditional PCR to monitor for disease because the viral load seems to correlate with signs of disease in affected fish.[7] Maintaining temperatures outside of the permissive range for the virus seems to limit clinical signs and may be an effective way to control outbreaks. In one case, bringing the temperature to more than 27°C stopped all mortalities at one breeding operation. Dropping and holding the temperature to 10°C slowed the replication of the virus.[7] Fish that recover from infection are considered carriers.

Cyprinid herpesvirus 3 (koi herpesvirus)

KHV (CyHV-3, carp interstitial nephritis, and gill necrosis virus) infects and causes massive mortality in koi and common carp (*Cyprinus carpio*).[12] KHV was first reported as a cause of massive fish mortality in Israel in 1998 and is now global in distribution.[13,14] It is listed as a reportable disease by the OIE.[15]

Clinical signs Clinical signs of KHV can be found in **Box 2**. On postmortem examination, all fish have gill necrosis, which often presents as patchy regions of white discoloration (**Fig. 3**). The necrosis can range from mild to severe; in more mild cases, you may just see the loss of gill epithelium with exposed lamellar cartilage. Other gross necropsy changes are nonspecific and may include darkening or mottling of internal organs (eg, the spleen, kidney, or liver), coelomic fluid accumulation, and adhesion formation.[14,15] Wet-mount examination of the gills shows necrosis with complete loss of normal lamellar architecture. Secondary skin and gill parasitic and bacterial infections are extremely common.

Virulent virus is shed via the feces, urine, and skin/gill mucus.[15] The main portal of entry for KHV in koi has recently been shown to be the skin,[16] with systemic spread of the virus from the skin and gills through the bloodstream (via white blood cells) to the kidney and other organs, such as the spleen, liver, and intestines.[17,18] Branchitis and interstitial nephritis are seen histologically as early as 2 days after infection, but mortality does not typically occur until 6 to 8 days after infection.[17,18] The virus causes lysis of infected cells (**Fig. 4**).[17] Different strains that vary in virulence have been reported but are thought to arise from the same KHV ancestor.[19]

Water temperature contributes significantly to the course of the disease, both directly by affecting viral replication and indirectly by modulating the fish's immune

---

Box 2
Clinical signs of KHV infection

- Piping (gasping at water surface)
- Elevated opercular rate
- Gathering near the surface and in well-aerated areas, such as near waterfalls/filter input
- Excessive mucus from the gills
- Mottled areas of gill necrosis/discoloration (see **Fig. 3**)
- Skin changes, including ulcers, hemorrhages, sloughing of scales, and increased or decreased mucus production
- Lethargy
- Anorexia
- Sunken eyes (enophthalmos)(see **Fig. 3**)
- Notched appearance dorsal to the nares (notched nose) (see **Fig. 3**)
- Erratic swimming
- Hanging with a head-down position in the water column
- High-level mortality (typically 70%–100%)

---

response.[15] The permissive range for clinical infection with KHV is 16°C to 28°C (61°F–82°F),[20] and clinical disease is only seen within this temperature range.[17] Fish seem most susceptible to clinical disease and mortality between 21°C and 27°C (72°F–81°F).[14] Typically, mortality approaches 70% to 100% over a course of 7 to 21 days.[20] The virus can replicate in common carp at 13°C (55°F) and in cell culture at 4°C (39°F), supporting the hypothesis that the virus can overwinter with the fish.[20,21] No growth occurs in cell culture at 30°C (86°F) or more.[20]

Fish surviving infection, including those subjected to elevated water temperatures following infection, develop partial or complete resistance to reinfection.[20] Fish that survive KHV infection are considered lifelong carriers of the virus, although it is currently unknown what percentage become carriers. In an effort to determine the site of latency, a recent publication evaluated normal fish from facilities with a history of KHV infection or exposure.[22] KHV DNA, but not infectious virus or mRNAs from lytic infection, were detected in white blood cells from investigated koi, suggesting that leukocytes are at least one possible site of latency for KHV.[22]

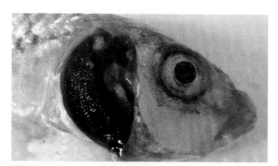

Fig. 3. Koi infected with KHV. Note patchy white areas of gill necrosis, notched nose, and hyphema. (*Courtesy of* Brian Palmeiro, VMD, DACVD, Allentown, PA.)

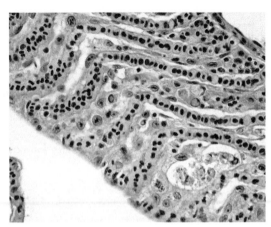

Fig. 4. Gill from koi infected with KHV. Note the intranuclear inclusion bodies and hyperplasia. (*Courtesy of* Thomas B. Waltzek, MS, DVM, PhD, Gainesville, FL.)

Common carp that recover from KHV infection can become persistently infected and may shed the virus to infect naïve fish at water temperatures greater than 20°C (68°F).[23] In one study, the virus became reactivated and infected naïve fish up to 30 weeks after the initial infection.[23] Given that persistently infected fish are created, exposing fish to KHV at nonpermissive temperatures is not considered a safe method of disease prevention.[23]

Diagnosis The diagnosis of KHV is based on clinical signs combined with the detection of the virus via virus isolation (on the KF-1 cell line) or DNA identification via PCR. PCR is considered the most sensitive diagnostic modality available[24]; in cases of an acute infection, PCR is the most practical and rapid method of diagnosis. Because KHV is most abundant in the gill, kidney, and spleen, these organs should be submitted for virologic testing.[15] The detection of KHV DNA via PCR is extremely difficult beyond 64 days after exposure.[21]

Currently, the most concerning and difficult aspect in the diagnosis of KHV is the ability to detect carrier fish. Detection of KHV antibodies is currently the only method of determining previous exposure to the virus if viral DNA is not detectable via PCR assays.[15] An enzyme-linked immunosorbent assay (ELISA) was shown to detect antibodies in the serum of koi for up to 1 year after previous exposure to the virus.[25] In a recent study, ELISA detected the antibody up to 65 weeks after exposure.[23] Serum antibodies have been shown to peak 3 to 4 weeks after infection with high levels of antibodies being maintained for several months, followed by a gradual and continuous decrease with time.[26] A quantitative KHV ELISA is currently commercially available at the University of California Davis Veterinary Teaching Hospital.

False-negative serology results may occur early in the course of exposure because the development of positive titers may take several weeks to develop. False positives may occur because of cross-reactions on ELISA testing between KHV and CyHV-1 but occur more commonly at lower serum dilutions.[23]

A KHV real-time PCR has been shown to detect DNA from white blood cells in 9 out of 10 fish previously exposed to KHV.[22] This test is currently under development for commercial use at Oregon State University and would provide another modality for detecting KHV carrier fish.

Treatment There is no effective treatment of KHV. Depopulation and disinfection is recommended because fish that survive infection are considered carriers. In private collections, some owners may elect to treat their pet fish. The water temperature can be increased to greater than 29°C (84°F) to help reduce morbidity and mortality. Secondary bacterial and parasitic infections are extremely common and must be treated accordingly. Prolonged bath immersion with salt (0.1%–0.3%) can be used to decrease osmotic stresses associated with gill necrosis and cutaneous ulceration. The owners must be thoroughly educated by the veterinarian that surviving fish are considered carriers and should not be mixed with naïve fish. If the owners wish to introduce new fish, it is recommended that only fish vaccinated for KHV be added to the system.

Prevention Methods to control and prevent KHV include avoiding exposure to the virus, good hygiene and biosecurity practices, and vaccination. Fish should be purchased from reputable sources and quarantined for a minimum of 4 to 6 weeks at permissive temperatures. Quarantine should be combined with blood testing to aid in the detection of carrier fish.

Goldfish housed with infected koi have been shown to harbor KHV without developing clinical disease, implicating their role as a possible vector in spreading of KHV.[27] Another study found that goldfish do carry the genome of KHV and that the genome can persist in goldfish for long periods following an outbreak.[28] An antemortem test to screen for the presence of the KHV carrier state in goldfish is not currently available, and the duration of carriage in goldfish is unknown; therefore, caution should be taken when introducing goldfish into any existing koi population.

The first report of successful vaccination of carp for KHV involved an attenuated virus that was created through serial transfer in cell culture; koi exposed to this attenuated virus were resistant to the disease.[29] The attenuated virus was then irradiated to decrease its pathogenicity and formulated into a modified live vaccine delivered by immersion.[29] Short-term immersion was found to be sufficient for infection/immunization, and the attenuated virus was found to be active in the water for at least 2 hours.[29]

A modified live KHV vaccine is approved by the US Department of Agriculture for use in koi. The vaccine is manufactured in Jerusalem, Israel and has been approved and used successfully by large koi producers in Israel since 2005. The virus was attenuated by 26 passages in cell culture followed by UV irradiation and selection by cloning.[17] The attenuated virus (referred to by the company as KV3) is reported to have more than 31 mutations in its DNA compared with the wild-type virus. The vaccine is available in 2 sizes: the smaller vial (10 mL) treats up to 20 kg of fish and the larger (100 mL) treats up to 200 kg of fish. During vaccination, the water temperature should be maintained between of 22°C and 26°C (71°F–79°F), with a pH of 6.8 to 7.4 and a dissolved oxygen of at least 6 ppm.[30] The vaccine is thawed and added into a defined volume of water (100 L/26.4 gal for smaller size, 1000 L/264 gal for larger size).[30] The fish are immersed into the well-aerated vaccine bath for 45 to 60 minutes. After vaccination, the fish should be placed back into water between 18°C and 28°C (64°F–82°F) for at least 5 days.[30] The duration of immunity with this vaccine is currently not known, but it is recommended that fish be revaccinated before periods of stress or exposure.[30] Some practitioners are recommending once yearly revaccination.

The vaccine has been shown to be safe in koi carp weighing greater than 90 g, with demonstrated mortality in smaller koi weighting 10 to 20 g. A recent study found that survival after vaccination was directly related to the fish body weight, with 100%

survival of fish weighing 87 g or greater.[31] Quantitative PCR for KHV peaked on day 14 in vaccinated fish and 94% tested negative/weak positive at day 28.[31] Naïve fish cohabitated with vaccinated fish did not develop any clinical signs of KHV.[31] The use in brood stock has not been evaluated.

Average survival of vaccinated fish after exposure to KHV is reported to be 88%.[30] One study found that mortality in vaccinated fish following KHV challenge only occurred in fish less than 70 g.[31] The survival rate was higher in the vaccinated group (97%) compared with the control (17%).[31]

Vaccinated koi have been shown to mount an antibody response to the virus.[26] The protection against KHV in recently vaccinated fish is proportional to the titer of anti-virus antibodies.[26] However, even vaccinated fish with no detectable antibodies have been shown to be resistant to infection with KHV, probably because of the subsequent rapid response of high affinity antivirus antibodies.[26] The fact that anti-virus antibodies neutralize the pathogenic effects of the virus in vitro emphasizes the central role probably played by the antibodies in anti–CyHV-3 protection in vivo.[26]

KHV can survive in pond water for at least 4 hours at temperatures of around 22°C (72°F)[26] and probably survives for much longer periods in feces and pond mud.[32,33] Its ability to survive in water likely plays an important role in its rapid spread between fish.[17] Common disinfectants that can be used on the system and equipment include chlorine (such as household bleach) at 200 mg/L and quaternary ammonium compounds.[14] Other disinfectants that are reported to inactivate the virus include iodophor at 200 mg/L for 20 minutes, benzalkonium chloride at 60 mg/L for 20 minutes, and 30% ethyl alcohol for 20 minutes.[17] Ponds and equipment can also be drained and dried, but the virus may survive in mud and pond sediment so complete drying for a minimum of 2 weeks is recommended.

Iridovirdae

Iridoviridae is a family of double-stranded DNA viruses currently comprised of 5 genera: *Iridovirus*, *Chloriridiovirus*, *Megalocytivirus*, *Ranavirus*, and *Lymphocystivirus*. *Iridovirus* and *Chloridiovirus* commonly infect invertebrate species. *Megalocytivirus*, *Ranavirus* and *Lymphocystivirus* infect lower vertebrates.[34] Lymphocystis disease virus 1 is the most common iridovirus in aquarium and pet fish. It causes a hypertrophy of dermal fibroblasts resulting in nodular tumorlike lesions in fresh and marine finfish. Infection is typically self-limiting and has been discussed in detail elsewhere.[35]

Ranavirus

Ranaviruses are major emerging diseases of fish and amphibians worldwide. Ranaviruses are large viruses ($\sim$150 nm in diameter) with an icosahedral structure. They contain a genome of approximately 105 kb and replicate in the cytoplasm and nucleus of host cells.[34] There are multiple ranaviruses reported in fish but only 3 are officially recognized by the ICTV in the *Ranavirus* genus: Epizootic hematopoietic necrosis virus (EHNV), European catfish virus (ECV), and Santee Cooper ranavirus (SCV, largemouth bass virus). Because EHNV and ECV are genetically close to one another and produce similar clinical signs and pathologic conditions, they will be considered together in further discussion. Santee Cooper virus and associated strains (guppy virus 6 and doctor fish virus) are more distantly related; although some investigators have suggested that they are not true ranaviruses, they are still considered part of the genera taxonomically by the ICTV.[36]

Ranaviruses, unlike the alloherpesviruses, lack host specificity. This lack of host specificity allows them to cause disease across many species, although the clinical signs of disease may vary by species. For example, EHNV, the first iridovirus to cause epizootic mortality in vertebrates, was discovered in Australia in 1985. Outbreaks of this disease caused mortality in wild redfin perch (*Perca fluviatilis*) but less severe disease in rainbow trout (*Oncorhynchus mykiss*).[37]

Clinical signs All ranaviruses in fish, except for SCV, produce a systemic necrotizing infection. Epizootic hematopoietic necrosis virus produces an often-fatal systemic disease in redfin perch and rainbow trout. On postmortem examination, there is often multifocal necrosis of the liver, spleen, and renal hematopoietic tissue. Grossly, the kidney and spleen may be swollen, and the liver will have miliary pale foci. There may be petechial hemorrhage at the base of the fins. If fish do survive the infection, they can be found to have extensive perivascular infiltrates of mononuclear cells.[34]

Santee Cooper ranavirus infection may be subclinical or cause mortalities. Clinical signs include erratic swimming or hyperbuoyancy caused by effects on the swim bladder, but this is uncommon.[38] Experimentally, the mortality rate of infection varies based on the isolate of SCV used and the route of infection. Inoculation of the virus into young largemouth bass seems to cause high mortalities, whereas exposure to the virus via bath or gavage shows lower mortality rates (less than 17%).[39] Natural transmission is assumed to be through direct contact with infected fish or ingestion of viral particles in food or water.

Diagnosis Histologically, basophilic intracytoplasmic inclusion bodies may be identified within the hepatocytes at the margins of necrotic foci or within splenic or renal interstitial cells. In some cases, the splenic foci may be diffuse and generalized.[34] Other variable signs have been described, including hyperplasia and multifocal necrosis of branchial epithelial cells, necrosis of atrial trabeculae and gastrointestinal (GI) epithelial cells, focal pancreatic necrosis of redfin perch, and ulcerative dermatitis and swim bladder edema and necrosis of rainbow trout.[40]

Diagnosis of ranavirus infections can be made from several tissue samples. The highest viral loads are typically found in the liver, spleen, and kidney.[34] The gold standard for diagnosis is virus isolation in cell culture monolayers.[34] When grown at 15°C to 22°C (59°F–72°F) on FTM, RTG, and BF–2 of CHSE–214, the virus produces a focal lytic cytopathic effect.[37,41] This effect is followed by the destruction of the monolayer in a few days. Viral presence is then confirmed by indirect fluorescent antibody stain, antigen-capture ELISA, electron microscopy, or PCR.[34]

In the cases of the SCV, there have been reports of low levels of wild largemouth bass with positive gill samples. Often, there are no obvious lesions on gross necropsy, aside from an overinflated swim bladder.[42] It has been suggested that the gills, swim bladder, and posterior kidney should be submitted for diagnosing SCV.[34]

Treatment/prevention There are no treatments currently available for ranavirus infections. Experimentally, redfin perch and rainbow trout develop antibody titers when injected with inactivated EHNV, but no vaccine is currently available.[34] Good husbandry practices are the best preventative measure for the disease. These practices include maintaining proper water quality, minimizing stress, and a proper quarantine protocol for bringing new fish into the collection because infection seems to be spread through the environment or ingestion of infected fish or tissues.[34] Stocking density may impact disease levels. It was found that juvenile largemouth bass in aquaria maintained under high stocking densities were 1.6 times more likely to show morbidity or mortality caused by SCV compared with those at lower stocking densities.[34]

Megalocytivirus

There are currently 3 well-described viruses within the *Megalocytivirus* genus, including infectious spleen and kidney necrosis virus (ISKNV), red sea bream iridovirus (RSIV), turbot reddish body iridovirus (TRBIV), or turbot iridiovirus.[43] ISKNV and closely related viral strains have caused disease in numerous species of freshwater and marine fish, including grouper, gourami, cichlid, red sea bream, angelfish, sea bass, and lampeye.[44] RSIV was first discovered in the early 1990s in Japan and has been reported in Asian marine finfish; it is a reportable disease to the OIE. TRBIV mainly affects Asian flounder species.[44] Other megalocytiviruses have been described based on molecular diagnostics and histologic diagnosis but are not placed in the family by the ICTV (**Table 1**). Megalocytivirus infections have been reported in several common ornamental fish, including Banggai cardinalfish *(Pterapogon kauderni)*,[45] freshwater angelfish *(Pterophyllum scalare)*, other freshwater cichlids, sailfin mollies *(Poecilia latipinna)*, other common live-bearers, and numerous gourami species.[44]

Clinical signs Fish infected with any of the megalocytiviruses show nonspecific signs of disease, including lethargy, loss of appetite, darkening, abnormal swimming or position in the water column, increased respiration, coelomic distension, ulceration/hemorrhages, pale gills/anemia, fin erosion, white feces, and death. Mortality may be up to 100% in some outbreaks.[44] On postmortem examination, there will be necrosis of internal organs, especially the spleen, kidney, and liver. Splenomegaly is common. Other affected organs include the muscles, gonad, heart, gills, and GI tract. There may be amber or hemorrhagic fluid in the coelomic cavity.[44]

The onset of clinical signs for megalocytiviruses has been correlated with environmental stressors that weaken the immune system and warmer temperatures. Megalocytiviruses have been reported to cause disease at water temperatures ranging from 20°C to 32°C (68°F–90°F).[44] In a study of RSIV in rock bream (*Oplegnathus fasciatus*), no infections were seen in temperatures less than 12°C (54°F), and the incubation period for disease decreased as the temperature was increased to 30°C (86°F).[46]

Diagnosis Megalocytivirus infection can be suspected with clinical signs and postmortem findings. Histologically, numerous distinctive hypertrophied cells can be

Table 1 ICTV-recognized megalocytiviruses of fish	
Viral Species Recognized by ICTV	**Viral Strains/Isolates**
ISKNV	Dwarf gourami iridovirus
	African lampeye iridovirus[a]
	Banggai cardinalfish iridovirus
	Mullet iridovirus
	Marble sleepy goby iridovirus
	Taiwan grouper iridovirus
RSIV	African lampeye iridovirus[a]
TRBIV	Flounder iridovirus
	Rock bream iridovirus
	Three-spine stickleback iridovirus

[a] African lampeye iridovirus may be placed in the ISKNV or RSBIV group based on differences in molecular analysis.

found throughout affected organs, namely, the spleen, kidney, GI tract, and less commonly in the liver, gills, and connective tissue. In affected cells, large foamy to granular basophilic inclusion bodies will fill the cytoplasm and may displace or compress nuclei (**Fig. 5**). These cells are often found along perivascular areas where they may occlude blood vessels resulting in ischemic necrosis.[44] A definitive diagnosis can be made by viral isolation, electron microscopy, or PCR testing (**Fig. 6**).[44]

Treatment/prevention There is no known treatment of fish infected with any of the megalocytiviruses. The treatment of concurrent diseases can be attempted but may only delay the mortality from the viral infection. The prevention of disease outbreaks may best be accomplished by good husbandry and biosecurity protocols. If there is concern of infection for new shipments of fish, a small number can be sacrificed and tested. A formalin-based vaccine has been developed and is commercially available in Japan for RSIV.[47]

Betanodavirus

Viruses in the family Nodaviridae are nonenveloped RNA viruses with an icosahedral capsid roughly 29 to 35 nm in diameter. Nodaviridae can be divided into 2 major genera or clades: *Alphanodavirus*, which primarily affect insects, and *Betanodavirus*, which primarily affect fish. The terms *viral nervous necrosis*, *encephalopathy*, and *vacuolating encephalopathy and retinopathy* (VER) have all been used to describe the signs of betanodaviral infections, although VER is the official term for the disease as proposed by the OIE in 2003.[48]

In the late 1980s, descriptions of brain lesions consistent with betanodoviral infections were described concurrently in barramundi in Australia and European sea bass in the Caribbean. In 1990, a virus with the structure of a nodavirus was found associated with nervous necrosis in Japanese parrot fish[49] and barramundi larvae.[50] The causative agent of VER in striped jack (striped jack nervous necrosis nirus) in Japan was identified as a new member of the family Nodaviridae in 1992.[51] Since then, several betanodaviruses have been described and have been found on all continents except Africa.[48] A list of betanodavirus species and several isolates can be found in **Box 3**.

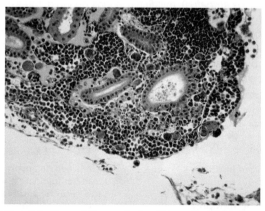

Fig. 5. Megalocytivirus infection of the posterior kidney in *Xiphophorus maculatus* (platy fish). Note the large basophilic cells and necrosis (H & E stain). (*Courtesy of* Roy P.E. Yanong, VMD, Ruskin, FL.)

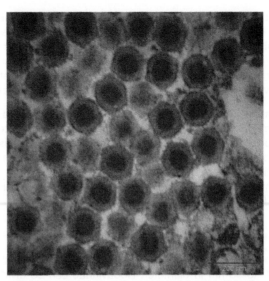

Fig. 6. Transmission electron microscopy of megalocytivirus in the spleen of a *Pterapogon kauderni* (Banggai cardinalfish). (*Courtesy of* Thomas B. Waltzek, MS, DVM, PhD, Gainesville, FL.)

Based on natural and experimental infections, betanodaviruses have been reported to infect numerous fish species, but are more common in marine fish.[48] Recently, freshwater ornamental guppies (*Poecilia reticulate*) were experimentally infected with a betanodavirus recovered from *Lates calcarifer*. Low mortality (11%) from 3 to 14 days after infection was observed, but the postmortem examination showed characteristic lesions of VER in the brain and retina. Virus was also found with reverse transcriptase PCR, proving infection of a freshwater species from a marine betanodavirus.[52] A survey of apparently healthy aquarium fish in South Korea tested for betanodavirus showed a 4.64% detection rate (11 out of 237 fish tested) in marine and freshwater fish and invertebrates using nested PCR.[53] Betanodavirus was detected in shrimp fish (*Aeoliscus strigatus*), milkfish (*Chanos chanos*), three-spot damsel (*Dascyllus trimaculatus*), Japanese anchovy (*Engraulis japonicus*), pinecone fish (*Monocentris japonica*), blue ribbon eel (*Rhinomuraena quaesita*), look down fish (*Selene vomer*), yellow tang (*Zebrasoma flavesenes*), South American leaf fish (*Monocirrhus polyacanthus*), red piranha (*Pygocentrus nattereri*), and spiny lobster (*Pamulirus versicolor*). Of the 11 positive fish, virus was cultured from 3 samples and shown to be the

---

Box 3
Betanodaviruses of fish—ICTV recognized and unclassified

Viral species recognized by ICTV	*Unclassified betanodaviral strains*
Barfin flounder nervous necrosis virus	Japanese flounder nervous necrosis virus
Respotted grouper nervous necrosis virus	*Lates calcarifer* encephalitis virus
Striped jack nervous necrosis virus	Atlantic halibut nodavirus
Tiger puffer nervous necrosis virus	Malabar grouper nervous necrosis virus
	Dicentrarchus labrax encephalitis virus

identical strain of red-spotted grouper virus.[54] There is evidence for vertical transmission in some species, notably in striped jack (*Pseudocaranx dentex*)[55]; but the true mode of transmission is still unknown.

Clinical signs Most fish are affected as larvae or juveniles, although outbreaks of disease have been seen in older fish in association with high water temperatures or other environmental stressors.[55] Mortality may be up to 100%. Infected fish will show signs correlated to the lesions in the brain and retina, including abnormalities in movement, sight, and coloration. Larval barramundi and halibut become pale, whereas groupers, juvenile halibut, European sea bass, and turbot become dark.[48] Fish will seem to be uncoordinated and darting can be seen. Flatfish may show looping swimming behavior and rest upside down.[48]

Diagnosis Tentative diagnosis is made on histologic examination of the central nervous system. The consistent finding on histology among all species is the vacuolization and necrosis of the central nervous system. Commonly, the anterior brain is more severely affected than the posterior brain and spinal cord. Intracytoplasmic vacuoles ranging from 1 to 5 μm depending on the species of fish are present in the gray matter of the brain. Other lesions include shrinkage and basophilia of affected cells, focal pyknosis and karyorrhexis of neural cells, granularity of the neutrophil, and the presence of mononuclear cell infiltrates. Retinal lesions have also been found in all instances when the eye has been examined.[48] Vacuolization of the bipolar and ganglionic nuclear layers and the rod and cone layer have been reported.[48] The presence of the virus can be confirmed by transmission electron microscopy, immunohistochemistry, or the use of indirect fluorescent antibodies. Reverse transcription PCR (RT-PCR) testing has been developed to test the presence of the virus in tissues of infected fish.[56,57]

Treatment/Prevention There is no treatment of betanodavirus infections. Prevention is aimed at keeping positive fish out of collections or breeding operations by implementing proper quarantine protocols and screening new shipments with nested RT-PCR looking for carriers. Disinfection of facilities and tanks between uses or new groups of fish can be achieved with 50 ppm sodium hypochlorite, benzalkonium chloride, or iodine for 10 minutes at 20°C.[55] Reducing environmental stresses and maintaining low stocking densities have also shown to decrease the incidence of disease.[48] Experimental vaccination with recombinant nodavirus coat proteins has shown some success, but DNA vaccines do not seem to be effective.[48]

BACTERIAL DISEASES
Rickettsial-like Organisms: Piscirickettsia salmonis and Francisella

Systemic infections caused by gram-negative intracellular bacteria that are difficult to culture on standard laboratory media have been recognized for many years in fish.[58] These infections have been commonly referred to as *Rickettsial-like* because of the morphologic similarities with the true *Rickettsia*.[58] Previous descriptions of Rickettsia-like organisms in fish may have been caused by *Piscirickettsia salmonis* or *Francisella spp. P salmonis* is the most commonly described rickettsial pathologic condition and infection in salmonids and has been reviewed elsewhere.[59] The genus *Francisella* is closely related to and similar in morphology and pathogenesis to *P salmonis*. Despite morphologic similarities, the genera *Francisella* and *Piscirickettsia* belong to the γ-proteobacteria and are, therefore, only distantly related to the true *Rickettsia* (α–proteobacteria).[58]

Francisella has been described in fish as early as the 1970s as an agent of tularemia; however, the species of *Francisella* that affect fish are genetically distinct from tularemia that affects humans and other mammals (*Francisella tularensis*).[60] The recent description and resurgence of *Francisella* in fish started with isolation of the bacteria in farmed saltwater and freshwater tilapia in Taiwan in 1994. In mortalities of blue-eyed plecostomus catfish (*Panaque suttoni*) shipped from Columbia, Khoo and colleagues[61] identified Rickettsial-like organisms from moribund specimens on transport. Since then, *Francisella* or *Francisella*-like bacteria have been described in numerous species of fish and invertebrates (**Box 4**). Molecular diagnostics have identified 2 major species of *Francisella* that affect fish: *F asiatica* (syn *F noatunensis subsp orientalis*)[62] and *F noaturensis*.[60] With better detection and reporting of this disease, the number and range of affected species are expected to increase.

Clinical signs Clinical signs of *Francisella* infections in fish are similar to other Rickettsial-like infections and include lethargy, anorexia, pale gills, anorexia, and abnormal swimming behavior.[60] Atlantic cod affected by *F noatunensis* may have raised hemorrhagic nodules on the skin.[60] On postmortem examination, white to cream-colored, partially raised nodules may be present on the spleen, heart, liver, and kidney with coelomic distension and serohemorrhagic effusion (**Fig. 7**).[60] Tilapia affected by *F asiatica* may not have these hemorrhagic nodules but may exhibit some petechiae, loss of scales, and erosions.[60] Splenomegaly and anterior renomegaly are consistent postmortem signs in tilapia.[60]

Diagnosis Histopathology of lesions shows a chronic, severe granulomatous host response. These granulomas consist of macrophages, fibroblasts, and lymphocytes of varying maturity depending on the chronicity of the disease. In addition to the granulomas, necrotizing vasculitis and thrombosis can be found throughout affected tissues.[60]

Cell culture is the gold standard of identifying an infection with *Francisella*. However, culture of *Francisella* can be difficult and requires a media with a source of iron and cysteine.[58] *Francisella* can also be grown in cell culture on various cell lines, with the maximum cytopathic effect occurring 5 to 7 days after inoculation.[60] Several PCR tests have been used experimentally to identify the bacteria to species, but the specificity and sensitivity varies based on the methodology.[58] In situ hybridization has also been described to identify *Francisella spp* in histologic samples.[63]

Treatment/Prevention As with other infectious diseases, good husbandry and biosecurity practices are key to prevention. Various antibiotics have been used to try and control infections, and Florfenicol has shown promise in controlling experimental infections in tilapia. Soto and colleagues[64] found that the use of Florfenicol in food at

---

Box 4
Summary of reported *Francisella spp* infections of fish and shellfish

Fish/shellfish species affected	*Primary Francisella species implicated*
Tilapia (*Oreochromis* sp)	*Francisella asiatica*
Atlantic cod (*Gadus morhua*)	*Francisella noatunensis*
Atlantic salmon (*Salmo salar*)	*Francisella sp*
Three-lined grunt (*Parapristipoma trilineatum*)	*Francisella sp*
Ornamental cichlids (various species)	Unknown (*Francisella*-like bacterium)
Hybrid striped bass (*Morone chrysops* × *M saxatilis*)	Unknown (*Francisella*-like bacterium)
Giant abalone (*Haliotis gigantea*)	*Francisella halioticida sp nov*

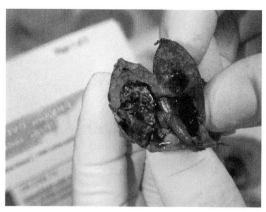

Fig. 7. Tilapia (*Oreochromis* sp) with Francisella infection. Note the pale, mottled, nodular kidney and spleen. This fish was cut dorsal to ventral approximately midway down the body and flapped open. (*Courtesy of* Roy P.E. Yanong, VMD, Ruskin, FL.)

a concentration of 15 or 20 mg/kg body weight per day for ten days significantly increased survivability compared with control groups. Florfenicol given at these concentrations was not able to completely clear infections in fish based on splenic cultures. An experimental vaccine based on an attenuated *iglC* mutant of *F noatunensis subsp orientalis* showed protective levels in experimentally challenged tilapia.[60] No vaccine is currently commercially available.

PARASITIC DISEASE
Cryptobia iubilans

Cryptobia (class Kinetoplastida, family Bononidae) is a genus that encompasses a wide variety of flagellated fish parasites. There are 52 currently identified species of *Cryptobia* in fish, including 5 species that infect the gills and skin (most commonly *Cryptobia branchialis*), 7 that infect the GI tract, and the remaining 40 that infect the blood (*Trypanoplasma spp.*).[65] It is speculated that because of their small size and structure, there may not be 52 individual species and these species may be combined with further studies. The species that affect the skin, gills, and GI tract have a direct life cycle, whereas the hemoparasitic species have an indirect life cycle most commonly spread by leeches.[65]

Cryptobia iubilans was first identified almost 30 years ago[66] but has received recent attention for the severity of disease found in captive populations in recent years.[67] *Cryptobia iubilans* is a small (10–13 μm long and 2 μm wide) protozoal parasite with 2 flagella of unequal lengths extending from the anterior end that move in slow, undulant movements. Organisms are characterized by having a prominent kinetoplast, paraxial rod, and cytoskeleton comprised of microtubules beneath the body surface on transmission electron microscopy. *C iubilans* has been described as causing disease in several East African and Central American cichlids and described in detail in discus (*Symphysodon spp.*).[67]

Clinical signs The clinical signs of *Cryptobia iubilans* infection are largely nonspecific and related to the granulomatous gastritis caused by the organism. Common clinical signs include anorexia, weight loss, abnormal appearing stools, darkening of the skin, lateral recumbency, lethargy, decreased fecundity, and hanging and moving slowly in the water column (**Fig. 8**). Morbidity and mortality are higher in younger fish (aged

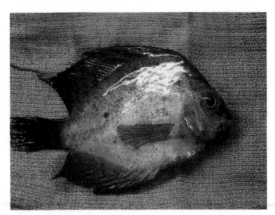

Fig. 8. Emaciated discus fish with *Cryptobia iubilans* infestation. (*Courtesy of* Brian Palmeiro, VMD, DACVD, Allentown, PA.)

<2 months old) when the mortality rate may be as high as 70% to 90%. Fish more than 2 months old suffer high morbidity but low mortality (2%–5%).[67] These older fish show an increased opercular rate and mucus production for up to 1 week before recovering. Coinfection with other parasites has been described.[67]

Diagnosis Presumptive diagnosis can be made on necropsy with the presence of granulomas found most commonly in the submucosa and mucosa of the stomach and intestines. Granulomas can also be found in other organs, including the liver, spleen, mesentery, mesenteric fat, heart, swim bladder, anterior and posterior kidneys, gall bladder, ovary, brain, and eye (**Fig. 9**).[67] Granulomas caused by *C iubilans* can be distinguished from granulomas caused by *Mycobacterium spp* via acid-fast staining. When the trophozoites are occasionally found on a wet-mount preparation of stomach/intestinal contents, they exhibit a slow, undulating movement.[67]

Tissues can be examined histologically for the parasite and surrounding inflammation. Single to coalescing granulomas can be seen in the mucosa or submucosal layer as large foci of macrophages surrounded by fibroblasts with cores of degenerative

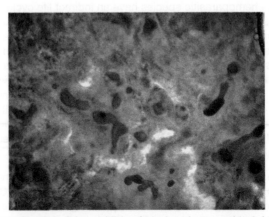

Fig. 9. Wet mount of spleen from cichlid infected with *Cryptobia iubilans*. (*Courtesy of* Roy P.E. Yanong, VMD, Ruskin, FL.)

cells and nuclear debris. Thickening of the submucosal layer can occur in severely affected cases. In some cases, elongate to ovoid flagellated structures can be found within vacuoles of the macrophages. Scanning or transmission electron microscopy is required to further visualize and speciate the protozoa based on structure.[67]

Treatment/Prevention There is no treatment of *Cryptobia iubilans*. Because of the granulomatous gastritis caused by the parasites, it may be difficult to impossible to completely eradicate in infected fish. Attempts have been made to treat affected fish with little to no response. Some farmers have reported decreased mortalities with sulfa drugs (eg, sulfadimethoxine), but this may just help with secondary infections or coinfections.[67] Yanong and colleagues[67] (2004) showed reduction of the prevalence of *C iubilans* in experimentally infected fish with treatments of dimetridazole and 2-amino-5-nitrothiazole, but more studies are needed to develop treatment recommendations.

FUNGAL DISEASE
Exophiala

Exophiala spp (order Chaetothyriales, family Herpotrichiellaceae) are ubiquitous melanized fungi found in both terrestrial and aquatic environments. The genus was first described in cutthroat trout (*Salmo clarkia*) in 1966.[68] In humans, they have been associated with numerous and varied clinical signs from superficial infections, subcutaneous infections, keratitis, pneumonia, and brain abscesses, to disseminated disease.[69] These infections are more often seen in immunocompromised individuals but can affect seemingly immunocompetent individuals.[69]

Since its first description in 1966, numerous species of *Exophiala* have been described in fish but have most recently been found in a wider variety of species, including several ornamental fish (**Table 2**). A new species of *Exophiala*, *Exophiala cancerae*, has also been implicated as a causative agent in lethargic crab disease in mangrove land crabs (*Ucides cordatus*).[70]

Clinical signs Clinical signs of infection with *Exophiala spp* vary based on the species affected and species of *Exophiala*. In weedy and leafy sea dragons, clinical signs included weakness, loss of appetite, lethargy, increased respiratory effort and rate,

Table 2
Summary of reported *Exophiala* infections in fish

Exophiala Species	Fish Species Affected	Symptoms/Gross Lesions
Exophiala salmonis	Atlantic salmon	Brain, eye, gill, kidney, and head granulomas
	Cutthroat trout	Cerebral mycetoma in fingerlings
Exophiala pisciphila	Channel catfish	Systemic mycosis, skin ulceration
	Atlantic salmon	Cranial mycosis
	Smooth dogfish	Cranial mycosis
Exophiala xenobiotica	Striped jack	Gill, heart, kidney infection
Exophiala angulospora	Weedy sea dragon, leafy sea dragon	Disseminated mycosis
Novel Exophiala (unclassified)	Japanese flounder	Ulcerative dermatitis
	King George whiting	Skin ulceration, kidney, and swim bladder granulomatous disease
	Weedy sea dragon, leafy sea dragon	Disseminated mycosis

abnormal buoyancy, listing, piping at the surface of the water, or death.[71] The duration of clinical signs was 1 week to 6 months, with a mean of 8 weeks before death.

In contrast to other *Exophiala* infections in fish, a novel *Exophiala* sp in Japanese flounder (*Paralichthys olivaceus*) causes ulcerative skin disease without systemic infection. The ulcerations were limited to the ocular side of the flounder without any internal lesions. Histologically, these ulcers extended laterally through the dermis with no evidence of inflammation or infection in the epidermis or musculature. There was a severe inflammatory response around the areas of hyphae growth with lymphocyte aggregation.[72]

Diagnosis A tentative diagnosis of *Exophiala* can be made during postmortem examination because the fungal plaques are a distinct olive to black-brown color. Lesions in sea dragons are most consistently found in the skeletal muscle, skin, and kidney, although they were also found in numerous locations (gill, swim bladder, heart, liver, spleen muscle coats and serosa of intestine, mesentery, and extradural sinus and spinal cord).[71] Concurrent infection with bacteria and parasites was observed. Infection of Atlantic salmon with *Exophiala salmonis* shows diffuse inflammation and necrosis, most commonly of the posterior kidney and liver.[73]

The cytologic examination of affected tissues and the histopathology of lesions show characteristic morphology associated with *Exophiala*. The presence of annelated zones with annelloconidia from nearly unidentified conidiogenous zones is characteristic for the genus. Colonies of *Exophiala* on fungal culture will appear as a velvety, olive or black-brown mold. Most *Exophiala* cultured from fish species have been shown to grow at an optimum temperature of 30°C to 33°C.[71,73] Identification to species level requires further molecular testing.[71]

Treatment/Prevention There is no treatment of *Exophiala* in fish. Several treatments have been described in weedy and leafy sea dragons, including fluconazole, voriconazole, itraconazole, terbinafine, formaldehyde, methylene blue, malachite green, acriflavine, and Virkon (Antec International Ltd., Sudbury, Suffolk, UK).[71] Response to these treatments is variable, but has not been curative for the *Exophiala* infection. Studies in the treatment of *Exophiala* in other species showed varied success with a combination of surgical and medical management.[74]

SUMMARY

New and emerging diseases of fish are being found and classified at an accelerated rate, partly because of the recent advances in pathogen identification and molecular diagnostics. These diseases all pose a threat to the current aquaculture and ornamental fish industry and highlight the need for further research into the proper prevention, detection, and treatment.

ACKNOWLEDGMENTS

The authors would like to thank Roy P.E. Yanong, VMD at the University of Florida Tropical Aquaculture Laboratory and Thomas B. Waltzek, MS, DVM, PhD at the University of Florida College of Veterinary Medicine for generously providing images for publication.

REFERENCES

1. Waltzek TB, Kelley GO, Alfaro ME, et al. Phylogenetic relationships in the family Alloherpesviridae. Dis Aquat Organ 2009;84:179–94.

2. van Beurden SJ, Bossers A, Voorbergen-Laarman MH, et al. Complete genome sequence and taxonomic position of anguillid herpesvirus 1. J Gen Virol 2010; 91(4):880–7.
3. Calle PP, McNamara T, Kress Y. Herpesvirus–associated papillomas in koi carp (Cyprinus carpio). J Zoo Wildl Med 1999;30(1):165–9.
4. Sano T, Morita N, Shima N, et al. Herpesvirus cyprini: lethality and oncogenicity. J Fish Dis 1991;14(5):533–43.
5. Jung SE, Miyazaki T. Herpesviral haematopoietic necrosis of goldfish, Carassius auratus (L.). J Fish Dis 1995;18(3):211–20.
6. Groff JM, LaPatra SE, Munn RJ, et al. A viral epizootic in cultured populations of juvenile goldfish due to a putative herpesvirus etiology. J Vet Diagn Invest 1998; 10:375–8.
7. Goodwin AE, Merry GE, Sadler J. Detection of the herpesviral hematopoietic necrosis disease agent (Cyprinid herpesvirus 2) in moribund and healthy goldfish: validation of a quantitative PCR. Dis Aquat Organ 2006;69: 137–43.
8. Chang PE, Lee SH, Chiang HC, et al. Epizootic of herpes–like virus infection in goldfish, Carassius auratus in Taiwan. Fish Path 1999;34(4):209–10.
9. Stephens FJ, Raidal SR, Jones B. Haematopoietic necrosis in a goldfish (Carassius auratus) associated with an agent morphologically similar to herpesvirus. Aust Vet J 2004;82(3):167–9.
10. Jeffery KR, Bateman K, Bayley A, et al. Isolation of a cyprinid herpesvirus 2 from goldfish, Carassius auratus (L.), in the UK. J Fish Dis 2007;30(11): 649–56.
11. Goodwin AE, Khoo L, LaPatra SE, et al. Goldfish hematopoietic necrosis herpesvirus (Cyprinid herpesvirus 2) in the USA: molecular confirmation of isolates from diseased fish. J Aquat Anim Health 2006;18(1):11–9.
12. Waltzek TB, Kelley GO, Stone DM, et al. Koi herpesvirus represents a third cyprinid herpesvirus (CyHV–3) in the family Herpesviridae. J Gen Virol 2005; 86(6):1659–67.
13. Gilad O, Yun S, Andree KB, et al. Initial characteristics of koi herpesvirus and development of a polymerase chain reaction assay to detect the virus in koi, Cyprinus carpio koi. Dis Aquat 2002;48:101–8.
14. Hartman KH, Yanong RP, Pouder DB, et al. Koi herpesvirus (KHV) disease. 2004;1–9. Available at: http://edis.ifas.ufl.edu/pdffiles/VM/VM11300.pdf. Accessed July 27, 2012.
15. Way K. Koi herpesvirus and goldfish herpesvirus: an update of current knowledge and research at Cefas. Fish Vet J 2008;10:62–73.
16. Costes B, Raj VS, Michel B, et al. The major portal of entry of koi herpesvirus in Cyprinus carpio is the skin. J Virol 2009;83(7):2819–30.
17. Walster C. Koi herpesvirus: the international perspective. In: WAVMA Conference/ 29th World Veterinary Congress. Vancouver (Canada). 2008.
18. Pikarsky E, Ronen A, Abramowitz J, et al. Pathogenesis of acute viral disease induced in fish by carp interstitial nephritis and gill necrosis virus. J Virol 2004; 78(17):9544–51.
19. Aoki T, Hirono I, Kurokawa K, et al. Genome sequences of three koi herpesvirus isolates representing the expanding distribution of an emerging disease threatening koi and common carp worldwide. J Virol 2007;81(10):5058–65.
20. Gilad O, Yun S, Adkison MA, et al. Molecular comparison of isolates of an emerging fish pathogen, koi herpesvirus, and the effect of water temperature on mortality of experimentally infected koi. J Gen Virol 2003;84(10):2661–7.

21. Gilad O, Yun S, Zagmutt-Vergara FJ, et al. Concentrations of a koi herpesvirus (KHV) in tissues of experimentally–infected Cyprinus carpio koi as assessed by real–time TaqMan PCR. Dis Aquat Organ 2004;60:179–87.

22. Eide KE, Miller-Morgan T, Heidel JR, et al. Investigation of koi herpesvirus latency in koi. J Virol 2011;85(10):4954–62.

23. St-Hilaire S, Beevers N, Way K, et al. Reactivation of koi herpesvirus infections in common carp Cyprinus carpio. Dis Aquat Organ 2005;67:15–23.

24. Haenen OLM, Way K, Bergmann SM, et al. The emergence of koi herpesvirus and its significance to European aquaculture. Bull Eur Assoc Fish Pathol 2004.

25. Adkison MA, Gilad O, Hedrick RP, et al. An enzyme linked immunosorbent assay (ELISA) for detection of antibodies to the koi herpesvirus (KHV) in the serum of koi Cyprinus carpio. Fish Path 2005;40(2):53–62.

26. Perelberg A, Ilouze M, Kotler M, et al. Antibody response and resistance of Cyprinus carpio immunized with cyprinid herpes virus 3 (CyHV–3). Vaccine 2008; 26(29):3750–6.

27. El-Matbouli M, Saleh M, Soliman H. Detection of cyprinid herpesvirus type 3 in goldfish cohabiting with CyHV–3–infected koi carp (Cyprinus carpio koi). Vet Rec 2007;161(23):792–3.

28. Sadler J, Marecaux E, Goodwin AE. Detection of koi herpes virus (CyHV–3) in goldfish, Carassius auratus (L.), exposed to infected koi. J Fish Dis 2008;31(1): 71–2.

29. Ronen A, Perelberg A, Abramowitz J, et al. Efficient vaccine against the virus causing a lethal disease in cultured Cyprinus carpio. Vaccine 2003;21(32):4677–84.

30. Cavoy product insert. Greensboro (NC): Novartis Animal Health; 2012.

31. Weber ES, Malm K, Yun, et al. Efficacy and safety of a modified live CyHV3 vaccine (Cavoy®) in koi carp. In: Proceedings 37th Eastern Fish Health Workshop. Lake Placid (NY): 2012. p. 45.

32. Hutoran M, Ronen A, Perelberg A, et al. Description of an as yet unclassified DNA virus from diseased Cyprinus carpio species. J Virol 2005;79(4):1983–91.

33. Dishon A, Davidovich M, Ilouze M, et al. Persistence of cyprinid herpesvirus 3 in infected cultured carp cells. J Virol 2007;81(9):4828–36.

34. Whittington RJ, Becker JA, Dennis MM. Iridovirus infections in finfish – critical review with emphasis on ranaviruses. J Fish Dis 2010;33(2):95–122.

35. Hossain K, Song JY, Kitamura SI, et al. Phylogenetic analysis of lymphocystis disease virus from tropical ornamental fish species based on a major capsid protein gene. J Fish Dis 2008;31(6):473–9.

36. Hyatt AD, Gould AR, Zupanovic Z, et al. Comparative studies of piscine and amphibian iridoviruses. Arch Virol 2000;145(2):301–31.

37. Langdon JS, Humphrey JD, Williams LM, et al. First virus isolation from Australian fish: an iridovirus–like pathogen from redfin perch, Perca fluviatilis L. J Fish Dis 1986;9(3):263–8.

38. Plumb JA, Zilberg D. The lethal dose of largemouth bass virus in juvenile largemouth bass and the comparative susceptibility of striped bass. J Aquat Anim Health 2011;11(3):246–52.

39. Woodland JE, Brunner CJ, Noyes AD, et al. Experimental oral transmission of largemouth bass virus. J Fish Dis 2002;25(11):669–72.

40. Langdon JS, Humphrey JD. Epizootic haematopoietic necrosis, a new viral disease in redfin perch, Perca fluviatilis L., in Australia. J Fish Dis 1987;10(4):289–97.

41. Crane MSJ, Young J, Williams LM. Epizootic haematopoietic necrosis virus (EHNV): growth in fish cell lines at different temperatures. Bull Eur Assoc Fish Patho 2005;25(5):228.

42. Hanson LA, Petrie-Hanson L, Meals KO, et al. Persistence of largemouth bass virus infection in a Northern Mississippi reservoir after a die–off. J Aquat Anim Health 2011;13(1):27–34.

43. Kurita J, Nakajima K. Megalocytiviruses. Viruses 2012;4(4):521–38.

44. Yanong RPE, Waltzek TB. Megalocytivirus infections in fish, with emphasis on ornamental species. 2011. Available at: http://edis.ifas.ufl.edu/fa182. Accessed July 24, 2012.

45. Weber ES, Waltzek TB, Young DA, et al. Systemic iridovirus infection in the Banggai cardinalfish (Pterapogon kauderni, Koumans 1933). J Vet Diagn Invest 2009; 21(3):306–20.

46. Jun LJ, Jeong JB, Kim JH, et al. Influence of temperature shifts on the onset and development of red sea bream iridoviral disease in rock bream Oplegnathus fasciatus. Dis Aquat Organ 2009;84:201–8.

47. Nakajima K, Maeno Y, Honda A, et al. Effectiveness of a vaccine against red sea bream iridoviral disease in a field trial test. Dis Aquat Organ 1999;36(1):73–5.

48. Munday BL, Kwang J, Moody N. Betanodavirus infections of teleost fish: a review. J Fish Dis 2002;25(3):127–42.

49. Yoshikoshi K, Inoue K. Viral nervous necrosis in hatchery–reared larvae and juveniles of Japanese parrotfish, Oplegnathus fasciatus (Temminck & Schlegel). J Fish Dis 1990;13(1):69–77.

50. Glazebrook JS, Heasman MP, de Beer SW. Picorna–like viral particles associated with mass mortalities in larval barramundi, Lates calcarifer Bloch. J Fish Dis 1990; 13(3):245–9.

51. Mori KI, Nakai T, Muroga K, et al. Properties of a new virus belonging to nodaviridae found in larval striped jack (Pseudocaranx dentex) with nervous necrosis. Virology 1992;187(1):368–71.

52. Hasoon MF, Daud HM, Arshad SS, et al. Betanodavirus experimental infection in freshwater ornamental guppies: diagnostic histopathology and nested RT–PCR. J Adv Med Res 2011;1(2):45–54.

53. Gomez DK, Lim DJ, Baeck GW, et al. Detection of betanodaviruses in apparently healthy aquarium fishes and invertebrates. J Vet Sci 2006;7(4):369–74.

54. Gomez DK, Baeck GW, Kim JH, et al. Genetic analysis of betanodaviruses in subclinically infected aquarium fish and invertebrates. Curr Microbiol 2008; 56(5):499–504.

55. Yanong RPE. Viral nervous necrosis (betanodavirus) infections in fish. 2011;1–7. Available at: http://edis.ifas.ufl.edu/fa180. Accessed July 24, 2012.

56. David R, Treguier C, Montagnani C, et al. Molecular detection of betanodavirus from the farmed fish, Platax orbicularis (Forsskal)(Ephippidae), in French Polynesia. J Fish Dis 2010;33(5):451–4.

57. Hodneland K, Garcia R, Balbuena JA, et al. Real–time RT–PCR detection of betanodavirus in naturally and experimentally infected fish from Spain. J Fish Dis 2011;34(3):189–202.

58. Colquhoun DJ, Duodu S. Francisella infections in farmed and wild aquatic organisms. Vet Res 2011;42(45):1–15.

59. Fryer JL, Hedrick RP. Piscirickettsia salmonis: a gram–negative intracellular bacterial pathogen of fish. J Fish Dis 2003;26(5):251–62.

60. Birkbeck TH, Feist SW, Verner-Jeffreys DW. Francisella infections in fish and shellfish. J Fish Dis 2011;34(3):173–87.

61. Khoo L, Dennis PM, Lewbart GA. Rickettsia–like organisms in the blue–eyed plecostomus, Panaque suttoni (Eigenmann & Eigenmann). J Fish Dis 1995;18(2): 157–64.

62. Soto E, Baumgartner W, Wiles J, et al. Francisella asiatica as the causative agent of piscine francisellosis in cultured tilapia (Oreochromis sp.) in the United States. J Vet Diagn Invest 2011;23(4):821–5.

63. Hsieh CY, Wu ZB, Tung MC, et al. PCR and in situ hybridization for the detection and localization of a new pathogen Francisella–like bacterium (FLB) in ornamental cichlids. Dis Aquat Organ 2007;75:29–36.

64. Soto E, Kidd S, Gaunt PS, et al. Efficacy of florfenicol for control of mortality associated with Francisella noatunensis subsp. orientalis in Nile tilapia, Oreochromis niloticus (L.). J Fish Dis 2012. [Epub ahead of print].

65. Floyd RF, Yanong RPE. Cryptobia iubilans in cichlids. 2003. Available at: http://edis.ifas.ufl.edu/document_vm077. Accessed July 27, 2012.

66. Nohynkova E. A new pathogenic Cryptobia from freshwater fishes: a light and electron microscopic study. Protistologica 1984;20(2):181–95.

67. Yanong RPE, Curtis E, Russo R, et al. Cryptobia iubilans infection in juvenile discus. J Am Vet Med Assoc 2004;224(10):1644–50.

68. Carmichael JW. Cerebral mycetoma of trout due to a Phialophora–like fungus. Med Mycol 1967;5(2):120–3.

69. Zeng JS, Sutton DA, Fothergill AW, et al. Spectrum of clinically relevant Exophiala species in the United States. J Clin Microbiol 2007;45(11):3713–20.

70. Orélis-Ribeiro R, Boeger WA, Vicente VA, et al. Fulfilling Koch's postulates confirms the mycotic origin of lethargic crab disease. Antonie Van Leeuwenhoek 2011;99(3):601–8.

71. Nyaoke A, Weber ES, Innis C, et al. Disseminated phaeohyphomycosis in weedy seadragons (Phyllopteryx taeniolatus) and leafy seadragons (Phycodurus eques) caused by species of Exophiala, including a novel species. J Vet Diagn Invest 2009;21(1):69–79.

72. Kurata O, Munchan C, Wada S, et al. Novel Exophiala infection involving ulcerative skin lesions in Japanese flounder Paralichthys olivaceus. Fish Path 2008; 43(1):35–44.

73. Richards RH, Holliman A. Exophiala salmonis infection in Atlantic salmon Salmo salar L. J Fish Dis 1978;1(4):357–68.

74. Gold WL, Vellend H, Salit IE, et al. Successful treatment of systemic and local infections due to Exophiala species. Clin Infect Dis 1994;19(2):339–41.

Selected Emerging Diseases of Amphibia

La'Toya V. Latney, DVM[a],*,
Eric Klaphake, DVM, Dip ABVP (Avian), DACZM, Dip ABVP (Reptile/Amphibian)[b]

KEYWORDS

• Amphibian • Viral • Fungal • Parasitic • Bacterial • Emerging • Disease

KEY POINTS

- *Batrachochytrium dendrobatidis* (Bd) and ranavirus are the most significant infectious diseases contributing to global population declines in amphibians.
- Fluid therapy and itraconazole are the mainstays of therapy for Bd infections.
- Ranaviruses infect several species of anurans, larval and adults, and disease susceptibility varies among species.
- Ranavirus polymerase chain reaction (PCR) results samples vary based on sampling methods.
- *Mycobacterium liflandii* and new noncommensal bacterial pathogens have been identified as causes of significant mortality in amphibian collections.
- Rana and Bd status can influence species susceptibility to parasitic disease.

Whether in private practice or in a zoologic setting, veterinarians of the exotic animal persuasion are asked to work on amphibians. As with most nondomestic species, many health issues in amphibians are traced back to problems with husbandry and/or nutrition. Because these areas are more adequately addressed in zoos and even by hobbyists and pet stores, however, veterinarians are able to evaluate more thoroughly for true medical issues, with infectious diseases at the forefront. Until recently, many infectious diseases were unknown or even misdiagnosed as caused by opportunistic secondary organisms. The days of a sick frog with hind leg erythema diagnosed as red leg caused by bacterial infection are becoming history. In a recent report, 4 species (*Dendrobates auratus*, *Phyllobates terribilis*, *Pyxicephalus adspersus*, and *Rhacophorus dennysi*) of captive anurans with a clinical history of lethargy and inappetence were found dead with irregular patches of sloughed skin and rare dermal ulcerations. Histologic findings of intracytoplasmic chytrid organisms and bacteria (cultured

[a] Exotic Companion Animal Medicine and Surgery, University of Pennsylvania Veterinary Teaching Hospital, 3900 Delancey Street, Office 2017, Philadelphia, PA 19104, USA; [b] Matthew J. Ryan Veterinary Hospital, University of Pennsylvania School of Veterinary Medicine, Cheyenne Mountain Zoo, 4250 Cheyenne Mountain Zoo Road, Colorado Springs, CO 80906, USA
* Corresponding author.
E-mail address: llatney@vet.upenn.edu

Aeromonas hydrophila) associated with the epidermal lesions and intracytoplasmic inclusion bodies in hepatocytes combined with Real-time-PCR–positive results for both ranavirus and Bd indicate that multiple infectious agents can occur in amphibians, and simply running a bacterial culture may have provided only a tiny part of the picture.[1] The challenge of convincing a client or even a curator to invest in diagnostic testing is often formidable. Likewise, it can be a challenge to collect samples from amphibians in useful quantities for such testing. Amphibians have been proposed as environmental sentinels, but the dearth of research on infectious amphibian diseases is remarkable in opposing support of that statement. This has been slowly changing, and this article is dedicated to exploring the known peer-reviewed research available for practitioners on the topic of emerging infectious amphibian diseases, including viruses, bacteria, fungi, and parasites. Two of these diseases require notification of the World Organisation for Animal Health (Office International des Epizooties [OIE])—Bd and ranaviruses (several species)—because of their contagious nature and capability of causing extinctions of entire species of amphibians.[2]

FUNGAL DISEASE
Batrachochytrid Dendrobatidis

Bd is a chytrid fungus that has been deemed responsible for causing extinction-level event population declines in amphibians worldwide since its first report in 1998.[3] At the 2005 Amphibian Conservation Summit, Bd was described as the "worst infectious disease ever recorded among vertebrates in terms of number of species impacted and its propensity to drive them to extinction." Ecologists consider Bd the largest infectious disease threat to biodiversity.[4] Bd has commissioned an immediate global response from the public, scientists, conservationists, and policy makers alike. Multiple conservation organizations share the universal goal of improving understanding of the fungi's ecology and pathogenesis to implement control of Bd's devastating effects on amphibian populations.

To understand Bd's impact, it is important to first appreciate where global amphibian population statistics stand. The International Union for Conservation of Nature (IUCN) has produced the first comprehensive assessment of the conservation status of amphibians (Global Amphibian Assessment: http://www.iucnredlist.org/initiatives/amphibians/analysis). The 2008 Global Amphibian Assessment updates reveal staggering data on amphibian population decline (**Box 1**). A global surveillance initiative has been launched to track the reports of Bd worldwide. More than 500 species of amphibians have been infected with Bd among 54 countries (www.spatialepidemiology.net/bd-maps/) and the highest numbers of reports come from North America. Since 2008, The OIE has listed Bd as a reportable disease and provides a freely accessible 2012 *Manual of Diagnostic Tests for Aquatic Animals* with a chapter outlining Bd history, surveillance, diagnostic tests, treatment, and control measures (http://www.oie.int/fileadmin/Home/eng/Health_standards/aahm/2010/2.1.01_INF_BATRACHOCHYRIUM.pdf).

History and Epidemiology

The origins of Bd were hypothesized two theories, the novel pathogen theory and the endemic pathogen theory. Many investigators propose that Bd was a novel pathogen introduced globally by the trade in infected *Xenopus laevis* frogs used for human pregnancy tests from Africa.[5] More recently, it has been implicated as a novel pathogen spread by the international trade of American bullfrogs (*Lithobates catesbeiana*). The endemic pathogen theory supports that Bd has always been endemic and the

---

Box 1
Key Findings of the IUCN Red List 2008 update on Amphibian Population Decline

- Among the world's amphibian species, 32% are threatened or extinct.

- The status of 25% of all species remains undetermined due to insufficient data.

- Among all species, 42% show population decline.

- Less than 1% of all species show population growth.

- There are 159 species extinct, 1 in the wild, and 120 are possibly extinct within recent years.

- The largest numbers of threatened species occur in Latin American countries, including Colombia (214), Mexico (211), and Ecuador (171).

- The highest levels of threat are in the Caribbean, where more than 80% of amphibians are threatened or extinct in the Dominican Republic, Cuba, and Jamaica and 92% in Haiti.

- Although habit loss poses the greatest threat to amphibians, a newly recognized fungal disease is seriously affecting an increasing number of species. Perhaps most disturbing, many species are declining for unknown reasons, complicating efforts to design and implement effective conservation strategies.

An analysis of amphibians on the 2008 IUCN Red List. www.iuncredlist.org/amphibians.

---

increased virulence seen currently is due to environmental changes in the host-pathogen dynamic.[6] The implications of either theory have far-reaching consequences for international law and policy change, biosecurity, and predictions of Bd's continued effect on amphibian diversity. In short, 2012 both theories have been proved, with new data that reshape previous assumptions about Bd diversity.

The results of Bd genomic proteinomic studies provide the following conclusions. First, there are multiple strains of Bd, consisting of endemic Bd strains and new highly virulent strains. Comparisons of Bd strains from multiple continents suggest recent intercontinental spread.[7] Second, through a global genomic survey, Farrer and colleagues[8] have shown that there are specific Bd genotypes associated with declining amphibian populations globally (global panzootic lineage [Bd-GPL] geno-types). Bd-GPL1 is a recent genotype that is replacing endemic Bd strains, which have had longer associations with their hosts.[8] Schloegel and colleagues[7] have recently identified hybrid virulent genotypes of Bd in American bullfrogs, which supports the hypothesis that there is a sexual reproductive stage in the Bd life cycle. Their article, furthermore, identifies a novel, highly divergent strain originating from Brazil (Bd-Brazil), which is now located on invasive bullfrogs in Japan. These eye-opening reports of Bd intercontinental gene flow[7] support the argument that this is a pandemic of anthropogenic cause. It strongly fuels the cry for international policy governed at improved biosecurity and amphibian importation restrictions from locales that harbor highly virulent Bd strains.

The scientific community has provided significant evidence that warns of the ability of Bd to cause extinction level events for Anura (frogs and toads), Caudata (salamanders, newts, and sirens), and Gymnophiona (caecilians). In a recent *Nature* review, emerging fungal diseases were proposed as the most important threat to plant and animal ecosystem health.[9] Many studies have provided mathematical models that predict the effects that emerging fungal pathogens will have on vertebrate biodiversity, including the predicted global impact Bd will continue to have on amphibian population declines.[9–13] One such study that evaluated the climatic sustainability of Bd alone proposed that one-sixth of all amphibian species are located in regions potentially suited for Bd susceptibility and more than 50% of all species overlap in areas of high Bd susceptibilities.[12] More than 379 species were identified as high risk for extinction. This report details that 40% of those species fall under the "Data Insufficient" category on the IUCN Red List. Remarkably, 94% of the proposed species fall on the same IUCN sufficient data list, where the species are categorized as threatened with extinction.[12] These alarming statistics, coupled with habit loss and ranavirus epidemic, heighten awareness to the frailty of the global amphibian population at large.

Bd Pathogenesis and Life Cycle

Bd is the single species of the monotypic genus *Batrachochytrium*, under the phylum Chytridiomycota, class Chytridiomycetes, and order Chytridiales.[14] It was first reported to cause fatal infections in amphibians in North and Central American frogs and in Australian frogs in 1998. The Bd life cycle has 2 main stages—substrate dependent and substrate independent. A sexual stage has recently been proposed.[7] In the substrate-independent stage (environmental), flagellated zoospores are waterborne, motile, and free living. They are short-lived (24 h) and travel distances of up to 2 cm in culture medium.[15] They exhibit chemotaxis, which assists the spore in finding a substrate characterized as the epidermis of adults or the mouthparts of tadpoles. In the substrate-dependent stage, the zoospore encysts in the epidermis; germlings develop into sporangia and produce more zoospores. These zoospores can reinfect the same host or move into the environment. The host reinfection contributes to high pathogen burdens and subsequent morbidity and mortality. The life cycle completes itself in 4 days' time, occurring at temperatures from 17°C to 22°C. A sexual stage has been recently suggested, because hybrid strains of the recently discovered Bd-GPL genotype can only originate from diploid generations of resting sporangia that are capable of sexual reproduction.[7] Although documented as rare, there are species within the phylum Chytridiomycota that have demonstrated sexual reproductive stages.[16]

The skin is the largest and most physiologically dynamic vital organ of amphibians. It serves as an innate immune barrier, produces antimicrobial peptides, and is largely responsible for respiration and osmoregulation. Zoospore invasion of the epidermis of adult frogs can induce peracute mortalities in infected individuals. There is evidence to support that Bd interferes with the sodium-potassium pump in the epidermis, inhibiting up to 50% of sodium and potassium plasma concentrations, which causes drastic declines in pH, bradycardia, and asystolic cardiac arrest.[17] In tadpoles, the loss of keratinized mouthparts decreases food intake, slows metamorphosis, and can contribute to sublethal morbidity and mortality. Bd can be transmitted within and between amphibian life stages[18] but it has not been documented to infect egg masses.

Host-pathogen influences that affect morbidity and mortality in all species include temperature, infective zoospore dose of Bd, and strain differences. Although interspecies variation in morbidity and mortality of amphibian species exists, fewer than 30 published experimental infections have been performed to estimate Bd species susceptibility and resulting mortality.[4] These studies show an extreme variation in host susceptibility and mortality, as is seen in nature.[19] As new evidence characterizing Bd strains continues to arise, studies correlating species-specific virulence will follow. Emerging proteinomic studies have implicated the American bullfrog (*Lithobates catesbeiana*),[20] Pacific chorus frog (*Pseudacris regilla*),[21] and eastern populations of northern leopard frogs (*Lithobates pipiens*)[22] as reservoir species in North America. In addition, Bd prevalence in feral African clawed frogs (*Xenopus laevis*)[23] and tiger salamanders (*Ambystoma tigrinum*)[24] is significant and these species are largely asymptomatic.

There are some basic observations with regard to assessing species susceptibility based on the climatic and environmental conditions alone for which Bd can be sustained.[25] Amphibian species that originate from upland regions where temperatures are cooler are highly susceptible because Bd is heat intolerant. The organism has been shown to die at temperatures above $32°C$.[25] In lowland areas, higher temperatures may be protective. Studies assessing the combined influences of infective zoospore dose, strain, and temperature are needed to accurately quantify and qualify species-specific morbidity and mortality.

Diagnostics and Treatment

Further studies are needed to characterize the nature of environmental influences, but current data provides us with some information necessary to implement control and guide treatment practices. For practitioners, attention to subtle clinical signs may afford quick detection and improve the treatment window for affected individuals. Clinical signs in adults can vary but include abnormal posture, abnormal behavior, increased time soaking in water resources, reflex loss, lethargy, excessive epidermal roughening or sloughing, epidermal hyperemia, and peracute death.[26,27] Tadpoles may be asymptomatic, have abnormal swimming behavior, or show discoloration of the mouthparts.

Diagnostic options include direct visualization in skin preparations and molecular detection of Bd DNA via PCR. Direct wet mounts of skin preparations (**Fig. 1**) or skin scrapings stained with lactophenol cotton blue can be used for cytologic diagnosis of zoospores in the epidermis. Old zoosporangia may be present in the epidermis and zoospores may also be noted. Histologic evidence of spherical zoosporangia may be seen on hematoxylin-eosin stain of tissue samples and periodic acid–Schiff stains on biopsy samples.[28] Quantitative PCR (qtPCR) techniques offer the most sensitive measure of detection than what has been reported for histologic confirmation[29] and qtPCR can be used to quantify zoospore burdens.[30] The Wildlife Disease Laboratories at the San Diego Zoo Institute for Conservation Research (http://www.sandiegozooglobal.org/News/Amphibian_Disease_Laboratory/) and Pisces Molecular laboratories (contact Dr John Wood at e-mail address: jwood@pisces-molecular.com web address: http://www.pisces-molecular.com/) offer commercial qtPCR testing.

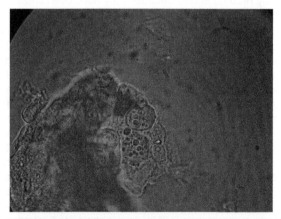

Fig. 1. Direct smear of dendrobatid skin with zoospores evident in epidermis. Magnification 40×. (*Courtesy of* C. Hatfield, MA, VetMB, MRCVS, Dipl ACZM, L.A. Clayton, DVM, DABVP [Avian and Reptile/Amphibian], National Aquarium, Baltimore, MD.)

Even if a laboratory is used that has a fast turnaround time, Bd pathogenesis necessitates immediate isolation, electrolyte replenishment, and treatment if patients are to recover from infection. Because peracute deaths can be observed, treatment should be implemented while awaiting PCR confirmation if immediate confirmation cannot be made from in-house wet mounts of skin samples.

Bd interferes with the sodium-potassium pump of the epidermis; therefore, electrolyte replenishment is the first line of treatment. Soaking affected individuals in shallow baths for 15 to 30 minutes daily in an electrolyte-balanced fluid replacement solution with pH 7.2 and osmolality of 200 mOsm/kg to 240 mOsm/kg is recommended. A 1:1 solution of lactated Ringer solution to 2.5% dextrose can be made for affected individuals.[31] Young and coauthors[32] report success with parental fluid therapy doses of 50 mL/kg subcutaneously every 8 hours for 3 days, then 50 mL/kg subcutaneously every 12 hours for 3 days, in treating terminally ill Bd-infected common green tree frogs.[32] Young and coauthors used Hartmann solution, which is a commercially available isotonic sodium lactate solution that contains sodium (129 mM/L), potassium (5 mM/L), calcium (2 mM/L), chlorine (109 mM/L), and H_2CO_3 (29 mM/L), and has an osmolality of 274 mOsm. Maintenance of cage humidity at levels appropriate for the species also helps prevent evaporate losses.

There are several studies that have evaluated the effectiveness of killing zoospores in the environment and in infected species. One clinical trial indicated that a shallow bath treatment of 0.0025% itraconazole for 5 minutes every 24 hours for 6 days reliably cured individuals from Bd and reduced the possible risk of drug toxicity.[33] Many practitioners use 0.01% itraconazole baths for 5 minutes daily for 11 days as an effective regimen for Bd treatment[34,35]; however, the 0.01% itraconazole dose is fatal to larvae and recent metamorphs in certain species, including the endangered Wyoming toad (Anaxyrus baxteri).[36,37] These itraconazole solutions are added to the electrolyte solutions used for fluid therapy in amphibians. One study revealed that environmental heat elevations to 37°C for 16 hours[38] resulted in clinical recovery for some species; however, increasing environmental heat may not be physiologically safe for many species. Chloramphenicol has also been shown effective and may also help treat secondary infections.[32] It has been shown, however, to cause aplastic anemia in a small subset of humans and unnecessary exposure should be prevented.[33,39] Formalin, malachite green, fluconazole, and benzalkonium chloride have also been assessed and are not currently recommended because they have been shown to have variable in vivo efficacy, species-dependent intolerance, and associated mortality.[33,40,41]

Biosecurity

Isolation of affected individuals, quarantine prior for new introductions, and disinfection are the mainstays of preventing the spread of this fungus in a collection. Affected individuals can be treated as discussed previously. Quarantine of new individuals to a collection should include qtPCR testing every 7 days for 2 consecutive negative PCR results before new exhibit introductions. The Association of Zoos and Aquariums recommends 30-day to 60-day quarantines for all new animals in their Amphibian Husbandry Resource Guide, which is available at http://205.251.117.60/uploadedFiles/Conservation/Commitments_and_Impacts/Amphibian_Conservation/Amphibian_Resources/AmphibianHusbandryResourceGuide.pdf. If the Bd status is undeterminable, the authors recommend isolation and treating newcomers with 0.0025% itraconazole for 5 minutes every 24 hours for 6 days. The Association of Zoos and Aquariums recommends 0.01% itraconazole for 5 minutes every 24 hours for 11 days. Disinfection protocols, as outlined in the OIE manual, include using heat at 37°C for 4 hours to inactivate zoospores. Additionally, common disinfectants can be used to clean hard surfaces and cages[28] and include quaternary ammonium compounds, didecyl dimethyl ammonium chloride (eg, Path-X, 1 in 500 dilution for 30 seconds), benzalkonium chloride (eg, F10, 1 in 1500 dilution for 1 minute), sodium hypochlorite (1% concentration for 20 seconds), ethanol (70% for 20 seconds), and Virkon (1 mg/mL for 20 seconds).[42]

VIRUSES

There are 2 major families of viruses that are common causes of disease in amphibians: Alloherpesviridae, which is now its own separate family containing herpesviruses of anurans and fish,[43–45] and Iridoviridae, specifically the genus *Ranavirus*.

Herpesviruses

Ranid herpesvirus 1 has been studied for many years in the northern leopard frog, *Rana pipiens*. It has a predictable life cycle that leads to a neoplasia called Lucke renal tumor, which is a papillary renal adenocarcinoma. Virus production within an infected frog is highest in the fall (viral production is enhanced by cooler temperatures). Ranid herpesvirus 1 is shed in spring during spawning; then, the adult frog develops clinical evidence of disease and dies postspawn of the fast-growing cancer during the summer (cancer growth is enhanced by higher temperatures). Ranid herpesvirus 2 has not been found pathogenic.[43] At this time, these are the only reported amphibian herpesviruses. There is no known treatment of the disease, and one of the authors (EK) has diagnosed a case antemortem by contrast radiographs showing a mass effect in the area of one of the kidneys, which was subsequently confirmed on histopathology.

Ranaviruses

Ranaviruses are of high enough concern that the OIE has them listed as a reportable disease.[2] As with Bd, another reportable disease, there is an OIE Web site summarizing current understanding of the pathogenenesis of ranaviruses in amphibians, although it has not been updated since 2007: http://www.oie.int/fileadmin/Home/eng/Internationa_Standard_Setting/docs/pdf/Ranavirus_card_final.pdf.

Previous to 1982, iridoviruses were reported only in fish and amphibians, with lymphocystis in fish the classic example. Several reptile species have been infected with ranavirus, and there is debate as to whether amphibians serve as a source of the infection or if subclinical reptiles and the environment serve as the reservoir. Ranaviruses have been implicated in frog, toad, and tiger salamander die-offs. Taxonomy of this genus of viruses can be confusing and seems to continue to undergo reclassification (merging in some cases), making which virus is discussed in many older publications challenging to ascertain. Those ranaviruses currently described include Ambystoma tigrinum virus (ATV), common midwife toad virus (CMTV), frog virus 3 (FV3), Rana grylio virus, Rana catesbeiana ranavirus, Mahaffey Road virus, Rana esculenta virus, Bohle iridovirus, and tiger frog virus.[46–49] Some of these viruses seem to affect the species of amphibian indicated by the name; in other cases, there is crossover. There also seem to be varying strains of the virus, with some benign to the host animal or species. Therefore, testing for the presence of ranavirus in pet, wild, or zoo amphibians that are clinically normal is of dubious benefit. In the face of mass mortalities, such testing is of benefit.

Mass mortality caused by ranavirus has occurred globally since at least the early 1990s. The pathogen infects multiple amphibian hosts, larval and adult cohorts, and may persist in reptile and fish reservoirs. Environmental persistence of ranavirus virions outside a host may be several weeks or longer in aquatic systems.

Transmission can be indirect or direct, including contaminated water or soil, casual or direct contact with infected individuals, and ingestion of infected tissue during predation, cannibalism, or necrophagy. Common gross lesions include swelling of the limbs or body, erythema, swollen friable livers, and hemorrhage. Susceptible amphibians usually die from chronic cell death in multiple organs, which can occur within a few days after infection or may take several weeks. The occurrence of recent widespread amphibian population die-offs from ranaviruses may be an interaction of suppressed and naive host immunity, anthropogenic stressors, and novel strain introduction. Biosecurity precautions include disinfecting footwear and equipment and testing commercially shipped amphibians for the pathogen.[49]

A mass die-off of imported red-tailed knobby newts (Tylototriton kweichowensis) occurred in Belgium and the Netherlands in 2004. In addition to massive infection with Rhabdias tokyoensis, FV3 was isolated. On experimental infection of axolotls (Ambystoma mexicanum) with this isolate, no marked pathology was noticed and the virus could not be reisolated at 9 weeks postinoculation. Apart from the possibility of exposure to a nonsensitive host, the mortality episode in the newts may be related to stress resulting from the importation of the newts in breeding condition. This possibility was supported by the presence of degenerating egg follicles in the female newts.[50]

A 4-year study of 4 geographically separated tiger salamander groups (Ambystoma tigrinum nebulosum) found that salamander populations were commonly infected with ATV. No morbidity or mortality was observed due to ATV, even with prevalence values from 0 to 57%. Infection prevalence across the landscape was more similar within a given year than between years. There was no statistically significant spatial pattern in prevalence across the landscape.[51] Temperature strongly influenced percent mortality and time to death of salamanders exposed to ATV. Most survived when exposed at 26°C, whereas all died at 18°C and nearly all died at 10°C. Some asymptomatic salamanders that survived 60 days at 10°C or 26°C were found to be carrying the virus. PCR was less sensitive than cell culture in detecting ATV at low concentrations. Virus titer, measured by cytopathic effect in homogenized tissue, was higher in salamanders held at 10°C than at 18°C but little virus, if any, was present in the small number of salamanders that died at 26°C. As with Bd, increased environmental temperatures may help amphibians fight off at least some ranavirus infections.[52]

When 6-week-old, larval, long-toed salamanders (Ambystoma macrodactylum) were exposed to ATV and sublethal concentrations of a commonly used herbicide, atrazine (2-chloro-4-[ethylamino]-6-[isopropylamino]-s-triazine), infection rates were lower than expected. Larvae exposed to both atrazine and ATV had lower levels of mortality and ATV infectivity compared with larvae exposed to virus alone, suggesting atrazine may compromise virus efficacy. The highest atrazine level accelerated metamorphosis and reduced mass and length at metamorphosis significantly. Exposure to ATV also significantly reduced length at metamorphosis. The study suggested moderate concentrations of atrazine may ameliorate effects of ATV on long-toed salamanders, whereas higher concentrations initiate metamorphosis at a smaller size, with potential negative consequences to fitness; however, atrazine is not recommended as a treatment option for ranavirus infections, because of its toxicity issues.[53]

Larval anurans can differ greatly in susceptibility to ranaviruses. Average mortality rates of Cope gray tree frogs (Hyla chrysoscelis) (66%) and pickerel frogs (Rana palustris) (68%) were similar but 3-fold higher than for eastern narrow-mouthed toads (Gastrophryne carolinensis). Direct ingestion of the viruses increased mean infection and mortality rates by 30% and caused death approximately 2 times faster compared with water bath exposure. Exposure duration did not have an impact, however, on mean infection or mortality rates. The isolate found at a ranaculture facility (a place that raises frogs in large numbers for food or research) increased mortality by greater than 34% compared with FV3.[54]

Ranaculture facilities seem to be a concerning source of ranaviruses introduced into naïve amphibians. Sick American bullfrog (*Lithobates catesbeianus*) tadpoles farmed in Brazil were confirmed to be naturally infected with Rana catesbeiana ranavirus and this is the first report of a ranaviral infection affecting aquatic organisms in Brazil.[47]

As previously implicated with introducing Bd, the African clawed frog (*Xenopus laevis*) is considered a concerning source of ranaviruses. *Xenopus* adults usually clear FV3 infection within a few weeks, but viral DNA can be detected in the kidneys several months after they had been experimentally infected. Additionally, this virus has been detected in seemingly healthy nonexperimentally infected adults. FV3 infects their peritoneal macrophages without harming those macrophages by the presence of FV3, suggesting that FV3 can become quiescent in resistant species, such as *Xenopus*, thereby making these species potential viral reservoirs.[55] In *Xenopus*, it has been found that FV3 infects the kidneys of adults but is cleared within 4 weeks, with faster clearance on reinfection with FV3 due to CD8$^+$ T-cell proliferation in the spleen and accumulation in infected kidneys. Earlier proliferation and infiltration associated with faster viral clearance were observed during secondary infection.[56] FV3 has a strong tropism for the proximal tubular epithelium of the kidney and is rarely disseminated elsewhere in *Xenopus*.[57]

One of the most recently discovered and published ranaviruses is CMTV in Europe. In 2010, a mass die-off of adult *Pelophylax* frogs and common newts (*Lissotriton vulgaris*) occurred in a pond in the Netherlands. Hemorrhagic disease with hepatomegaly and splenomegaly was evident. Microscopically, multiple organs presented cells with multifocal intracytoplasmic inclusion bodies. All specimens examined tested positive for ranavirus by PCR, with sequencing indicating CMTV.[58] CMTV was also associated with mortalities in juvenile alpine newts (*Mesotriton alpestris cyreni*) and common midwife toad tadpoles (*Alytes obstetricans*) in Northern Spain. The kidneys' glomeruli had the most severe histologic lesions in common midwife toad tadpoles whereas both glomeruli and renal tubular epithelial cells exhibited foci of necrosis in juvenile alpine newts. Viral antigens were detected by immunohistochemical labeling mainly in the kidneys of common midwife toad tadpoles and in ganglia of juvenile alpine newts.[59]

FV3 is the cause of tadpole edema syndrome with adults as subclinical carriers. A new clinical presentation of FV3 found a free-ranging American bullfrog metamorph with the right eye approximately 50% the size of the left, and 2 granulomas within the orbit. Electron microscopic examination revealed FV3 virus particles.[60] Bohle-like iridovirus has been identified in Australian frogs. Captive magnificent tree frogs (*Litoria splendid*) and green tree frogs (*L caerulea*) in Australia either died or were euthanized after becoming lethargic or developing skin lesions. A Bohle-like ranavirus, tentatively named Mahaffey Road virus, was isolated.[48]

PCR results may vary between tissue samples obtained by antemortem versus postmortem procedures. Testing liver samples for infection is a common lethal sampling technique to estimate ranavirus prevalence because the pathogen often targets this organ and the liver is easy to identify and collect. Tail clips or skin swabs may be more practicable for ranavirus surveillance programs, however, compared with collecting and euthanizing animals, especially for uncommon species. Using PCR results from American bullfrog tadpoles with liver samples for gold standard comparison, the false-negative and false-positive rates were 20% and 6%, respectively, for tail samples, and 22% and 12%, respectively, for skin swabs. False-negative rates were constant over time, but false-positive rates decreased with postexposure duration.

Thus, the prevalence of infection when using tail clips or skin swabs may be underestimated when compared with results obtained with liver samples.[61]

A study compared the persistence of amphibian and reptilian ranaviruses in a pond habitat. All 4 tested viruses (FV3, an unidentified isolate from a frog, and 2 ranaviruses of reptilian origin [tortoise and gecko]) were resistant to drying. Viral persistence was highest in the sterilized pond water (PW), followed by unsterilized PW, and was lowest in soil. There were no significant differences in the survival times between the amphibian and reptilian viruses. The study suggested that ranaviruses can survive for long periods of time in pond habitats at low temperatures, because T90 values (values where 90% of virus infectivity is gone) at 4°C were 102 days to 182 days in sterile PW, 58 days to 72 days in unsterile PW, and 30 days to 48 days in soil versus at 20°C; T90 values of the viruses were 22 days to 31 days in sterile PW and 22 days to 34 days in unsterile PW.[62] In cases of ranavirus mortalities in captivity, aggressive sterilization/removal of substrate and cleaning is advised. Cleansers that are effective at inactivating ranaviruses after 1 minute of exposure include chlorhexidine (0.75%), sodium hypochlorite (3.0%), and Virkon S (1.0%). Potassium permanganate at 2 ppm or 5 ppm is not recommended because it was ineffective at inactivating the virus at 5 ppm.[63]

BACTERIA

Few studies have attempted to identify the natural microflora of amphibian skin. One study evaluated apparently healthy, free-ranging adult eastern newts (*Notophthalmus viridescens*), larval American bullfrogs, and redback salamanders (*Plethodon cinereus*) and found 5 bacterial species from the newts, 3 from the bullfrogs, and 4 bacterial species and 1 yeast from the redback salamanders. Profiles of bacterial communities at 6 sites with newt and bullfrog tadpole populations were also evaluated. The result suggested that only a subset of bacteria in the environment are able to successfully colonize amphibian skin.[64] Enteric bacterial communities from southern toads (*Bufo terrestris*) and spring peepers (*Pseudacris crucifer*) found higher levels of enteric gram-negative bacteria during metamorphosis in each species' intestines. Gut content had no effect on bacterial levels in the toads. Much higher bacterial levels were recorded in smaller metamorphs. The results of this research suggest that enteric microflora may play an ecological role in anuran development and metamorphosis.[65]

Classically, frogs presenting for signs, such as bloating, erythema of the skin and underlying muscles, ascites, anorexia, lethargy, sometimes open sores, convulsions, and sudden death were referred to as having red leg. There are several caveats that need to be considered with this term. First, many frog species are naturally red on the ventrum of the legs. When it was believed to be a clinical sign of disease, the cause had been relegated to a bacterial infection, most likely due to gram-negative staining rods—usually *Aeromonas* sp. In retrospect, many of these infections involving die-offs may have had primary bacterial or fungal components that were overlooked due to lack of diagnostics or funds. Because the immune system was overwhelmed by the primary infection, the secondary gram-negative rod infection took advantage of the opportunity.

There can be primary bacterial infections in frogs, and most are due to poor husbandry and water quality. These infections cause erythema due to rupture and dilation of capillaries from disseminated septic thrombi—the red leg. Hydrops and hydrocoelom often follow, coining the term, red leg syndrome. Both *Flavobacterium* sp and *Aeromonas* sp have high epizootic potential. It is important to treat for secondary bacterial infections with any viral or fungal infection for this reason. Red leg syndrome causes huge economic losses in American bullfrog hatcheries, usually due to *Citrobacter freundii*. Antibiotic or chemical treatment/prevention results in modifications of the indigenous microbiota, development of antibiotic resistance, presence of their residues in food, and enhancement of production costs. *Lactococcus lactis* subsp *lactis* CRL 1584 was found to have potential as a probiotic used in the prevention of red leg syndrome in ranaculture.[66] *Elizabethkingia meningoseptica* was frequently isolated from tiger frogs (*Rana tigerina rugulosa*) with cataract disease, the most common disease of unknown origin of frogs in Hainan, China. The organisms were only susceptible to vancomycin and moderately susceptible to cefoperazone among the 20 investigated chemotherapeutic agents. Virulence test with strain W0702 was conducted and pathogenicity was demonstrated in the tiger frog.[67] Fifteen cases of a newly recognized spinal arthropathy in adult cane toads (*Chaunus* [*Bufo*] *marinus*), an invasive species in Australia, were reported, with ventral proliferation of bone and cartilage that resulted in ankylosis and lesions found at multiple intervertebral sites. Bacterial culture grew *Ochrobactrum anthropi,* and it was proposed that there was an interaction between degenerative and bacterial etiologies in the pathogenesis of this condition. Invasive toads may be predisposed to this condition because of their large size, increased rates of movement, and, possibly, immunosuppression resulting from inhabiting a novel environment.[68]

Chlamydiae

Chlamydophila sp is a common organism of concern in birds and more recently in reptiles. In amphibians, it was reported as causing red leg in *Xenopus* sp and Solomon Island eyelash frogs (*Ceratobatrachus guentheri*). The diagnosis was based on lack of bacterial growth plus the presence of intracytoplasmic inclusions resembling elementary bodies and reticular bodies. Generally, if *Chlamydophila* is present, other pathology indicates a granulomatous response, so *Mycobacterium* sp and certain systemic fungal diseases need to be ruled out.[69] Some isolated strains from amphibians have been identified as *Cp pneumoniae*. Whether these strains of *Cp pneumoniae* are zoonotic remains to be determined but may provide further insights into the relationship of this common respiratory infection with its human host.[70] 210 frog samples originating either from a mass mortality or from routine postmortem investigations were examined retrospectively for possible involvement of Chlamydiae. Using PCR, 14.8% of the samples from the mass mortality were positive for *C suis*. A control group of healthy *Xenopus laevis* had 3 of 38 positive samples, sequenced as *C suis*. In this same study, *Cp pneumoniae* was detected from exotic frogs kept in a zoo. Of those frogs collected for a prevalence study, 2.5% tested positive, 1 each for *C suis*, *Cp pneumonia*, and uncultured Chlamydiales, and the remaining 3 revealed *C abortus*.[71]

Mycobacterium

Mycobacterium spp identified in amphibians include *M marinum*, *M xenopi*, and *M ranae*. As with *Chlamydophila* spp, however, *Mycobacterium* ssp are likely to undergo significant reclassification in the years ahead as DNA PCR technology continues to progress and be refined. Most are believed to be from a water or soil source, with a clinical sign of weight loss despite good appetite. Identification of the organism is as standard for *Mycobacterium* ssp. Zoonotic potential is assumed but ultimately unknown.[69] A research colony of *Xenopus* (*Silurana*) *tropicalis* frogs presented with nodular and ulcerative skin lesions, splenomegaly, and multiple tan-yellow nodular foci in the spleen and liver. Copious acid-fast–positive bacteria were present in touch impression smears of spleen, skin, and livers of diseased frogs.

Histologically, necrotizing and granulomatous dermatitis, splenitis, and hepatitis with numerous acid-fast bacilli were consistently present, indicative of systemic mycobacteriosis. Infrequently, granulomatous inflammation was noted in the lungs, pancreas, coelomic membranes, and rarely reproductive organs. *M liflandii* was identified by PCR and is significant because this is a mycobacterium that has had a devastating impact on research frog colonies throughout the United States.[72] In another study, *M marinum* was identified as the etiologic agent in a commercial breeding farm of American bullfrogs in Brazil, with skin lesions on the head and extremities and necropsy findings, including disseminated granulomatous lesions that were observed to have that bacteria that stained acid-fast positive.[73]

There are many articles evaluating naturally occurring antimicrobial peptides from amphibians and their effectiveness against Bd. Researchers have also looked into them, however, as a novel antimicrobial against multidrug-resistant clinical isolates belonging to species often involved in nosocomial infections (*Staphylococcus aureus*, *Enterococcus faecium*, *Pseudomonas aeruginosa*, *Stenotrophomonas maltophilia*, and *Acinetobacter baumannii*). They assessed antimicrobial peptides from *Rana temporaria*, *Rana esculenta*, and *Bombina variegata*. When they were tested in buffer, all the peptides were bactericidal against all bacterial species tested (3 strains of each species).[74]

PARASITES

The final group of potential infectious organisms in amphibians is parasites. Most parasites have evolved to be a minimal drain on their host, to avoid killing the goose with the golden egg. There are many articles on normal parasites found in amphibians, discussion of which is beyond the scope of this article. Many parasites can be commensal and treatment of those may cause more harm than good. Pathology can also occur when concurrent infections with Bd or ranavirus occur. Northern red-legged frog (*Rana aurora aurora*) tadpoles with oral disc, integumentary, and cloacal abnormalities were infected with Bd and 7 parasites, including trematodes, leeches, and protozoa. Infection was associated with some environmental and coinfection risk factors. *Apiosoma* sp was the most prevalent and widespread. Tadpoles infected with Bd had a lower diversity of oral parasites than those that were uninfected.[75]

Protozoa

Amebiasis has been reported in amphibians, with *Entamoeba ranarum* reported in anurans. The anuran ingests the infective cyst in a direct life cycle, which, like many amoeboid cysts, is durable in environment. Once infected, trophozoites mature in the colon to cyst form. A renal form in *Bufo marinus* occurs as an ascending infection and hepatic abscessation has also been reported. Clinically, most infected amphibians have general illness signs, some with gastrointestinal manifestation, and possible edema and coelomic fluid. Some amphibians may have commensal amoebas, which can be difficult to differentiate from pathogenic ones, but if high numbers of amoeba and clinical signs are seen, pathogenic disease should be highly suspected. Treatment usually involves metronidazole, even as a bath.[69]

Only one species of *Cryptosporidium* has been identified in amphibians.[76] Ciliated protozoa are in that category of possible commensal status with uncertain pathogenicity, in both the gastrointestinal tract and urinary bladder (for amphibians with bladders). General beliefs are to treat if Cryptosporidia are found in high density with inflammation or clinical signs. For aquatic species, external pathogenic ciliates can cause cloudy skin patches/gills and ulcers. This often indicates a water filtration problem rather than a ciliate problem.[69]

Microsporidia caused septicemia and ulcerative dermatitis in *Phyllomedusa* sp, a South American tree frog genus. Recommended treatment was chloramphenicol.[69] Fatal renal myxosporean infection caused by *Chloromyxum* sp was reported in a collection of Asian horned frogs, *Megophrys nasuta.*[77] A proliferous, polycystic, and sometimes fatal kidney disease due to an infection with myxosporidia *H. anurae* n sp, called frog kidney enlargement disease, was reported in wild African hyperohid frogs (*Afrixalus dorsalis, Hyperolius concolor, Hyperolius* sp).[78] The mesomycetozoan, *Amphibiocystidium ranae*, is known to infect several European amphibian species and was associated with a recent decline of frogs in Italy. *Amphibiocystidium viridescens* was reported in the eastern red-spotted newt (*Notophthalmus viridescens*) with evidence of mortality due to infection.[79]

An *Ichthyophonus* sp–like organism that affects red-spotted newts and several frog species has been associated with several mass mortalities. The organism used to be considered a fungal organism but is now classified as a protist. The amphibian leech (*Placobdella picta*) acquires *Ichthyophonus* sp infection when inserting its proboscis into the muscles beneath the skin of infected newts and transmits the infection to other newts in subsequent feeding bouts. The number of leeches attached to newts was strongly related to the proportion of newt habitat containing emergent vegetation, suggesting that anthropogenic eutrophication might lead to more frequent or severe outbreaks of *Ichthyophonus* sp infection in amphibians.[80]

Hemoprotozoa are being more thoroughly evaluated in terms of their role in disease.[81] Diagnostically, it is important to differentiate these parasites from viral or chlamydophilic inclusions. Trypanosomes and *Lankesterella* sp are common in the blood, are often subclinical, and, when they are clinical, cause anemia, sudden death, and splenomegaly. In captivity, these are introduced into the amphibian by feeder fish or other live foods. Preventative recommendations include dipping food items in a hypertonic bath for approximately 5 minutes, then rinsing.[69]

Nematodes

Nematodes are another parasitic group, where the question becomes, How many is too many? *Rhabdias* spp are the most common lungworms in anurans. Having a direct life cycle, the larvae penetrate the anuran skin, molt, and travel to the lungs to mature, with embryonated eggs passed up the airway to be swallowed and shed in feces. A heavy infection can cause pathology. Recommended treatment and management include isolating infected animals and administering ivermectin/levamisole baths. *Strongyloides* spp also have a direct life cycle and have been reported to cause gastrointestinal lesions. *Pseudocapillaroides* sp has been reported to be pathologic in *Xenopus* sp, causing cutaneous hemorrhage and exfoliation, found in mucous/skin scrapings.[69]

Trematodes and Cestodes

Most trematodes and cestodes are usually larval forms in anurans that serve as intermediate hosts, causing minimal clinical sign and focal pathology once encysted but clinically relevant pathology and disease during migration through tissues. In Australian white-lipped tree frogs (*Litoria infrafrenata)* a retrospective found 28% prevalence of visible *Spirometra erinacei* infection in emaciated frogs, but this was not statistically different from 25% prevalence in nonemaciated frogs. Emaciated specimens, however, all had heavy *Spirometra erinacei* infections when present and the odds of visible sparganosis were statistically greater in emaciated frogs.[82]

Adult trematodes can be found in the lungs, urinary bladder, kidney, gastrointestinal tract, and skin. Recent concern and research has centered around *Ribeiroia* sp and a relationship with the formation of supernumery limbs in *Bufo boreas*, the boreal toad.[83,84] The widely used herbicide, atrazine, was the best predictor of the abundance of larval trematodes in the declining northern leopard frog *(Rana pipiens)*. The combination of atrazine and phosphate—principal agrochemicals in global corn and sorghum production—accounted for 74% of the variation in the abundance of these often debilitating larval trematodes (atrazine alone accounted for 51%). Analysis of field data supported a causal mechanism whereby both agrochemicals increase exposure and susceptibility to larval trematodes by augmenting snail intermediate hosts and suppressing amphibian immunity.[85]

Ectoparasites

External parasites are the final grouping of parasites. Most leeches are ectoparasites, although one species has been reported to get into the lymphatics of anurans. Recommended treatment of external leeches is a hypertonic saline bath. Likewise, external copepods are treated with salt baths. Small freshwater mussels are sometimes found attached to the toes of aquatic phase amphibians and were found to have caused local tissue and bone damage to their host and may interfere with egg laying. The mussels may benefit from the interaction through enhanced dispersal, which represents a novel form of parasitism.[86]

Cutaneous trombidiosis (*Vercammenia gloriosa* and *V zweifelorum*) in the skin of a wild tree frog, *Litoria wilcoxii,* manifested as small, domed vesicular lesions on the dorsal and lateral surfaces posterior to the eyes. The lesions contained small, orange trombiculid mites, with a surrounding minimal inflammatory reaction. The general health and behavior of the frog seemed unaffected.[87] Three plethodontid salamanders (*Desmognathus fuscus, Eurycea cirrigera,* and *Plethodon cylindraceus*) were found parasitized by *Hannemania dunni. Desmognathus fuscus* harbored mites more frequently, had higher parasite loads, and were found more frequently on their limbs compared with the other 2 species. Salamander habitat preferences and edaphic or climatic differences among study sites may influence patterns of *Hannemania* sp parasitism of salamanders.[88] With trombiculid mites, larvae are the only problem; all other life stages of chiggers live in the environment. Reptiles and amphibians are the natural host of these larvae, which can lead to blood depletion and erythematous vesicles on those hosts. Treatment options in amphibians include ivermectin or hypertonic salt baths. For infested exhibits, soil heated in the oven kills the other life stages.

SUMMARY

Ranavirus and Bd are the largest emerging infectious disease threats of amphibians worldwide and ample evidence supports that both are largely responsible for realtime amphibian extinction events. Species-specific morbidity and mortality varies for both pathogens and the most sensitive method of detection at present is PCR. There are few studies that describe natural bacterial flora of amphibians; however, *Flavobacterium* sp, *Aeromonas* sp, *Citrobacter freundii*, *Chlamydophila* sp, *C suis*, *Elizabethkingia meningoseptica*, and *Ochrobactrum anthropi* have been noted to cause disease and losses in ranaculture and in invasive species.

The clinical significance of amoeboid, cryptosporidial, microsporidial, and hemoprotozoal infections varies; however, treatment is warranted in the face of clinical signs and heavy parasite burdens. Myxosporean infections caused by *Chloromyxum* sp can cause fatal polycystic renal disease in amphibian species. The lung nematode *Rhabdias* spp have a rapid, direct life cyle and can cause significant mortalities in collections. Amphibians usually serve as intermediate hosts for cestodes and trematodes; however, heavy *Spirometra erinacei* burdens can result in severe migration-associated tissue damage in amphibian hosts.

The trematode, *Ribeiroia* sp, is responsible for causing supernumery limbs in *Bufo* spp, and the effects of atrazine and phosphate herbicides seem to augment disease susceptibility in amphibian hosts that were once unaffected as intermediate hosts. Leeches and the larvae of orange trombiculid mites can cause significant cutaneous disease. The virulence of Bd and ranavirus is changing the disease susceptibility of amphibia to historically nonpathogenic organisms. The importance of testing for multiple pathogens for any clinical amphibian cannot be overstated, because multiple infectious agents can and will continue to occur.

REFERENCES

1. Miller DL, Rajeev S, Brookins M, et al. Concurrent infection with Ranavirus, Batrachochytrium dendrobatidis, and Aeromonas in a captive anuran colony. J Zoo Wildl Med 2008;39(3):445–9.
2. Schloegel LM, Daszak P, Cunningham AA, et al. Two amphibian diseases, chytridiomycosis and ranaviral disease, are now globally notifiable to the World Organization for Animal Health (OIE): an assessment. Dis Aquat Org 2010;92(2–3): 101–8.
3. Berger L, Speare R, Daszak P, et al. Chytridiomycosis causes amphibian mortality associated with population declines in the rain forests of Australia and Central America. Proc Natl Acad Sci U S A 1998;95(15):9031–6.
4. Kilpatrick AM, Briggs CJ, Daszak P. The ecology and impact of chytridiomycosis: an emerging disease of amphibians. Trends Ecol Evol 2010;25(2):109–18.
5. Weldon C, Du Preez LH, Hyatt AD, et al. Origin of the amphibian chytrid fungus. Emerg Infect Dis 2004;10(12):2100.
6. Fisher MC, Bosch J, Yin Z, et al. Proteomic and phenotypic profiling of the amphibian pathogen Batrachochytrium dendrobatidis shows that genotype is linked to virulence. Mol Ecol 2009;18(3):415–29.
7. Schloegel LM, Toledo LF, Longcore JE, et al. Novel, panzootic and hybrid genotypes of amphibian chytridiomycosis associated with the bullfrog trade. Mol Ecol 2012;21(21):5162–77.
8. Farrer RA, Weinert LA, Bielby J, et al. Multiple emergences of genetically diverse amphibian-infecting chytrids include a globalized hypervirulent recombinant lineage. Proc Natl Acad Sci U S A 2011;108(46):18732–6.
9. Fisher MC, Henk DA, Briggs CJ, et al. Emerging fungal threats to animal, plant and ecosystem health. Nature 2012;484(7393):186–94.
10. McCallum H. Disease and the dynamics of extinction. Philos Trans R Soc Lond B Biol Sci 2012;367(1604):2828–39.
11. Collins JP. Amphibian decline and extinction: what we know and what we need to learn. Dis Aquat Org 2010;92(2–3):93–9.
12. Rödder D, Kielgast J, Lötters S. Future potential distribution of the emerging amphibian chytrid fungus under anthropogenic climate change. Dis Aquat Org 2010;92(2–3):201–7.
13. Vredenburg VT, Knapp RA, Tunstall TS, et al. Dynamics of an emerging disease drive large-scale amphibian population extinctions. Proc Natl Acad Sci U S A 2010;107(21):9689–94.

14. Hyatt AD, Boyle DG, Olsen V, et al. Diagnostic assays and sampling protocols for the detection of Batrachochytrium dendrobatidis. Dis Aquat Org 2007;73:175–92.

15. Rosenblum EB, Stajich JE, Maddox N, et al. Global gene expression profiles for life stages of the deadly amphibian pathogen Batrachochytrium dendrobatidis. Proc Natl Acad Sci U S A 2008;105(44):17034–9.

16. Miller CE. A developmental study with the SEM of sexual reproduction in Chytriomyces hyalinus. Bull Soc Bot Fr 1977;124:281–9. Available at: http://openagricola.nal.usda.gov/Record/CAIN789078432.

17. Voyles J, Young S, Berger L, et al. Pathogenesis of chytridiomycosis, a cause of catastrophic amphibian declines. Science 2009;326(5952):582–5.

18. Rachowicz LJ, Vredenburg VT. Transmission of Batrachochytrium dendrobatidis within and between amphibian life stages. Dis Aquat Org 2004;61:75–83.

19. Spitzen–van der Sluijs AM, Zollinger R. Literature review on Batrachochytrium. 2010. Available at: http://www.ravon.nl/Portals/0/Pdf/Lit%20studie%20Bd%20Def.pdf. Accessed February 23, 2013.

20. Daszak P, Strieby A, Cunningham AA, et al. Experimental evidence that the bullfrog (Rana catesbeiana) is a potential carrier of chytridiomycosis, an emerging fungal disease of amphibians. Herpetol J 2004;14(4):201–7. Available at: http://cat.inist.fr/aModele=afficheN&cpsidt=16329306.

21. Reeder NM, Pessier AP, Vredenburg VT. A reservoir species for the emerging amphibian pathogen batrachochytrium dendrobatidis thrives in a landscape decimated by disease. PLoS One 2012;7(3):e33567.

22. Paetow LJ, Daniel McLaughlin J, Cue RI, et al. Effects of herbicides and the chytrid fungus Batrachochytrium dendrobatidis on the health of post-metamorphic northern leopard frogs (Lithobates pipiens). Ecotoxicol Environ Saf 2012;80:372–80.

23. Solís R, Lobos G, Walker SF, et al. Presence of Batrachochytrium dendrobatidis in feral populations of Xenopus laevis in Chile. Biol Invasions 2010;12(6):1641–6.

24. Davidson EW, Parris M, Collins JP, et al. Pathogenicity and transmission of chytridiomycosis in tiger salamanders (Ambystoma tigrinum). Copeia 2003;2003(3):601–7.

25. Hyatt AD, Speare R, Cunningham AA, et al. Amphibian chytridiomycosis. Dis Aquat Org 2010;92:89–91.

26. Simoncelli F, Fagotti A, Dall'Olio R, et al. Evidence of Batrachochytrium dendrobatidis infection in water frogs of the Rana esculenta complex in central Italy. Ecohealth 2005;2(4):307–12.

27. Cunningham AA, Garner TW, Aguilar-Sanchez V, et al. Emergence of amphibian chytridiomycosis in Britain. Vet Rec 2005;157(13):386–7.

28. World Organization for Animal Health. Chapter 8.1. Infection with Batrachochytrium dendrobatidis. vol. 2012. Available at: http://www.oie.Int/index.php?id=171&L=0&htmfile=chapitre_1.8.1.htm. Accessed February 23, 2013.

29. Kriger KM, Hines HB, Hyatt AD, et al. Techniques for detecting chytridiomycosis in wild frogs: comparing histology with real-time Taqman PCR. Dis Aquat Org 2006;71(2):141.

30. Ruthig GR, DeRidder BP. Fast quantitative PCR, locked nucleic acid probes and reduced volume reactions are effective tools for detecting Batrachochytrium dendrobatidis DNA. Dis Aquat Org 2012;97:249–53.

31. Hatfield C. Fluid therapy osmolality recommendations for anurans. 2012.

32. Young S, Speare R, Berger L, et al. Chloramphenicol with fluid and electrolyte therapy cures terminally ill green tree frogs (Litoria caerulea) with chytridiomycosis. J Zoo Wildl Med 2012;43(2):330–7.

33. Brannelly LA, Richards-Zawacki CL, Pessier AP. Clinical trials with itraconazole as a treatment for chytrid fungal infections in amphibians. Dis Aquat Org 2012;101(2):95.
34. Nichols DK, Lamirande E, Pessier A, et al. Experimental transmission and treatment of cutaneous chytridiomycosis in poison dart frogs (Dendrobates auratus and Dendrobates tinctorius). Paper presented at: Annual Conference-American Association of Zoo Veterinarians. New Orleans (LA), 2000.
35. Forzán MJ, Gunn H, Scott P. Chytridiomycosis in an aquarium collection of frogs: diagnosis, treatment, and control. J Zoo Wildl Med 2008;39(3):406–11.
36. Pessier A. Management of disease as a threat to amphibian conservation. Int Zoo Yearbk 2008;42(1):30–9.
37. Pessier A, Mendelson J. A manual for control of infectious diseases in amphibian survival assurance colonies and reintroduction programs. Apple Valley: IUCN/SSC Conservation Breeding Specialist Group 2010. Available at: http://www.cbsg.org/cbsg/workshopreports/26/amphibian_disease_manual.pdf. Accessed February 23, 2013.
38. Woodhams DC, Alford RA, Marantelli G. Emerging disease of amphibians cured by elevated body temperature. Dis Aquat Org 2003;55:65–7.
39. Malik S, Sarwar I, Mehmood T, et al. Aetiological considerations of acquired aplastic anaemia. 20101008 DCOM- 20101102. J Ayub Med Coll Abbottabad 2009;21(3):127–30.
40. Berger L, Speare R, Marantelli G, et al. A zoospore inhibition technique to evaluate the activity of antifungal compounds against Batrachochytrium dendrobatidis and unsuccessful treatment of experimentally infected green tree frogs (Litoria caerulea) by fluconazole and benzalkonium chloride. Res Vet Sci 2009;87(1):106–10.
41. Berger L, Speare R, Pessier A, et al. Treatment of chytridiomycosis requires urgent clinical trials. Dis Aquat Org 2010;92(2):165.
42. Phillott AD, Speare R, Hines HB, et al. Minimising exposure of amphibians to pathogens during field studies. Dis Aquat Org 2010;92(2–3):175–85.
43. Davison AJ, Cunningham C, Sauerbier W, et al. Genome sequences of two frog herpesviruses. J Gen Virol 2006;87(12):3509–14.
44. Davison AJ, Eberle R, Ehlers B, et al. The order herpesvirales. Arch Virol 2009; 154(1):171–7.
45. Waltzek TB, Kelley GO, Alfaro ME, et al. Phylogenetic relationships in the family Alloherpesviridae. Dis Aquat Org 2009;84:179–94.
46. Holopainen R, Ohlemeyer S, Schutze H, et al. Ranavirus phylogeny and differentiation based on major capsid protein, DNA polymerase and neurofilament triplet H1-like protein genes. Dis Aquat Org 2009;85(2):81–91.
47. Mazzoni R, de Mesquita AJ, Fleury LFF, et al. Mass mortality associated with a frog virus 3-like Ranavirus infection in farmed tadpoles Rana catesbeiana from Brazil. Dis Aquat Org 2009;86(3):181.
48. Weir RP, Moody NJ, Hyatt AD, et al. Isolation and characterisation of a novel Bohle-like virus from two frog species in the Darwin rural area, Australia. Dis Aquat Org 2012;99(3):169.
49. Gray MJ, Miller DL, Hoverman JT. Ecology and pathology of amphibian ranaviruses. Dis Aquat Org 2009;87(3):243–66.
50. Pasmans F, Blahak S, Martel A, et al. Ranavirus-associated mass mortality in imported red tailed knobby newts (Tylototriton kweichowensis): a case report. Vet J 2008;176:257–9.
51. Greer AL, Brunner JL, Collins JP. Spatial and temporal patterns of Ambystoma tigrinum virus (ATV) prevalence in tiger salamanders Ambystoma tigrinum nebulosum. Dis Aquat Org 2009;85:1–6.

52. Rojas S, Richards K, Jancovich JK, et al. Influence of temperature on Ranavirus infection in larval salamanders Ambystoma tigrinum. Dis Aquat Org 2005;63: 95–100.

53. Forson D, Storfer A. Effects of atrazine and iridovirus infection on survival and life history traits of the long toed salamander (Ambystoma macrodactylum). Environ Toxicol Chem 2006;25(1):168–73.

54. Hoverman JT, Gray MJ, Miller DL. Anuran susceptibilities to ranaviruses: role of species identity, exposure route, and a novel virus isolate. Dis Aquat Org 2010; 89(2):97–107.

55. Robert J, Abramowitz L, Gantress J, et al. Xenopus laevis: a possible vector of ranavirus infection? J Wildl Dis 2007;43(4):645–52.

56. Morales HD, Robert J. Characterization of primary and memory CD8 T-cell responses against ranavirus (FV3) in Xenopus laevis. J Virol 2007;81(5): 2240–8.

57. Robert J, Morales H, Buck W, et al. Adaptive immunity and histopathology in frog virus 3-infected Xenopus. Virology 2005;332(2):667–75.

58. Kik M, Martel A, Sluijs AS, et al. Ranavirus-associated mass mortality in wild amphibians, The Netherlands, 2010: a first report. Vet J 2011;190(2):284–6.

59. Balseiro A, Dalton KP, Del Cerro A, et al. Outbreak of common midwife toad virus in alpine newts (Mesotriton alpestris cyreni) and common midwife toads (Alytes obstetricans) in Northern Spain: a comparative pathological study of an emerging ranavirus. Vet J 2010;186(2):256–8.

60. Burton EC, Miller DL, Styer EL, et al. Amphibian ocular malformation associated with frog virus 3. Vet J 2008;177(3):442–4.

61. Gray MJ, Miller DL, Hoverman JT. Reliability of non-lethal surveillance methods for detecting ranavirus infection. Dis Aquat Org 2012;99.1–6.

62. Nazir J, Spengler M, Marschang RE. Environmental persistence of amphibian and reptilian ranaviruses. Dis Aquat Org 2012;98(3):177–84.

63. Bryan LK, Baldwin CA, Gray MJ, et al. Efficacy of select disinfectants at inactivating Ranavirus. Dis Aquat Org 2009;84:89–94.

64. Culp CE, Falkinham Iii JO, Belden LK. Identification of the natural bacterial microflora on the skin of eastern newts, bullfrog tadpoles and redback salamanders. Herpetologica 2007;63(1):66–71.

65. Fedewa LA. Fluctuating gram-negative microflora in developing anurans. J Herpetol 2006;40(1):131–5.

66. Pasteris SE, Guidoli MG, Otero MC, et al. In vitro inhibition of Citrobacter freundii, a red-leg syndrome associated pathogen in raniculture, by indigenous Lactococcus lactis CRL 1584. Vet Microbiol 2011;151(3):336–44.

67. Xie ZY, Zhou YC, Wang SF, et al. First isolation and identification of Elizabethkingia meningoseptica from cultured tiger frog, Rana tigerina rugulosa. Vet Microbiol 2009;138(1):140–4.

68. Shilton CM, Brown GP, Benedict S, et al. Spinal arthropathy associated with Ochrobactrum anthropi in free-ranging cane toads (Chaunus [Bufo] marinus) in Australia. Vet Pathol 2008;45(1):85–94.

69. Wright K. Reptile medicine and surgery, vol. 2. St Louis (MO): Elsevier; 2006.

70. Bodetti TJ, Jacobson E, Wan C, et al. Molecular evidence to support the expansion of the hostrange of chlamydophila pneumoniae to include reptiles as well as humans, horses, koalas and amphibians. Syst Appl Microbiol 2002;25(1): 146–52.

71. Blumer C, Zimmermann DR, Weilenmann R, et al. Chlamydiae in free-ranging and captive frogs in Switzerland. Vet Pathol 2007;44(2):144–50.

72. Fremont-Rahl JJ, Ek C, Williamson HR, et al. Mycobacterium liflandii Outbreak in a Research Colony of Xenopus (Silurana) tropicalis Frogs. Vet Pathol 2011;48(4): 856–67.
73. Ferreira R, Fonseca LS, Afonso AM, et al. A report of mycobacteriosis caused by Mycobacterium marinum in bullfrogs (Rana catesbeiana). Vet J 2006;171(1): 177–80.
74. Mangoni ML, Maisetta G, Di Luca M, et al. Comparative analysis of the bactericidal activities of amphibian peptide analogues against multidrug-resistant nosocomial bacterial strains. Antimicrobial Agents Chemother 2008;52(1):85–91.
75. Nieto NC, Camann MA, Foley JE, et al. Disease associated with integumentary and cloacal parasites in tadpoles of northern red-legged frog Rana aurora aurora. Dis Aquat Org 2007;78(1):61.
76. Plutzer J, Karanis P. Genetic polymorphism in Cryptosporidiumi species: an update. Vet Parasitol 2009;165(3):187–99.
77. Duncan AE, Garner MM, Bartholomew JL, et al. Renal myxosporidiasis in Asian horned frogs (Megophrys nasuta). J Zoo Wildl Med 2004;35(3):381–6.
78. Mutschmann F. Pathological changes in African hyperoliid frogs due to a myxosporidian infection with a new species of Hoferellus (Myxozoa). Dis Aquat Org 2004;60(3):215–22.
79. Raffel TR, Bommarito T, Barry DS, et al. Widespread infection of the Eastern red-spotted newt (Notophthalmus viridescens) by a new species of Amphibiocystidium, a genus of fungus-like mesomycetozoan parasites not previously reported in North America. Parasitology 2008;135(02):203–15.
80. Raffel TR, Dillard JR, Hudson PJ. Field evidence for leech-borne transmission of amphibian Ichthyophonus sp. J Parasitol 2006;92(6):1256–64.
81. Stenberg PL, Bowerman WJ. Hemoparasites in Oregon spotted frogs (Rana pretiosa) from central Oregon, USA. J Wildl Dis 2008;44(2):464–8.
82. Young S, Skerratt LF, Mendez D, et al. Using community surveillance data to differentiate between emerging and endemic amphibian diseases. Dis Aquat Org 2012;98(1):1.
83. Schotthoefer AM, Labak KM, Beasley VR. Ribeiroia ondatrae cercariae are consumed by aquatic invertebrate predators. J Parasitol 2007;93(5):1240–3.
84. Peterson NA. Seasonal prevalence of Ribeiroia ondatrae in one population of Planorbella trivolvis (= Helisoma trivolvis), including notes on the larval trematode component community. Comp Parasitol 2007;74(2):312–8.
85. Rohr JR, Schotthoefer AM, Raffel TR, et al. Agrochemicals increase trematode infections in a declining amphibian species. Nature 2008;455(7217):1235–9.
86. Wood LR, Griffiths RA, Groh K, et al. Interactions between freshwater mussels and newts: a novel form of parasitism? Amphibia-Reptilia 2008;29(4):457–62.
87. Mendez D, Freeman AB, Spratt DM, et al. Pathology of cutaneous trombidiosis caused by larval trombiculid mites in a wild Lesueur's tree frog (Litoria wilcoxii). Aust Vet J 2010;88(8):328–30.
88. Westfall MC, Cecala KK, Price SJ, et al. Patterns of trombiculid mite (Hannemania dunni) parasitism among plethodontid salamanders in the western piedmont of North Carolina. J Parasitol 2008;94(3):631–4.

Emerging Infectious Diseases of Chelonians

Paul M. Gibbons, DVM, MS, DABVP (Reptiles and Amphibians)[a],*,
Zachary J. Steffes, DVM[b]

KEYWORDS

- Testudines • Chelonians • Adenovirus • *Iridovirus* • *Ranavirus* • Coccidiosis
- Cryptosporidiosis

KEY POINTS

- Intranuclear coccidiosis of Testudines is a newly emerging disease found in numerous chelonian species that should be on the differential list for all cases of systemic illness and cases with clinical signs involving multiple organ systems. Early diagnosis and treatment is essential, and PCR performed on conjunctival, oral and choanal mucosa, and cloacal tissue seems to be the most useful antemortem diagnostic tool.
- *Cryptosporidium* spp have been observed in numerous chelonians globally, and are sometimes associated with chronic diarrhea, anorexia, pica, decreased growth rate, weight loss, lethargy, or passing undigested feed. A consensus PCR can be performed on feces to identify the species of *Cryptosporidium*. No treatments have been shown to clear infection, but paromomycin did eliminate clinical signs of disease in a group of *Testudo hermanni*.
- Iridoviral infection is an emerging disease of chelonians in outdoor environments that usually presents with signs of upper respiratory disease, oral ulceration, cutaneous abcessation, subcutaneous edema, anorexia, and lethargy. The disease can be highly fatal in turtles, and can be screened for with PCR of oral and cloacal swabs, and whole blood.
- Adenoviral disease is newly recognized in chelonians and presents most commonly with signs of hepatitis, enteritis, esophagitis, splenitis, and encephalopathy. Death is common in affected chelonians. PCR of cloacal and plasma samples has shown promise for antemortem detection, although treatment has proved unsuccessful to date.

Several infectious diseases continue to be prevalent in captive and wild chelonians. Important diseases that have been well described include mycoplasmosis and herpesvirus in tortoises, and herpesvirus-associated fibropapillomas in sea turtles. Diseases that are currently emerging as important pathogens include intranuclear coccidiosis of Testudines, cryptosporidiosis in tortoises, *Iridovirus*, and adenovirus.

[a] Turtle Conservancy Behler Chelonian Center, PO Box 1289, Ojai, CA 93023, USA; [b] Pet Hospital of Peñasquitos, 9888 Carmel Mountain Road, Suite F, San Diego, CA 92129, USA
* Corresponding author.
E-mail address: paul@turtleconservancy.org

Vet Clin Exot Anim 16 (2013) 303–317
http://dx.doi.org/10.1016/j.cvex.2013.02.004
1094-9194/13/$ – see front matter © 2013 Elsevier Inc. All rights reserved.
vetexotic.theclinics.com

This article describes each of these emerging pathogens by its biology, epidemiology, clinical signs, diagnosis, treatment, gross pathology, histopathologic changes, and any anticipated future trends.

INTRANUCLEAR COCCIDIOSIS OF TESTUDINES
Biology and Epidemiology

A disease-causing, primarily intranuclear, coccidian parasite of Testudines (TINC) was first identified in radiated tortoises in 1990.[1] Subsequently, the same pathogen (Gen-Bank accession number AY728896), determined by sequencing of a coccidial 18S rRNA consensus polymerase chain reaction (qPCR) product, has caused systemic disease in impressed tortoises (*Manouria impressa*); leopard tortoises (*Stigmochelys* [*Geochelone*] *pardalis*); Forsten tortoises (*Indotestudo forstenii*); bowsprit tortoises (*Chersina angulata*); spider tortoises (*Pyxis arachnoides*); flat-tailed tortoises (*Pyxis planicauda*); Galapagos tortoises (*Chelonoidis nigra becki*); eastern box turtles (*Terrapene carolina carolina*); and Arakan forest turtles (*Heosemys depressa*).[2–5] The authors have also confirmed the disease in several other chelonian species (Paul M. Gibbons, DVM, unpublished data, 2013) postmortem by histopathology usually after severe acute illness. Cases have been reported in Germany and the United States including New York, Louisiana, Florida, Georgia, Texas, California, and Hawaii, although no systematic prevalence study has been undertaken to date.[1–7] Most of these cases occurred in zoologic collections and a few had been recently imported from Indonesia.

The life cycle and method of transmission of the TINC organism are unknown and the organism has not been studied in vitro. Although it has not been assigned to a genus, the phylogenetic position of the organism has been characterized by sequencing an 18S small ribosomal unit. It is most closely related to *Eimeria arnyi*, a species identified by oocysts in the feces of the eastern ringneck snake (*Diadophis punctatus arnyi*).[3,8] Life stages of the TINC organism including trophozoites, meronts, merozoites, macrogametocytes, microgametocytes, and nonsporulated oocysts have been found in the nucleus, cytoplasm, and extracellularly in tissues by histology and electron microscopy. Reports have failed to describe TINC oocysts in feces, and the authors have been unable to find oocysts on fecal flotation from several polymerase chain reaction (PCR) test-positive animals with clinical signs of illness. The TINC organism has not been identified outside of cells or tissues, and samples of various invertebrates and substrate from the enclosures of affected tortoises during an outbreak of TINC at a zoologic facility were negative when tested by quantitative PCR.[4]

Clinical Signs

Although the organism is often reported in highest number in the kidney or pancreas, infection is frequently disseminated to an array of organs so clinical signs vary among cases and are not specific to TINC. Clinical signs range from mild chronic conjunctival or nasal erythema or discharge to severe gasping, subcutaneous edema, and ulceration of the cloacal mucosa. Additional clinical signs can include anorexia, lethargy, lack of normal diurnal behavior patterns, increased respiratory effort, mouth breathing, and rapid weight gain or loss. Rapid weight gain is common, and results from ascites or retention of urine in the urinary bladder (Paul M. Gibbons, DVM, personal communication, 2013). Death can occur within a few days of initial clinical signs, or after months of clinical management including improved husbandry and anticoccidial drug therapy (Paul M. Gibbons, DVM, personal communication, 2013). Stress and thermoregulatory challenges (eg, insufficient heat or evaporative heat loss) seem to enhance progression of disease, probably because of reduced immune response. In groups housed together, morbidity and mortality vary from a few to all of the individuals showing signs of disease (Paul M. Gibbons, DVM, personal communication, 2013). Often a proportion of the animals in an affected group survives and apparently recovers (Paul M. Gibbons, DVM, personal communication, 2013).[5,7] Some cases have survived after a positive diagnostic test, and some of these have become test-negative after treatment (Paul M. Gibbons, DVM, personal communication, 2013).[5] Animals that recover from clinical signs of illness could become carriers; clinical signs can recrudesce, and recovered animals can become test-positive again (Paul M. Gibbons, DVM, personal communication, 2013). It is likely, but not proved, that test-positive animals shed infectious stages of the organism. No systematic study has been undertaken to determine the likelihood that recovered or exposed individuals become carriers or reservoirs. It is unknown whether the organism is directly transmitted or requires an intermediate host, but most of the animals in an affected group usually become test-positive (Paul M. Gibbons, DVM, personal communication, 2013).[5]

Diagnosis

Antemortem diagnosis is possible and TINC should be included in the differential diagnosis of all cases of Testudinoidea (Chelonia) with systemic signs of illness or clinical signs involving multiple organ systems. The organism can sometimes be identified on cytologic examination of nasal discharge stained by Wright-Giemsa, Fite acid-fast, or periodic acid–Schiff techniques (**Fig. 1**).[3] Cytologic examination of nasal discharge also generally shows a mononuclear inflammatory response.[3] Biopsy and histologic examination of affected tissues may also be diagnostic, particularly in cases with rhinitis or cloacitis, and renal or pancreatic biopsies may also be examined in cases with systemic signs of illness. At this time, however, the most useful clinical diagnostic tool is quantitative PCR performed on swabs from the conjunctiva, oral and choanal mucosa, and cloaca.[4]

Treatment

Treatment is focused on providing optimal husbandry and minimizing stress. Isolate affected individuals and remove fecal matter promptly to minimize the presence of potentially infectious material. Provide appropriate live plants (shelter and browse); natural substrates; surface duff; refuges; and an array of species-specific options for thermoregulation including diurnal temperature fluctuation and presence or absence of a basking lamp. Many species benefit from providing background temperatures in the upper one-third of the species-specific range during treatment, in addition to the usual basking site. Provide moisture as appropriate for the species, which may include regular misting, diurnal humidity fluctuation, morning dew, fog, and a humid refuge. Provide species-appropriate light spectrum, intensity, and diurnal cycles. Handle the animal infrequently, preferably only during administration of therapeutic agents. Nutritional therapy may not be indicated in many cases, because placing feed in the gastrointestinal tract could worsen disease in the presence of ileus or diffuse pancreatic, hepatic, or intestinal necrosis. It may be better to simply provide favorite feed items fresh daily and allow the tortoise to eat voluntarily when appetite returns. Consider fluid therapy only if not drinking or if more than 5% dehydrated. Administer broad-spectrum anthelmintic, antiprotozoal, and antibiotic therapy if animals exhibit signs of systemic illness including abnormal diurnal behavior patterns, lethargy, or anorexia. Toltrazuril (Baycox 5% oral suspension; Bayer Vital GmbH, Deutschland) 15 mg/kg by mouth (gavage) every 48 hours for 30 days might eliminate

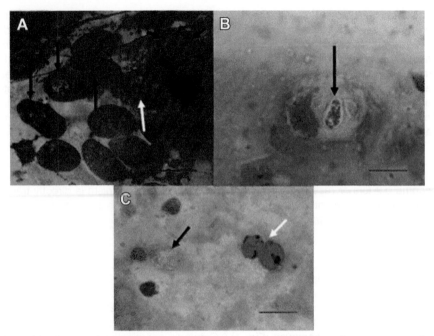

Fig. 1. Nasal mucosal smear, Sulawesi tortoise, Case no. 4. (*A*) Cluster of respiratory epithelial cells, many of which contain single intranuclear gametes (*long black arrows*), one that contains multiple gametes (*short black arrows*). A meront (*white arrow*) is noted in the nucleus of one cell. Modified Wright-Giemsa. (*B*) Intranuclear gamete (*arrow*) stains positive for the periodic acid–Schiff reaction. (*C*) Single intranuclear acid-fast gamete (*black arrow*) and two extracellular unsporulated acid-fast oocysts (*white arrow*). Fite acid-fast. Bar = 8 um. (*From* Innis CJ, Garner MM, Johnson AJ, et al. Antemortem diagnosis and characterization of nasal intranuclear coccidiosis in Sulawesi tortoises (*Indotestudo forsteni*). J Vet Diagn Invest 2007;19(6):660–7; with permission.)

infection, and shorter durations seem to reduce clinical signs without clearing the organism (Paul M. Gibbons, DVM, personal communication, 2013). Ponazuril, the active metabolite of toltrazuril, has also been used and may be equally effective at a similar dosage for similar duration.[5] Chronic TINC-associated conjunctivitis has been observed in some cases (Paul M. Gibbons, DVM, personal communication, 2013). Abbreviated treatments (2 weeks) with toltrazuril have been followed by chronic infection (particularly brain) and death many months later (Paul M. Gibbons, DVM, personal communication, 2013). After the organism was apparently eliminated by treatment (absent on histopathology), one of the authors (PMG) has observed several cases with organ damage caused by TINC (present on histopathology) that was sufficient to cause chronic maldigestion, weight loss, subcutaneous edema, urine retention (urinary bladder distended with urine and urates), and death many months later. Taken together, this case information suggests that delayed or abbreviated treatment is less likely to be effective than early prolonged treatment.

Gross Pathology and Histopathologic Changes

Death occurs in many cases. Gross pathologic abnormalities may include thick oral mucus, severely distended urinary bladder, firm gray kidneys, pericloacal erythema,

red lungs, epicardial petechiae, gastrointestinal mucosal pseudomembrane formation, erythematous and edematous intestinal serosa and submucosa, and voluminous
pale yellow to red translucent coelomic fluid.[5] Histopathologic changes in all body
tissues generally include necrosis and lymphocytic or lymphoplasmacytic inflammation associated with various stages of coccidia in the nucleus and rarely in cytoplasm
or extracellular spaces.[2] Lesions suggestive of coccidiosis (necrosis and inflammation) are sometimes detected in the heart and central nervous system without
coccidia.[2] Coccidia are best observed in sections stained with hematoxylin and eosin
(H&E), and the organism is not observed in sections stained by periodic acid–Schiff or
Fite acid-fast techniques.[2] Cases that die after treatment often have fibrosis that is
distributed in a pattern matching the distribution of lesions in cases with coccidia
present. This suggests that treatment can eliminate the organism, but tissue sclerosis
can have a long-term effect on organ function, which emphasizes the importance of
early diagnosis and treatment (Paul M. Gibbons, DVM, personal communication,
2013).

CRYPTOSPORIDIOSIS
Biology and Epidemiology

Cryptosporidiosis has been recognized in snakes and lizards for many years.[9–11]
Cryptosporidia are now being reported with increasing frequency in chelonians
including Indian star tortoise (G elegans); pancake tortoise (Malacochersus tornieri);
Russian tortoise (Agrionemys horsfieldii); radiated tortoise (Astrochelys [Geochelone]
radiata); gopher tortoise (Gopherus polyphemus); an Indotestudo-like tortoise (probably I forstenii); and several species of tortoise in the genus Testudo.[12–18] Cases
have been reported in Italy; Germany; Spain; Switzerland; the Czech Republic; Ghana;
Australia; and the United States including North Carolina, Georgia, Missouri,
Kentucky, Washington DC, Maryland, and Kansas. At least two distinct novel species
have recently been identified in tortoises, one with intestinal tropism and a proposed
name of "C ducismarci" (GenBank accession numbers EF519704 and EF547155), and
another with gastric tropism that is yet unnamed, but is referred to as "Cryptosporidium sp. tortoise 750" (GenBank accession number AY120914).[13,15,19]

Life cycles and methods of transmission for these novel Cryptosporidium sp have
not been described, but direct, fecal-oral transmission is likely because oocysts can
be identified in feces and in the gastrointestinal tract on histopathology, and this is
the usual mode of transmission for cryptosporidia. Several surveys have been
reported, and cryptosporidia were found in a proportion of the sample group in
each report.[13,15,17,18]

Clinical Signs

Clinical signs of gastrointestinal disease occur in some cases in which cryptosporidial
organisms are found. Clinical signs, when they occur, can include chronic diarrhea,
decreased appetite, pica, decreased growth rate, weight loss, lethargy, and passing
undigested feed.[12,15,20] Concurrent infection with additional pathogens has been
reported, and concomitant infections may enhance disease progression.

Diagnosis

Several clinical diagnostic tests are available. Fecal flotation techniques may be useful
to prepare samples for microscopy and Ziehl-Neelsen or Fite acid-fast staining, car-
bolfuchsin staining, and immunoassay.[15–18,20] Oocysts are round and range from
3.4- to 6.3-μm diameter on fecal examination or cytologic examination of mucosal

smears.[15,16] On histopathology, oocysts range from 1- to 5-µm diameter.[12] The most specific, readily available fecal test consists of DNA extraction and consensus PCR with sequencing of the *Cryptosporidium* 18S rRNA gene to identify the species.[13,17]

Treatment

Treatment is focused on providing optimal husbandry as described previously for TINC. A few anticoccidial drugs have been used, but none is proved to eliminate infection. Suggested chemotherapeutics include paromomycin, toltrazuril, ponazuril, and possibly halfuginone or spiramycin.[9,20,21] Paromomycin, 100 mg/kg by mouth every 24 hours for 7 days, eliminated clinical signs and led to negative test results for 9 months in a group of Herman tortoises (*Testudo hermanni*).[20] Supportive care can include fluid therapy for dehydrated tortoises, and some authors suggest immunostimulants.[20] Nutritional supplementation is important for tortoises with chronic anorexia.

In general, cryptosporidia are resistant to most disinfectants and survive well in the environment for many months. Equipment should be discarded when no longer needed for infected individuals. Temperatures greater than 65°C (149°F) can be applied with steam or a flame thrower. Formalin (10%), glutaraldehyde (2.65%), and possibly 5% to 10% ammonia solution may be effective on clean, smooth, impermeable surfaces, but must be used with care to prevent toxicity to humans or animals in the vicinity.

Gross Pathology and Histopathologic Changes

The pathologic changes associated with cryptosporidiosis in tortoises have been described in few cases.[12] Few, if any, gross changes occur. The stomach-associated species (*Cryptosporidium* sp tortoise 750) is found in gastric mucosal cells and may be associated with mild lymphocytic and heterophilic inflammation of the lamina propria of the mucosa.[12] The species with a proposed name of *Cryptosporidium ducismarci* is associated with intestinal mucosal cells and may elicit a mixed inflammatory response in the lamina propria of the mucosa or in the submucosa.[12] Cryptosporidia appear on H&E-stained histopathologic preparations as 1- to 5-µm diameter amphophilic round organisms with an eccentrically located dense basophilic internal structure.[12]

IRIDOVIRUS
Biology and Epidemiology

Iridoviruses are rapidly gaining notoriety as a serious emerging pathogen causing morbidity and mortality in turtle and tortoise populations. Iridoviruses of the genus *Ranavirus*, well known for causing mass mortality events in fish and amphibians, have increasingly been determined to be the cause of disease and mass mortality events in turtle and tortoise populations worldwide.[22] *Ranavirus* causes high mortality in exposed turtle populations.[23,24]

Iridoviruses are large, double-stranded, enveloped DNA viruses with a diameter of 120 to 200 nm, and an icosahedral nucelocapsid.[25–27] Replication initially occurs in the nucleus, and is followed by replication in the cytoplasm.[26] In vertebrates, eosinophilic and basophilic intracytoplasmic inclusions may be seen in H&E-stained tissue sections[26] and have also been visualized in circulating leukocytes[28] and circulating red blood cells.[29,30] The family Iridoviridae consists of four genera: *Chloriridovirus* and *Iridovirus*, which both infect insects; *Lymphocystivirus*, which infects fish; and

Ranavirus, which has been shown to be capable of infecting fish, amphibians, and reptiles.[26]

Before 2003 there were few cases of iridoviral infection noted in chelonians worldwide. In 1982, a Hermann tortoise (*T hermanni*) that died after 2 days of anorexia was found to have cytoplasmic inclusions in hepatocytes consistent with iridoviral infection.[31] In 1996, a free-living gopher tortoise (*G polyphemus*) presented with clinical signs associated with upper respiratory disease and was subsequently euthanized because of poor response to therapy. It was shown to have iridoviral particles in epithelial cells of the trachea, lung, and necrotic cells of the tracheal lumen.[32] In 1999, an *Iridovirus* was shown through experimental viral infection studies to be the cause of "red-neck disease" in soft-shelled turtles (*Trionyx sinensis*)[33] and two Hermann tortoises (*T hermanni*) that died of systemic disease.[27] In 2002, five eastern box turtles (*T carolina carolina*) died after showing acute signs of cutaneous abcessation, oral ulceration or abcessation, respiratory distress, anorexia, and lethargy, with an *Iridovirus* being isolated in two of the five turtles.[25]

Since 2003, additional outbreaks and infections have been diagnosed in free-ranging and captive chelonians. In 2006, a free-ranging eastern box turtle was presented for suspected trauma and blindness, and subsequently became anorexic, lost weight, had increased clear ocular and nasal discharges, became progressively depressed, and died 6 days postpresentation. Iridoviral intracytoplasmic inclusions were discovered in circulating leukocytes.[28] In 2008, *Iridovirus* was described in a gopher tortoise, numerous eastern box turtles, a Florida box turtle (*Terrepene carolina bauri*), and a Burmese star tortoise (*Geochelone platynota*).[24] A free-ranging gopher tortoise was euthanized after presenting for palpebral swelling and ocular and nasal discharge, and was positive for *Ranavirus* by PCR and viral isolation.[24] A captive female Burmese star tortoise died 3 days after presenting with nasal discharge, conjunctivitis, severe subcutaneous edema of the neck, and yellow-white cutaneous plaques observed on the tongue, and was positive for *Ranavirus* by PCR, virus isolation, and transmission electron microscopy (TEM).[24] Numerous eastern box turtles died or were euthanized after presenting from various locations with palpebral edema, ocular discharge, fluid draining from the mouth, with or without caseous plaques in the oral cavity, and were *Ranavirus* positive by PCR, virus isolation, and TEM in the cases where those tests were performed.[24] A free-living Florida box turtle was euthanized after not responding to therapy on exhibiting palpebral edema, nasal and ocular discharge, and yellow-white caseous plaques in the oral cavity, and was positive for *Ranavirus* by PCR and viral isolation.[24]

Clinical Signs

The most common clinical signs associated with *Ranavirus* infection include upper respiratory tract disease, including respiratory distress and nasal discharge, oral ulceration, cutaneous abcessation, subcutaneous edema, anorexia, and lethargy.[23,29,31,32] Less common clinical signs include red skin lesions on the neck in moribund 4- to 6-g soft-shelled turtles,[33] and severe unilateral conjunctivitis and cellulitis of the head and neck.[25]

Few clinical pathology reports exist from turtles and tortoises with confirmed iridoviral infection, but consistently elevated values from box turtles in one study included urea (three of five), aspartate aminotransferase (three of five), creatine kinase (four of five), lactate dehydrogenase (five of five), and anemia,[28] and toxic changes to the heterophils were noted in all turtles.[25] Bloodwork abnormalities are likely the result of moderate to severe dehydration and tissue damage associated with infection.

Histopathologic Changes

Histopathologic lesions have been described for many of the confirmed cases of *Ranavirus* infection. Lesions include fibrinoid vasculitis of the integument, mucous membranes, liver, and lungs[25]; severe necrotizing conjunctivitis with cytoplasmic inclusions; severe acute necrotizing glossitis; esophagitis; tracheitis; multifocal acute necrotizing pneumonia with cytoplasmic inclusions; moderate multifocal random acute hepatocellular necrosis with cytoplasmic inclusions; moderate multifocal acute necrotizing enteritis and glomerulonephritis; mild focal acute necrotizing pancreatitis; mild multifocal acute necrotizing cystitis; and intramural gastric nematodes of unde-termined species.[28] Multifocal necrosis and heterophilic infiltration is commonly found in the mucosa of the oral cavity, tongue, pharynx, esophagus, small and large intes-tine, and cloaca.[27] Additional findings can include multicentric fibrinoid vasculitis and formation of fibrin thrombi in small blood vessels in numerous tissues[23]; focal necrotizing hepatitis, focal necrotizing enteritis, and confluent necrotizing splenitis[31]; and necrotizing and ulcerative stomatitis or esophagitis, fibrinous and necrotizing splenitis, and multicentric fibrinoid vasculitis.[24]

Viral cytoplasmic inclusions consistent with *Ranavirus* infection appear most commonly in hepatocytes,[27,31] trachea,[24] lung,[27] tongue,[24] esophagus,[24] spleen,[24] endothelial cells,[24] stomach,[24] and leukocytes.[28] There are cases of experimentally induced infection[27,32] and case reports of naturally occurring infection[24,25] where no viral inclusions were noted in tissues with light microscopy. Because inclusion bodies do seem to be an inconsistent finding, their lack of discovery in tissues should not be used to rule out possible *Ranavirus* infection.[23,25] TEM examination of tissues revealing no viral inclusions with light microscopy did reveal icosahedral particles 150 to 190 nm in diameter consistent with *Iridovirus* virions in two cases.[23,25] TEM evaluation of tissues in cases suggestive of *Ranavirus* infection based on clinical signs is recommended, because it does seem to be able to detect viral particles even in the absence of visible inclusions on histologic section.

Diagnosis

Diagnosis is initially based on suggestive clinical signs, and intracytoplasmic viral particles of appropriate diameter (120–200 nm) observed with TEM. Virus isolation has been used to successfully confirm *Ranavirus* infection.[23–25,27,28] Virus was cultured from 4- to 6-g soft-shelled turtles and identified with TEM. Cultured virus was then used to experimentally challenge unexposed soft-shelled turtles.[33] An enzyme-linked immunosorbent assay has shown the ability to detect IgM and IgY anti-*Iridovirus* antibodies in gopher tortoises and eastern box turtles.[29] The enzyme-linked immunosorbent assay seems to be able to detect recent infections (IgM) and longer standing infections (IgY), but it is unknown how long anti-*Iridovirus* antibodies remain at detectable levels in chelonians or if all animals mount an immune response.[29] PCR analysis has been used successfully in numerous studies to detect *Iridovirus* infections.[22–25,27,28] PCR was used to detect *Ranavirus* infection from oral, cloacal, and urine samples in ornate box turtles (*Terrepene ornata ornata*) and red-eared sliders (*Trachemys scripta elegans*) with success.[23] Recently, PCR analysis was performed on whole blood samples and oral swabs in free ranging eastern box turtles, with both samples showing the ability to detect the presence of virus.[22] Oral and cloacal swabs and whole blood may be reasonable samples to submit for PCR until further information is obtained.

The mechanism of transmission of iridoviruses is still unknown. Because iridoviral particles were observed in circulating leukocytes it has been postulated that transmission by blood-feeding parasites or biting insects may be possible.[23,28] Other thoughts include cannibalism of infected animals[24]; common environmental sources of virus (eg, bodies of water)[23]; fomites[28]; and amphibian and fish reservoirs.[28] In one study ornate box turtles and red-eared sliders were inoculated with Burmese star tortoise *Ranavirus* orally and intramuscularly. All intramuscularly inoculated turtles in this study showed clinical signs, and three died as a result of infection. No orally inoculated turtles showed signs of infection or died. Based on these findings the authors hypothesized that turtles may not become exposed to *Ranavirus* through ingestion of infected animals or water sources, and that abrasions naturally acquired from ingesting bones or other material may be necessary for the virus to be introduced systemically. It is also possible that the amount of virus provided orally needs to be in greater quantity, or repeated exposure may be necessary.[23] One of the intramuscularly inoculated turtles did seem to recover from disease, and this makes the possibility of asymptomatic carriers in turtle populations as vectors.[23] Reports of disease outbreak in turtles have noted the presence of frogs in or near the enclosures,[24,25] but at this time it is not clear whether they are the source of the virus, or just also susceptible to disease and coincidentally noted.

Treatment

Most case reports show limited success with treatment of turtles and tortoises with *Ranavirus* infection. General treatment with systemic antibiotics (ceftazidime, enrofloxacin, clindamycin),[24,25,28,32] warm water soaks,[24] intracoelomic fluid therapy,[24] parenteral fluid therapy,[25] nutritional support,[25,32] analgesics,[24,25] topical antibiotics (triple antibiotic ointment),[25] antiviral therapy (acyclovir, interferon),[24,25] and vitamin A and D supplementation[28] has been attempted. The only report showing any treatment success involved Burmese star tortoises where antiviral therapy and intracoelomic fluids were administered.[24] Based on cases in the literature it seems that antiviral therapy and fluid therapy are indicated, and it is recommended to provide nutritional and fluid support. Systemic antibiotics, analgesics, topical antibiotics, and vitamin supplementation did not seem to alter the course of the disease, but because there are still a small number of proved cases in the literature these treatments should be used on a case by case basis.

Anticipated Future Trends

Numerous cases of *Ranavirus* infection are being reported, and chelonian species not previously documented are being shown susceptible to infection.[24] *Ranavirus* seems to be a fatal viral disease capable of causing high mortality in wild chelonian populations. Infection has been observed in wild populations in Florida, Tennessee, Georgia, New York, Pennsylvania, and Texas. Because more cases of *Ranavirus* infection in wild populations are being encountered, it is important to pay close attention to how affected turtles are handled, and eventually released. Current studies show the prevalence of *Ranavirus* infection in the wild is low, but because the disease has high mortality, many that have succumbed to disease in the wild likely were probably not found.[22] The methods of transmission are not yet clear, and questions remain about whether the disease is arthropod-borne, acquired by ingestion of infected materials, or acquired by direct contact. Because diagnostic evaluation performed on collected turtles could miss infection in asymptomatic carriers of disease, it is especially important for rehabilitators to release turtles as close to the site of capture as possible even if *Iridovirus* is not detected. Because the possibility remains that chelonians may be capable of serving as asymptomatic carriers,[23] *Iridovirus*-positive animals should not be released into the wild until more is learned about carrier status and disease transmission. Infection in chelonians, and more specifically box turtles, in the United States seems to be a significant threat to populations, particularly those undergoing environmental stress, such as that expected with climate change, and this disease needs to be monitored closely in wild populations moving forward.

ADENOVIRUS
Biology and Epidemiology

Adenoviruses have received increasing attention in tortoises since 2009. Before 2009, the only reported case of adenovirus in a chelonian was from a leopard tortoise (S [Geochelone] pardalis) with biliverdinuria, wasting, and episodes of hemorrhage.[34] Since 2009, there have been reports of adenovirus infection in an ornate box turtle (T ornata ornata),[35] Sulawesi tortoises (I forstenii),[36] impressed tortoises (M impressa),[37] and a Burmese star tortoise (G platynota).[37]

Adenoviruses are double-stranded, linear, nonenveloped DNA viruses with a diameter of 80 to 110 nm, a 26- to 45-kbp genome and an icosahedral nucleocapsid. Replication of the virus is within the nucleus of host cells, and intranuclear inclusions can be visualized during stages of reproduction in H&E-stained tissue sections. Viral inclusions are typically basophilic with H&E stain, but eosinophilic inclusions have also been reported.[26,35] Adenoviruses have been described in all tetrapod classes and a sturgeon, and are classified into five genera: (1) Siadenovirus, (2) Mastadenovirus, (3) Aviadenovirus, (4) Atadenovirus, and (5) Icthadenovirus.[37] There are numerous reports of adenovirus-related disease in reptiles[38–48] but it currently seems to be an emerging pathogen in chelonians.

Adenoviruses are often host specific and transmitted by the fecal-oral route or direct contact by oronasal secretions.[43] Adenovirus-related disease most often occurs in young and immunocompromised animals.[43] The wild-caught Sulawesi tortoises had recently been confiscated, the result of illegal importation. Tortoises intended for the pet trade are often exposed to other animals and pathogens not in their normal environment, and being exposed to such conditions as overcrowding, poor sanitation, poor nutrition, and other physiologic stresses.[37] The ornate box turtle was an adult; age and exposure status to conspecifics was not reported.[35] One impressed tortoise was a wild-caught adult that had been healthy for the 2.5 previous years in the collection. The other impressed tortoise was a previously healthy, 5-year-old captive hatched tortoise. The Burmese star tortoise was a previously healthy, 4-year-old captive bred tortoise.[37]

It does seem that Sulawesi tortoise adenovirus-1 can be horizontally transmitted between tortoise species because the virus was found in three previously healthy tortoises with known exposure to infected tortoises.[37] Vertical transmission has not been described in tortoises. It is suspected in the case of the impressed tortoises and Burmese star tortoise that the virus was spread by fomites, aerosols, or animal caretakers.[37] Adenoviruses are very environmentally persistent, and disinfection of adenovirus contamination is challenging.[37] Because this does seem to be an emerging and important pathogen of tortoises it should be considered when introducing newly acquired tortoises to collections. Spatial separation of quarantined tortoises from established collections, ideally in separate buildings with separate caretakers, should be considered especially critical in captive assurance colonies of endangered species.[37]

Concurrent disease may also make tortoises more susceptible to severe systemic disease the result of adenoviral infection.[36] Coinfections with intranuclear coccidiosis,[37] amoeba,[36] nematodes,[36] Escherichia coli,[36] Aeromonas hydrophila,[36]

Chlamydophila sp,[36] and a *Mycoplasma* sp were observed.[35] Some of the diseases noted as coinfections can cause morbidity and mortality in tortoises alone, and the relationship between adenoviral infection and concurrent infections remains to be better described.

The first brief report of adenoviral-related disease involved a leopard tortoise in 2004.[34] In 2009, a case of systemic *Siadenovirus* infection in a group of 105 illegally imported Sulawesi tortoises was reported. Thirty of the tortoises died before veterinary examination, and 62 of the 75 remaining tortoises died despite aggressive therapy at various institutions.[36] In 2009, an ornate box turtle was reported to have died the result of a mixed adenoviral and mycoplasmal infection.[35] In 2012, two impressed tortoises and one Burmese star tortoise were determined to have died with Sulawesi tortoise adenovirus-1 infections after being in the same facility as confiscated Sulawesi tortoises.[37]

Clinical Signs

The most common lesions in reptiles presenting with adenoviral infections include hepatitis, enteritis, esophagitis, splenitis, and encephalopathy.[48] The ornate box turtle had no premonitory signs of disease described and was found deceased[35]; the Sulawesi tortoises presented with anorexia, lethargy, mucosal ulcerations and palatine erosions of the oral cavity, nasal and ocular discharge, and diarrhea[36]; the impressed tortoises both died without premonitory signs[37]; and the Burmese star tortoise died after a 2-week period of lethargy and anorexia.[37]

Diagnosis

Clinical pathology was only reported for the Sulwesi tortoises (N = 19), with the most common complete blood count results being anemia (33% of affected animals), leukopenia (21%), leukocytosis (21%), heteropenia (21%), heterophilia (31%), lymphopenia (37%), lymphocytosis (10%), eosinophilia (5%), and azurophilic monocytosis (11%), and were consistent with abnormalities expected with a chronic inflammatory response.[36] Plasma biochemical abnormalities were elevated aspartate aminotransferase activity (28%), elevated creatine phosphokinase activity (5%), hypoglycemia (21%), hyperglycemia (58%), elevated blood urea nitrogen (92%), hyperkalemia (22%), and elevated uric acid concentration (21%), and were suspected to be secondary to muscle and possibly liver damage, and moderate to severe dehydration.[36]

PCR was effective at detecting adenoviral nucleic acid in most turtles and tortoises from which samples were submitted. Adenovirus PCR amplicons were detected from 97.6% of Sulwesi tortoise samples submitted during a multi-institutional disease outbreak (N = 42)[36]; all samples submitted from two impressed tortoises and one Burmese star tortoise that had been exposed to adenovirus-infected Sulawesi tortoises[37]; and from the adult ornate box turtle in Hungary.[35] All nasal flush, nasal mucosa, choanal and choanal-cloacal swab, colon, liver, lung, kidney, and spleen samples were PCR positive, and 19 of 20 plasma samples were PCR positive.[36] Sample collection for PCR is generally noninvasive and practical in conscious animals, and thus seems to be useful for antemortem diagnosis of active adenoviral infection. Until more is known about adenovirus infection in chelonians, cloacal and plasma samples should be submitted for testing by PCR.[36] In situ hybridization using a riboprobe specific for Sulawesi tortoise adenovirus-1 did detect hybridization signals using a fluorescein-labeled riboprobe (RNA probes).[37] As more sequence data become available, development of additional probes may improve the ability to develop sensitive and specific diagnostic in situ hybridization techniques that can be used to complement PCR, TEM, and histopathologic findings when evaluating for the presence of adenovirus.[37]

Treatment

Sulawesi tortoise adenovirus-1 caused severe systemic disease with a mortality rate of 87.6% (92 of 105 animals).[35] Medical therapy varied based on the institution where the Sulawesi tortoises were treated, but all tortoises were treated with systemic antibiotics, antiparasitics, fluid therapy, and nutritional support.[36] Most of the other cases were found deceased so no treatment was attempted, although the Burmese star tortoise was treated for 2 weeks before dying, without success. Based on previous cases, owners should be warned of the poor prognosis of adenoviral disease in chelonians. As of now supportive therapy with fluids, nutritional support, antibiotics for secondary infections, thermal support, and antiparasitics (because parasites were commonly noted in the previous tortoises) can be attempted.[36]

Histopathologic Changes

Histopathologic lesions were described for most of the turtles and tortoises that died as the result of adenoviral infection. Most commonly affected organ systems were liver,[35–37] intestinal tract,[35–37] bone marrow,[36,37] and spleen.[36,37] Less common findings were interstitial pneumonia, myocarditis, renal tubular necrosis, focal ulcerative stomatitis, facial dermatitis, and nonsuppurative meningoencephalitis.[37]

Viral intranuclear inclusions consistent with adenovirus infection in tortoises seem to be most commonly found in the liver,[35–37] but also occurred in bone marrow,[36] reticuloendothelial cells of the spleen,[36,37] biliary epithelium,[37] pancreas,[36] testis,[36] ovary,[36] respiratory epithelium,[36] renal epithelium,[36] vascular and cardiac epithelium,[36] cerebral glia and choroid plexus,[36] and colon.[37] The intranuclear inclusions were evaluated by TEM, which confirmed the presence of nonenveloped, 70- to 90-nm diameter, viral particles in nuclei with marginated chromatin and abnormal nuclear sizes and shapes, which are consistent with an adenovirus.[36,37]

Anticipated Future Trends

The mortality of the initial outbreak in Sulawesi tortoises (87.6%), along with the pathology seen in the cases of adenoviral infections, indicates that this virus has the potential to affect tortoise popluations.[35–37] Wild-imported tortoises were the first reported to show evidence of adenoviral infection.[36] It is not known if these animals had adenoviral disease before collection for the pet trade, or were exposed during the importation process. The origin of the disease is not known, but it may be present in wild animals. Adenoviral-related disease in tortoises is still not completely understood. When considering release of animals back into a wild population a decision tree analysis has been previously developed.[49] Until more is known about this disease, adenovirus-positive tortoises should not be considered for release into wild populations, and should be kept separate from other chelonians.

SUMMARY

Numerous pathogens have been described in chelonians and of these TINC, cryptosporidiosis, Ranavirus, and adenovirus are emerging as important diseases. Much remains to be learned about the biology and epidemiology of these organisms, and continuing research is needed to fully characterize them. In general, disease caused by these organisms is associated with stressors that can include changing environmental conditions, inappropriate care in captivity, shipping, and translocation.

Chelonians that exhibit signs of systemic disease must be isolated to reduce the risk of transmission to additional individuals. Diagnostic tests are available, and together with quarantine are essential to prevent movement of pathogens into new populations. Collections must be managed with strict biosecurity, and conservation introductions must include thorough diagnostic testing, health evaluation, and quarantine before movement to the release site. Fortunately, these tools can be effective and sufficient to prevent outbreaks if applied in the context of appropriate environmental conditions.

REFERENCES

1. Jacobson ER, Schumacher J, Telford SR, et al. Intranuclear coccidiosis in radiated tortoises (*Geochelone radiata*). J Zoo Wildl Med 1994;25(1):95–102.
2. Garner MM, Gardiner CH, Wellehan JF, et al. Intranuclear coccidiosis in tortoises: nine cases. Vet Pathol 2006;43(3):311–20.
3. Innis CJ, Garner MM, Johnson AJ, et al. Antemortem diagnosis and characterization of nasal intranuclear coccidiosis in Sulawesi tortoises (*Indotestudo forsteni*). J Vet Diagn Invest 2007;19(6):660–7.
4. Alvarez WA, Gibbons PM, Rivera S, et al. Development of a quantitative PCR for rapid and sensitive diagnosis of an intranuclear coccidian parasite in Testudines (TINC), and detection in the critically endangered Arakan Forest Turtle (*Heosemys depressa*). Vet Parasitol 2013;193(1-3):66–70.
5. Praschag P, Gibbons P, Boyer T, et al. An outbreak of intranuclear coccidiosis in Pyxis spp. tortoises. Presented at the 8th Annu Symp Conserv Biol Tortoises Freshwater Turtles. Orlando (FL): Turtle Survival Alliance; 2010. p. 42–3.
6. Schmidt V, Dyachenko V, Aupperle H, et al. Case report of systemic coccidiosis in a radiated tortoise (*Geochelone radiata*). Parasitol Res 2008;102(3):431–6.
7. Reavill DR, Okimoto B, Barr BC, et al. Proliferative pneumonia due to intracellular protozoa in radiated tortoises (*Geochelone radiata*). In: Proc Joint Conf Am Assoc Zoo Vet, Am Assoc Wildl Vet, Wildl Dis Assoc. San Diego (CA): American Association of Zoo Veterinarians; 2004. p. 614–5.
8. Upton SJ, Oppert CJ. Description of the oocysts of *Eimeria arnyi* n. sp. (Apicomplexa, Eimeriidae) from the eastern ringneck snake *Diadophis punctatus arnyi* (Serpentes, Colubridae). Syst Parasitol 1991;20(3):195–7.
9. Cranfield MR, Graczyk TK. Cryptosporidiosis. In: Mader DR, editor. Reptile medicine and surgery. 2nd edition. St Louis (MO): Saunders Elsevier; 2006. p. 756–62.
10. Brownstein DG, Strandberg JD, Montali RJ, et al. Cryptosporidium in snakes with hypertrophic gastritis. Vet Pathol 1977;14(6):606–17.
11. Upton SJ, McAllister CT, Freed PS, et al. Cryptosporidium spp. in wild and captive reptiles. J Wildl Dis 1989;25(1):20–30.
12. Griffin C, Reavill DR, Stacy BA, et al. Cryptosporidiosis caused by two distinct species in Russian tortoises and a pancake tortoise. Vet Parasitol 2010;170(1–2):14–9.
13. Xiao L, Ryan UM, Graczyk TK, et al. Genetic diversity of *Cryptosporidium* spp. in captive reptiles. Appl Environ Microbiol 2004;70(2):891–9.
14. Alves M, Xiao L, Lemos V, et al. Occurrence and molecular characterization of *Cryptosporidium* spp. in mammals and reptiles at the Lisbon Zoo. Parasitol Res 2005;97(2):108–12.
15. Traversa D, Iorio R, Otranto D, et al. Cryptosporidium from tortoises: genetic characterisation, phylogeny and zoonotic implications. Mol Cell Probes 2008;22(2):122–8.

16. Graczyk TK, Cranfield MR, Mann J, et al. Intestinal *Cryptosporidium* sp. infection in the Egyptian tortoise, Testudo kleinmanni. Int J Parasitol 1998;28(12):1885–8.

17. Pedraza-Diaz S, Ortega-Mora LM, Carrion BA, et al. Molecular characterisation of *Cryptosporidium* isolates from pet reptiles. Vet Parasitol 2009;160:204–10.

18. Raphael B, Calle P, Gottdenker NL, et al. Clinical significance of *Cryptosporidia* in captive and free-ranging chelonians. In: Proc Am Assoc Zoo Vet. Houston (TX): American Association of Zoo Veterinarians; 1997. p. 19–20.

19. Traversa D. Evidence for a new species of *Cryptosporidium* infecting tortoises: *Cryptosporidium ducismarci*. Parasit Vectors 2010;2010(3):21.

20. Richter B, Rasim R, Vrhovec MG, et al. Cryptosporidiosis outbreak in captive chelonians (*Testudo hermanni*) with identification of two *Cryptosporidium* genotypes. J Vet Diagn Invest 2012;24(3):591–5.

21. Grosset C, Villeneuve A, Brieger A, et al. Cryptosporidiosis in juvenile bearded dragons (*Pogona vitticeps*): effects of treatment with paromomycin. J Herp Med Surg 2011;21(1):10–5.

22. Allender MC, Abd-Eldaim M, Schumacher J, et al. PCR prevalence of ranavirus in free-ranging eastern box turtles (*Terrapene Carolina Carolina*) at rehabilitation centers in three southeastern US states. J Wildl Dis 2011;47:759–64.

23. Johnson AJ, Pessier AP, Jacobson ER. Experimental transmission and induction of ranaviral disease in western ornate box turtles (*Terrapene ornata ornate*) and red-eared sliders (*Trachemys scripta elegans*). Vet Pathol 2007;44:285–97.

24. Johnson AJ, Pessier AP, Wellehan JF, et al. Ranavirus infection of free-ranging and captive box turtles and tortoises in the United States. J Wildl Dis 2008;44:851–63.

25. De Voe R, Geissler K, Elmore S, et al. Ranavirus-associated morbidity and mortality in a group of captive eastern box turtles (*Terrapene carolina carolina*). J Zoo Wildl Med 2004;35:534–43.

26. Jacobson ER. Infectious disease and pathology of reptiles. Boca Raton (FL): CRC Press; 2007. p. 404–5.

27. Marschang RE, Becher P, Posthaus H, et al. Isolation and characterization of an iridovirus from Hermann's tortoises (*Testudo hermanni*). Arch Virol 1999;144:1909–22.

28. Allender MC, Fry MM, Irizarry AR, et al. Intracytoplasmic inclusions in circulating leukocytes from an eastern box turtle (*Terrapene carolina carolina*) with an iridoviral infection. J Wildl Dis 2006;42:677–84.

29. Johnson AJ, Wendland L, Norton TM, et al. Development and use of an indirect enzyme-linked immunosorbent assay for detection of iridovirus exposure on gopher tortoises (*Gopherus polyphemus*) and eastern box turtles (*Terrapene carolina carolina*). Vet Microbiol 2010;142:160–7.

30. Telford SR, Jacobson ER. Lizard erythrocytic virus in east African chameleons. J Wildl Dis 1993;29:57–63.

31. Heldstab A, Bestetti G. Viral hepatitis in a spur-tailed Mediterranean land tortoise (*Testudo hermanni*). J Zoo Wildl Med 1982;13:113–20.

32. Westhouse RA, Jacobson ER, Harris RK, et al. Respiratory and pharyngo-esophageal iridovirus infection in a gopher tortoise (*Gopherus polyphemus*). J Wildl Dis 1996;32:682–6.

33. Chen Z, Zheng J, Jiang Y. A new iridovirus isolated from soft-shelled turtle. Virus Res 1999;63:147–51.

34. McArthur S, Wilkinson R, Meyer J. Medicine and surgery of tortoises and turtles. Oxford (United Kingdom): Blackwell Publishing; 2004.

35. Farkas SL, Gal J. Adenovirus and mycoplasma infection in an ornate box turtle (*Terrapene ornata ornata*) in Hungary. Vet Microbiol 2009;138:169–73.
36. Rivera S, Wellehan JF, McManamon R, et al. Systemic adenovirus infection in Sulawesi tortoises (*Indotestudo forsteni*) caused by a novel Siadenovirus. J Vet Diagn Invest 2009;21:415–26.
37. Schumacher VL, Innis CJ, Garner MM, et al. Sulawesi tortoise adenovirus-1 in two Impressed tortoises (*Manouria impressa*) and a Burmese Star tortoise (*Geochelone platynota*). J Zoo Wildl Med 2012;43:501–10.
38. Frye FL, Munn RJ, Gardner M, et al. Adenovirus-like hepatitis in a group of related Rankin's dragon lizards (*Pogona henrylawsoni*). J Zoo Wildl Med 1994;25:167–71.
39. Heldstab A, Bestetti G. Virus associated gastrointestinal disease in snakes. J Zoo Anim Med 1984;14:118–28.
40. Jacobson ER, Gardiner CH. Adeno-like virus in esophageal and tracheal mucosa of a Jackson's chameleon (Chameleo jacksoni). Vet Pathol 1990;27:210–2.
41. Jacobson ER, Kollias GV. Adenovirus-like infection in a Savannah Monitor. J Zoo Wildl Med 1986;17:149–51.
42. Jacobson ER, Kopit W, Kennedy FA, et al. Coinfection of a bearded dragon, *Pogona vitticeps*, with adenovirus- and dependovirus-like viruses. Vet Pathol 1996;33:343–6.
43. Kim DY, Mitchell MA, Bauer RW, et al. An outbreak of adenoviral infection in inland bearded dragons (*Pogona vitticeps*) coinfected with dependovirus and coccidial protozoa (*Isospora* sp). J Vet Diagn Invest 2002;14:332–4.
44. Kinsel MJ, Barbiers RB, Manharth A, et al. Small intestinal adeno-like virus in a Mountain Chameleon (*Chameleo montium*). J Zoo Wildl Med 1997;28:498–500.
45. Ramis A, Fernandez-Bellon H, Majo N, et al. Adenovirus hepatitis in a boa constrictor (Boa constrictor). J Vet Diagn Invest 2000;12:573–6.
46. Raymond JT, Lamm M, Nordhausen R, et al. Degenerative encephalopathy in a coastal mountain kingsnake (*Lampropeltis zonata multifasciata*) due to adenoviral-like infection. J Wildl Dis 2003;39:431–6.
47. Schumacher J, Jacobson ER, Burns R, et al. Adenovirus-like infection in two Rosy Boas (Lichanura trivirgata). J Zoo Wildl Med 1994;25:461–5.
48. Wellehan JFX, Johnson AJ, Harrach B, et al. Detection and analysis of six lizard adenoviruses by consensus PCR provides further evidence of a reptilian origin for the atadenoviruses. J Virol 2004;78:13366–9.
49. Jacobson ER, Behler JL, Jarchow JL. Health assessment of chelonians and release into the wild. In: Fowler ME, Miller RE, editors. Zoo and wild animal medicine, vol. 4. Philadelphia: W.B. Saunders; 1999. p. 232–42.

Selected Emerging Infectious Diseases of Squamata

La'Toya V. Latney, DVM[a],*,
James Wellehan, DVM, MS, PhD, DACZM, DACVM[b]

KEYWORDS

- Reptile • Viral • Fungal • Parasitic • Bacterial • Emerging • Disease

KEY POINTS

- Polymerase chain reaction (PCR) products should be validated with the use of DNA sequencing or probe hybridization to appropriately diagnose infectious disease agents.
- Diverse adenoviruses are strongly implicated in chronic enteric disease in a variety of squamates.
- Arenaviruses are strongly implicated as the cause of inclusion body virus of boid snakes.
- Diverse paramyxoviruses infect squamates; serologic methods are fraught with problems and PCR-based diagnostics are preferred.
- *Chrysosporium ophiodiicola* causes severe facial disfiguration and systemic mycosis in North American snakes.
- Site of infection is more important than exact host species for *Cryptosporidium*; *Cryptosporidium varanii* is the most common intestinal species in squamates and *Cryptosporidium serpentis* is the most common gastric species.

In comparative medicine, we often lack information in a given species, including which infectious agents are present and their clinical significance. When information is lacking in a given species, the best model to use is typically the closest relative from which data are available. This model requires knowledge of species relationships; many commonly used terms, such as reptile or lizard, can lead to erroneous understanding of relationships.

A common error is the idea of lizards as a group distinct from snakes. In squamate evolution, the earliest divergence is the geckos, followed by the divergence of the skinks, night lizards, plated lizards, and girdled lizards. The next groups to branch off were the teiids, lacertids, and amphisbaenids, and the remaining group, containing

[a] Exotic Companion Animal Medicine & Surgery, Veterinary Teaching Hospital, University of Pennsylvania, 3900 Delancey Street, Office 2017, Philadelphia, PA 19104, USA; [b] Zoological Medicine Service, University of Florida College of Veterinary Medicine, PO Box 100126, 2015 Southwest 16th Avenue, Gainesville, FL 32608-0125, USA
* Corresponding author.
E-mail address: llatney@vet.upenn.edu

Vet Clin Exot Anim 16 (2013) 319–338
http://dx.doi.org/10.1016/j.cvex.2013.01.003
1094-9194/13/$ – see front matter © 2013 Elsevier Inc. All rights reserved.

snakes, iguanids, agamids, chameleons, monitors, helodermatids, and anguids, is known collectively as the Toxicofera, named for the commonality of the presence of venom glands.[1] Snakes diverge in the middle of the squamates, and if snakes are removed, then lizards are not a monophyletic group. Snakes are a group of lizards, and a corn snake is a better model than a leopard gecko for a bearded dragon.

Within the past decade, several important advances have identified novel causes of significant emerging diseases of captive squamates. These advances have led to the development of diagnostic tools that are essential for squamate practitioners. It is important that reptile clinicians have an appreciation for the epidemiology, clinical signs, pathology, diagnostic options, and prognostic parameters for those diseases that have recently flooded the primary literature. This article provides an update on emerging squamate diseases reported in the primary literature within the past decade. For a comprehensive overview of reported infectious diseases, consultation of Jacobson E, editor, *Infectious Diseases and Pathology of Reptiles: A Color Atlas and Text* (Boca Raton, FL: CRC Press; 2007) is recommended.

CLINICAL APPROACHES TO INFECTIOUS DISEASES
Diagnostics

Because of the extensive list of organisms that may be normal flora in many contexts in diverse squamate species, it is imperative not to misinterpret culture and sensitivity reports and molecular diagnostic test results. The host-pathogen interaction can be definitively diagnosed only with the aid of histopathologic or sometimes cytologic analysis. Biopsies are therefore strongly recommended to diagnose, confirm, and characterize the nature of clinical infections in reptiles.

For microbial infections, culture and sensitivity of fresh biopsy tissue samples can be coupled with polymerase chain reaction (PCR) and sequencing to confirm specific pathogens and guide treatment approaches. Immunohistochemistry and in situ hybridization can be performed on formalin-fixed tissue sections to identify disease-causing agents and can subsequently guide therapeutic practices. However, samples should be processed into paraffin blocks quickly, and tissues that spend more than a few days in formalin become unsuitable for in situ hybridization. Cytology and special stains can aid in the quick ascertainment of potential diagnoses and guide clinician treatment recommendations pending receipt of PCR, biopsy, and culture/sensitivity results. Gram stains of impression smears can aid in characterizing bacterial pathogens. Wright-Giemsa and lactophenol cotton blue can be used to characterize yeasts and fungal hyphae. Acid-fast stains (Ziehl-Neelson or Fite) can be used to identify mycobacterial infections, *Nocardia*, and some parasitic infections, such as *Cryptosporidium*. *Cryptosporidium* stains acid-fast on fresh smears only and not in formalin-fixed tissues.

There are 2 major approaches to testing for infectious agents. These tests are based on (1) the animal's acquired immune response to an agent or (2) the presence of the agent.[2] Acquired immune responses can be further subdivided into 2 categories. Tests that evaluate antibody production against specific pathogens assess the lizard's humoral immune response. Some of these tests include enzyme-linked immunosorbent assays, hemagglutination inhibition, virus neutralization, and agarose gel immunodiffusion. Tests that evaluate the presence of cellular immunity, which is centered around the T-cell receptor, are not commonly available; assays that are used in human medicine include T-cell proliferation assays. It is important to consider when assaying humoral immunity that it is only part of the acquired immune response, and generally the less important aspect for defense against intracellular pathogens such as viruses. Several factors can affect both types of immune response, including seasonal variation, reproductive status, endogenous cortisol levels, age, and exogenous administration of corticosteroids.[3]

Electron microscopy (EM), PCR, and culture are tools that are used to look for the presence of the infectious agent. EM is a cost-effective, underused tool that can help characterize viral agents isolated in tissues and fecal samples. Negative-staining EM is offered at low cost by many state diagnostic laboratories and can aid in assessing which subsequent diagnostic is recommended for confirmation. Culture requires a live infectious agent, and its usefulness depends on collection of appropriate samples and known culture techniques for the agent. Knowledge of the biology of the agent is needed to determine appropriate sample selection. Appropriate culture conditions have yet to be determined for many infectious agents. PCR requires intact nucleic acid; the agent can be dead or alive. Because PCR is highly sensitive, contamination of samples is a significant concern and significant care needs to be taken with sample collection and transport.[2] PCR products need to be identified after amplification. Older techniques for this procedure may have consisted of gel electrophoresis alone or restriction enzyme digestion; these often fail to differentiate nonspecific products and should no longer be considered sufficient. Better techniques for product validation are now affordable and should be used; these include use of specific probe hybridization (used in TaqMan [but not SYBR Green] quantitative PCR]) and DNA sequencing.

When interpreting testing, evidence of an infectious agent or an immune response does not mean that the agent is causing disease, and the absence of an infectious agent in a sample does not mean that it is not elsewhere in the animal. Animals may show exposure to pathogens and not develop clinical disease. Others may show clinical disease only after a viremia has occurred and sample selection becomes imperative for identifying the underlying causative agent.

Guidelines for Therapy and Control

Initial stabilization of the patient requires an assessment of the underlying factors contributing to the reptile's medical condition. Thermal support largely influences clinical recovery, because the reptile's immune response, metabolism of drugs, and use of fluid therapy are heat dependent. For ambulatory poikilothermic patients, it is always best to supply a thermal gradient appropriate for the species, and let the animal choose. For nonambulatory patients, thermal support is more challenging, and temperature selection needs to be based on species and context. For some species, cooling may be indicated. Stabilization of the patient should include supportive fluid therapy, analgesics if indicated, and a reduction of exposure to environmental stressors. Careful selection of appropriate antimicrobial or antiparasitic medications is warranted after diagnostic samples have been collected. The inappropriate administration of antifungal or antiparasitic medications can cause significant side effects. Nutritional support can be carefully administered when there is confirmation that the gastrointestinal system is functional. This procedure is best performed after dehydration deficits have been corrected. A routine minimum database can be collected, and advanced diagnostics should be pursued to help confirm a clinical diagnosis.

Husbandry and continued care should be optimized to improve the patient's recovery and to control the spread of infectious agents to other animals. Biosecurity protocols should be reviewed for collections. Specific therapeutics may be modified based on results of diagnostic testing.

VIRAL DISEASES
Adenoviruses

Adenoviruses are linear, double-stranded DNA viruses with a genome of 25 to 45 kpb.[3] They have an icosahedral capsid composed of 3 major antigenic viral proteins: the fiber, penton, and hexon.[4] Adenoviruses have been described in 5 classes of vertebrates and their corresponding families are based on phylogenic origin: Mastadenovirus (mammals), Aviadenovirus (dinosauria), Atadenovirus (squamates, mammals, dinosauria), Siadenovirus (amphibians, dinosauria, testudine species), and Icthadenovirus (fish).[4] A fifth clade found in turtles and tortoises likely represents a sixth genus. Although *Atadenovirus* is found in avian and mammal species, it likely evolved in squamate hosts.[3]

Reported *Atadenovirus* infections in squamates include snake adenovirus 1 (SnAdV1) in a boa constrictor (*Boa constrictor*), a royal python (*Python regius*), and a corn snake (*Elaphe guttata*); snake adenovirus 2 (SnAdV2) in milksnakes (*Lampropeltis triangulum*), California kingsnakes (*Lampropeltis getulus californiae*), a European asp (*Vipera aspis aspis*), and an Indonesian pit viper (*Parias hageni*); snake adenovirus 3 (SnAdV3) in milksnakes and a bull snake (*Pituophis catenifer sayi*); agamid adenovirus 1 (AgAdV1) in inland bearded dragons (*Pogona vitticeps*) and a central netted dragon (*Ctenophorus nuchalis*); eublepharid adenovirus 1 (EuAdV1) in leopard geckos (*Eublepharis macularis*) and fat-tailed geckos (*Hemitheconyx caudicinctus*); gekkonid adenovirus 1 (GeAdV1) in a tokay gecko (*Gekko gecko*); chameleonid adenovirus 1 (ChAdV1) in a mountain chameleon (*Chameleo montium*); scincid adenovirus 1 (ScAdV1) in blue-tongued skinks (*Tiliqua scincoides intermedia*); helodermatid adenovirus 1 (HeAdV1) in Gila monsters (*Heloderma suspectum*); helodermatid adenovirus 2 (HeAdV2) in beaded lizards (*Heloderma horridum*), Gila monsters, a western bearded dragon (*Pogona minor*), and an inland bearded dragon; and varanid adenovirus 1 in green tree monitors (*Varanus prasinus*).[3] There have also been reports of uncharacterized adenoviruslike particles in a variety of additional squamate species.

AgAdV1 has been recognized as a serious cause of mortality in captive bearded dragons in the United States,[5,6] Europe,[7] and New Zealand.[8] The first report of severe hepatitis caused by adenovirus infection in a squamate was identified in a coastal bearded dragon (*Pogona barbata*).[8] Several reports subsequently followed supporting adenovirus as a serious infectious disease of captive *Pogona* species.[3] The most common clinical signs reported in association with AgAdV1 infections include weight loss, anorexia, and diarrhea secondary to hepatic necrosis. However, many dragons can be asymptomatic. Lymphohistiocytic interstitial nephritis,[6] pancreatitis,[6] encephalopathy, splenitis, pneumonia, and esophagitis have also been reported.[7] Hemorrhagic urates, coelomic effusion secondary to severe vasculitis, hindlimb weakness, central nervous signs, and sudden death may be seen. Signs of the central nervous system (CNS), including circling, abrupt paresis, and opisthotonus, have been reported[9] and observed by the first author (LL). On histopathologic evaluation of infected agamid lizards, basophilic intranuclear viral inclusions and severe coagulative necrosis are noted in the liver, intestine, and bile duct.[8] Concurrent coccidial and dependovirus infections have also been described.[10] It is not known whether dependoviruses, which are a genus in the family Parvoviridae that require adenoviral coinfection to replicate, play a role in disease causation. Although a causal role for disease is possible, it is also plausible that their parasitism of adenoviruses may mitigate disease. The genomic diversity of the AgAdV1 hexon capsid analyzed in 17 bearded dragons housed in 4 different collections has since shown that there are multiple genotypes of AgAdV1 and some dragons can carry multiple strains.[11] The stability of adenoviruses in the environment and the poor biosecurity that is typical in reptile breeding facilities has made this pathogen common in North American and European populations of bearded dragons. Ball and Marschang[12] have successfully isolated AgAdV1 in culture, which serves to enable further essential research. In 2011, Hyndman and Shilton[13] characterized AgAdV1 from a captive central netted dragon (*Ctenophorus nuchalis*), which is the first time AgAdV1 was reported in the native range of *Pogona* (Australia). Histopathologic lesions in the central netted dragon included necrotizing hepatitis and rare epithelial inclusions.

Papp and colleagues[7] isolated HeAdV2 from Mexican beaded lizards in 2009. This virus is closely related to HeAdV1 from Gila monsters, which are in turn close relatives of beaded lizards. Being large DNA viruses with intranuclear replication, adenoviruses show high host fidelity, so this finding was not unexpected. However, in 2011, Hyndman and Shilton[13] identified HeAdV2 in a captive western bearded dragon in Australia. More recently, HeAdV2 was identified in a captive inland bearded dragon in the United States.[14] These reports of HeAdV2 in nonhelodermatid hosts bring into question the degree of host fidelity of these viruses.

Adenoviruses are strongly associated with chronic enteritis in snakes.[15] Disease is especially common in the colubrid genera *Lampropeltis* and *Pituophis*. Basophilic or eosinophilic intranuclear inclusions have been found in hepatocytes,[3] enterocytes,[16] myocardium,[17] renal tubule cells,[17] endocardium,[17] spinal cord and brain,[18] and oral mucosa.[18] Severe hepatitis, enteritis, splenitis, vasculitis, gliosis, endocarditis, stomatitis, and nephritis have been clinically associated with ophidian adenovirus infections. Antibody titers to SnAdV1 have been reported in symptomatic and asymptomatic snakes.[16] Pees and colleagues[19] have recently reported the prevalence of viral infections in Germany through a survey of 100 boid snakes among 14 different collections. Of 86 blood samples submitted, 4 contained titers for adenovirus.

Closely related adenoviruses may differ greatly in clinical significance. As 1 example, canine adenovirus 1 often results in a fatal hepatitis in dogs; the closely related canine adenovirus 2 generally causes bronchitis with minor morbidity and virtually no mortality. Several academic and private molecular diagnostic laboratories offer conventional PCR tests and EM for antemortem diagnosis. EM is useful but does not identify adenoviral genus or species. It is crucial, when submitting PCR testing, to understand how a PCR product is validated. Any test capable of identifying more than 1 agent needs to be validated by sequencing; a diagnosis of atadenovirus without specific identification is not clinically actionable data. The other acceptable method of product identification is probe hybridization. The most common way this is implemented is in TaqMan (but not SYBRGreen) quantitative PCR (formerly known as real-time PCR) assays. However, assay design to ensure that the probe provides specific product identification is critical.

There are no formal studies evaluating disinfection and contact times, but adenoviruses are stable in the environment and there is some evidence that suggests that some adenoviruses are heat labile at 56°C.[20] Adenoviruses are commonly spread through fecal-oral transmission. In addition, aerosolized viral transmission via respiratory inhalation occurs in humans. Current recommendations for disinfection include removal of organic debris with soap and water followed by use of a 10% bleach solution on cages and hard surfaces, allowing for a 10-minute contact time.[21] Extended contact with direct unfiltered sunlight or other intense ultraviolet sources may also aid disinfection. It is imperative that all bleached supplies and cages be thoroughly rinsed afterward, because the solution can be corrosive and cause respiratory irritation.

Symptomatic lizards should be isolated and afforded supportive care. New additions should be quarantined for PCR screening for adenovirus before introduction to established colonies/collections, and proper biosecurity protocols need to be in place.

Knowledge of collection infection status is important for management. It is important to resolve or treat concurrent illness in infected patients to reduce morbidity.

Rhabdoviruses

The family Rhabdoviridae, along with the Paramyxoviridae, Filoviridae, and Bornaviridae, belongs to the order Mononegavirales. They are enveloped, single-strand negative-sense RNA viruses with bullet-shaped virions. Rhabdoviridae are divided into 6 genera; a large clade of arboviral rhabdoviruses known as the dimarhabdoviruses contains the genera *Vesiculovirus* and *Ephemerovirus*. Many dimarhabdoviruses are responsible for causing devastating disease including vesicular stomatitis virus, Chandipura encephalitis virus, spring viremia of carp virus, and bovine ephemeral fever virus, which profoundly affect both the veterinary and human communities.[22]

There have been isolations of rhabdoviruses from squamates, including skinks, geckos, and teiid lizards, although rhabdoviruses have been conspicuously absent from the Toxicofera despite surveillance.[3] Marco, Timbo, Chaco, and Sena Madureira viruses were isolated from *Ameiva ameiva ameiva* and *Kentropyx calcaratus* in Brazil and were further classified as rhabdoviruses by EM in 1979.[23,24] Both the Chaco and Marco viruses have been shown to replicate in the salivary glands of the mosquito *Aedes egypti*.[23] Charleville and Almpiwar viruses were isolated in Australia from geckos (*Gehrya australis*) and skinks (*Cryptoblepharus [Ablepharus] virgatus*), respectively. However, until recently, nothing was known about the behavior of these viruses in their squamate hosts. Recently, a rhabdovirus was identified by EM in the intracytoplasmic inclusions in the erythrocytes of a caiman lizard (*Dracaena guianensis*).[25] This virus, along with PCR consequence techniques, were used to show that the virus genetically clustered with all known squamate rhabdoviruses, except for Marco virus cluster, in a dimarhabdovirus clade termed the Almpiwar group, which are homologous on a level similar to that in named genera. The Almpiwar group contains only viruses using squamate hosts and Humpty Doo virus, which was isolated from hematophagous insects and whose vertebrate hosts are yet unknown. This finding suggests that the Almpiwar group specializes in using squamate hosts. The intraerythrocytic inclusions would be an advantageous site for hematophagous insect transmission, and the more metabolically active erythrocytes of reptiles enable viruses to use this niche in a way not possible in nonnucleated mammalian red cells.

Marco virus clusters with Hart Park subgroup, a dimarhabdovirus group that also contains viruses that use cattle, macropods, and birds as vertebrate hosts. The ability to use diverse hosts indicates that the degree of zoonotic risk may be higher with Marco virus than with other squamate rhabdoviruses. The significance of rhabdoviral infections for their squamate hosts needs further study.

Reoviruses

Reoviridae are nonenveloped double-stranded segmented RNA viruses and are approximately 60 to 80 nm in diameter. The family contains 12 genera and all of the squamate reoviruses have been classified in the genus *Orthoreovirus*.[26,27] Orthoreoviruses can cause severe pneumonia, neurologic disease, and gastrointestinal disease in squamates. Lesions include cytolysis and giant syncytial cell formation within host cells, and isolates are frequently recovered from oral and cloacal swabs, lung, liver, brain, and small intestinal tissue. Several of the reported clinical signs mirror those caused by paramyxovirus infections.

Orthoreovirus isolation, PCR and sequencing, or antibody production has been documented in the following squamate species: corn snakes (*Pantherophis guttatus*),[28] rough green snakes (*Opheodrys aestivus*),[29] green iguana (*Iguana iguana*),[30] chameleons,[30] leopard gecko (*Eublepharis macularis*),[31] *Xenosaurus grandis*,[32] *Abronia graminea*,[32] green lizards (*Lacerta viridis*),[33] Moellendorff rat snake (*Elaphe moellendorffi*),[34] beauty snake (*Elaphe taenuris*),[34] black rat snake (*Pantherophis [Elaphe] obselta obsoleta*),[34] brown tree snakes (*Boiga irregularis*), *Ctenosaura bakeri*,[35] *Ctenosaura similis*,[36] *Iguana iguana rhinopha*,[36] *Uromastyx hardwickii*,[37] prairie rattlesnake (*Crotalus viridis*),[38] Mojave rattlesnakes (*Crotalus scutulatus*),[39] emerald tree boa (*Corallus caninus*),[40] boa constrictors (*Boa constrictor*), aesculapian snake (*Elaphe longissima*),[41] Chinese vipers (*Azemiops feyi*),[42] variable bush vipers (*Atheris squamigera*), carpet pythons (*Morela viridis*), and ball pythons (*Python regius*).[43]

Clinical disease has been documented in several squamate species. Experimental infection has been shown, using a reovirus isolate recovered from a Moellendorff rat snake and beauty snake both suffering from severe respiratory disease. These reovirus isolates were inoculated into black rat snakes and produced severe proliferative pneumonia and tracheitis.[34] Most recently, a triple infection of reovirus, paramyxovirus, and atadenovirus has been reported in a collection of largely asymptomatic corn snakes. One corn snake in the collection had clinical signs of dyspnea and vomiting before death.[28] An orthoreovirus was the causative agent of syncytial cell enteropathy and hepatopathy in leopard geckos.[31]

Iridoviruses

Iridoviruses are large 120-nm to 200-nm double-strand cytoplasmic DNA viruses.[44] Both are capable of infecting a diverse range of hosts, and iridoviruses have been implicated in multiple recent interclass and cross-class host shifts.[26,45] The family Iridoviridae currently consists of 5 genera. *Chloriridovirus* and *Iridovirus* infect insects, although the genus *Iridovirus* has also been found to infect squamates. *Megalocytivirus* and *Lymphocystivirus* infect nontetrapod bony fish, and *Ranavirus* infects fish, amphibians, and reptiles.[46] A clade of intraerythrocytic iridoviruses characterized from squamates likely represents a sixth genus.[47,48] Until 1966, iridoviral intracytoplasmic inclusions found within erythrocytes were mistaken for a protozoal pathogen and named *Pirhemocyton*.[49] The 3 genera of iridioviruses known to infect squamates are summarized in **Table 1**.

The importance of ranaviruses cannot be understated, because frog virus 3 (FV3) infection in amphibians is now a reportable disease to the World Organization for Animal Health. The epidemiology and pathogenesis of ranaviruses in fish, testudines, and amphibians is covered, see the articles by Latney and Gibsons elsewhere in this issue. The ranaviruses are major pathogens of nonavian reptiles, as shown by the epidemic in wild box turtle populations of North America. FV3, a ranavirus, has been isolated from a gecko (*Uroplatus fimbriatus*).[50] The histologic examination was limited because of autolysis of the patient, which revealed a severe ulcerative necrotizing glossitis and had a focal area of hepatic necrosis. Despite viral isolation from the liver, the lack of pathology data calls into question the role of FV3 in disease in this animal. A ranavirus was found in 2 illegally imported green tree pythons (*Morelia viridis*), which died.[51] Histologic lesions included an ulcerative pharyngitis and hepatic necrosis. Concurrent nematode and bacterial infections of the sinuses were present in the 2 snakes that underwent histopathologic evaluation. Immunohistochemical staining confirmed the presence of the virus in the affected tissues. The ranavirus isolate shared 97% nucleotide homology with FV3 and 98% with epizootic hematopoetic virus of fish and Bohle virus. It was subsequently named Wamena virus, after the location in Irian Jaya where the snakes had originated.

Erythrocytic iridoviruses have been reported in squamates and likely represent a novel genus. Previously believed to be protozoal hemoparasites *Toddia* and

Table 1
Overview of Iridoviridae genera found to infect squamata

Genera of Iridoviridae	Infected Species	Viral Agent	Reference
Ranavirus	Uroplastus fimbriatus (giant leaf-tailed gecko)	Frog virus 3 (FV3)	Marschang et al,[50] 2005
	Lacerta monticola (Iberian rock lizard)	Related to frog virus 3, novel	Alves de Matos et al,[48] 2011
	Chrondropython viridis (green python)	Wamena virus	Hyatt et al,[51] 2002
Invertebrate iridovirus	Chameleo quadricornis (four-horned chameleon)	EM evaluation consistent with iridovirus morphology	Drury et al,[37] 2002
	Chameleo hoehnelli (high-casqued chameleon)		
	Chameleo hoehnelli (high-casqued chameleon)	Invertebrate iridescent virus 6	Weinmann et al,[54] 2007
	Pogona Vitticeps (bearded dragon), Chamycosaurus kingii (frilled dragon), Chameleo quadricornis (four-horned chameleon)	Invertebrate iridescent virus 6	Just et al,[53] 2001
Erythrocytic virus (EV)	Lacerta monticola (Iberian rock lizard)	Lucerne enation virus	Alves de Matos et al,[52] 2002
	Lacerta schreiberi (Schreiber green lizard)		
	Thamnophis sauritus sackenii (peninsula ribbon snake)	TsEV	Wellehan et al,[47] 2008
	Bothrops moojeni (lancehead viper)	Snake erythrocyte virus	Johnsrude et al,[94] 1997
	Thamnophis nadix (Plains garter snake)	Snake erythrocyte virus	Jacobson,[26] 2007
	Thamnophis sauritus (peninsula ribbon snake)		
EV previously diagnosed as Toddia and Pirhemocyton	Agkistrodon piscivorus leucostoma (cottonmouths)	Snake erythrocyte virus	Marquardt and Yager,[95] 1967
	Nerodia sipedon (northern water snake)	Snake erythrocyte virus	Brooker and Yongue,[96] 1982, Smith et al,[97] 1994

Pirhemocyton, the cause of the intracytoplasmic eosinophilic inclusions associated with square-shaped crystalline viral structures has been confirmed as iridoviral. The first sequence characterization of an erythrocytic iridovirus was from a ribbon snake (*Thamnophis sauritus sackenii*) in Florida.[47] On the blood sample obtained from the wild ribbon snake, 60% of the erythrocytes were hypochromic and showed frequent polychromasia, and 95% of these erythrocytes contained 1 of 2 types of intracytoplasmic inclusions. The leukogram revealed a moderate heteropenia, toxicity, and a left shift, azurophilia, and monocytosis, suggestive of severe chronic inflammation. Occasionally, azurophils and monocytes contained phagocytized erythrocytes. The histopathologic examination revealed parasite burdens, poor body condition, and hepatic necrosis, but viral inclusions were noted only in erythrocytes. In an experimental infection of *Lacerta monticola* lizards with an erythrocytic iridovirus,[52] clinical disease was not apparent in lizards until the environmental temperature was decreased to 2°C to 15°C, when crystalloid inclusions were noted in circulating leukocytes and the animals died. Inclusions were also identified in the endothelial cells and hepatocytes of the same animals. Infected lacertids maintained at preferred environmental temperatures had erythrocytic inclusions up 98% of circulating red blood cells but did not develop clinical disease and recovered. Coinfection with a ranavirus was identified in the *Lactera monticola* as well.[48] The erythrocytic iridovirus of *Lactera monticola* shared significant sequence homology with the ribbon snake erythrocytic iridovirus.

The genus *Iridovirus* has traditionally been considered to infect arthropod hosts. Just and colleagues[53] isolated an iridovirus from a 4-horned chameleon (*Chamaeleo quadricornis*), a frilled dragon (*Chlamydosaurus kingii*), and bearded dragon. This finding was confirmed in a study that experimentally infected crickets with an iridovirus isolated from a high-casqued chameleon.[54] The isolate caused 20% to 25% mortality in infected crickets and was confirmed on nested PCR, in situ hybridization, and EM of the fat bodies of cricket carcasses.

Arenavirus

The family Arenaviridae are single-stranded, negative-sense enveloped RNA viruses with bipartite genomes.[44,55] There is only 1 genus, *Arenavirus,* and rodents are believed to be their natural hosts. Until recently, arenaviruses had been known to infect only mammals. They are responsible for severe zoonotic diseases, including Guanarito virus (Venezuelan hemorrhagic fever), Junin virus (Argentine hemorrhagic fever), lymphocytic choriomeningitis virus (lymphocytic choriomeningitis), Lassa virus (Lassa fever), Machupo virus (Bolivian hemorrhagic fever), and Sabiá virus.[56]

Inclusion body disease (IBD), a highly infectious, fatal viral disease of boid snakes, had eluded etiologic confirmation for more than 30 years. In the late 1970s, IBD became recognized as a disease that caused fatal CNS disease in boid snakes.[17] It has also been reported in palm vipers (*Bothriechis marchi*)[26] and an eastern kingsnake (*Lampropeltis getulus*).[18] Although it has since been reported in several python and boa species, it was initially commonly reported in Burmese pythons (*Python molurus bivittatus*). Clinical signs can vary; however, it seems that pythons rapidly decline from CNS clinical signs, which include opisthotonus, loss of righting reflex, head tilt, disequilibrium, head tremors, incoordination, and sudden death. In boa species, these signs may or may not be seen, and some boas may remain asymptomatic or survive for months to years with supportive care.[26] Secondary infections are common, and viral immunosuppression is a significant component of this disease.

On histologic examination, the disease is characterized by the eosinophilic to amphophilic intracytoplasmic inclusions identified on hematoxylin-eosin–stained tissue sections. Inclusions are composed of a 68-kDa protein, now known to be arenaviral nucleoproteins, which are mainly found within the CNS. IBD inclusions are also visualized on hematoxylin-eosin stain of the esophageal tonsils, respiratory epithelium, mucosal epithelium of the gastrointestinal tract, hepatocytes, renal tubular epithelial cells, and pancreas.[26] Viral inclusions are occasionally identified within circulating lymphocytes.[19]

A retrovirus was formerly suspected as the cause of IBD,[26] but recent developments from Stenglein and colleagues[56] provide strong evidence that arenaviruses are the cause of IBD. Using high-throughput metagenomic analysis, 2 viruses that caused disease in annulated tree boas (Corallus annulatus) (California Academy of Sciences [CAS] virus) and 2 species of boa constrictors from (Golden Gate virus [GGV]) were completely sequenced. A third partially characterized virus was isolated from a moribund boa (Collierville virus). A culture system for CAS was established using boa constrictor kidney cells, and reverse transcriptase PCR was developed as a screening test for detecting the viruses. The isolated viral proteins were detected in 6 of 8 confirmed IBD-positive cases. Labeled antibodies to the GGV nucleoprotein stained the inclusions of IBD-positive snakes. Experimental challenge studies are needed to fulfill Koch's postulates, but the evidence for an arenaviral cause for IBD is strong.

Paramyxovirus

The family Paramyxoviridae, along with the Rhabdoviridae, Filoviridae, and Bornaviridae, belongs to the order Mononegavirales. Paramyxoviridae contains negative-sense, enveloped single-stranded RNA viruses that are pleomorphic. The family is divided into 2 subfamilies. The subfamily Paramyxovirinae contains the genera Rubulavirus, Avulavirus, Respirovirus, Henipavirus, Morbillivirus, Aquaparamyxovirus, and Ferlavirus. The Pneumovirinae subfamily contains the genera Pneumovirus and Metapneumovirus.[44] Sunshine virus does not fall into either subfamily. Paramyxoviridae are the causative agents of several important pathogens, including human parainfluenza, measles, canine distemper, rinderpest, Nipah virus, Newcastle disease, mumps, and human respiratory syncytial virus.[26]

Members of the genus Ferlavirus are recognized as significant causes of severe pulmonary disease in snakes. It was first recognized in 1976 in lancehead vipers (Bothrops moojeni) associated with a die-off at a snake farm in Switzerland.[57] In addition to pneumonia, clinical signs include head tremors, regurgitation, anorexia, and sudden death.[27] Reports of ferlavirus disease in squamates other than snakes are limited to caiman lizards (Dracaena guianensis),[58] although serologic evidence is present in a wide variety of squamates.[3] Ferlaviruses are classified into subgroups A, B, and C, along with a tortoise ferlavirus isolate that is distinct from the other 3 groups.[28,30] Group C seems to be the most prevalent in the United States (Wellehan, unpublished data). Serologic responses to the 3 squamate subgroups differ, with limited cross-reactivity (Wellehan, unpublished data, 2013). Marschang and colleagues[30] reported that there was no host species specificity in grouping isolates from several snake and lizard species. Specific diagnosis of ferlaviruses is best accomplished via consensus PCR and sequencing. The polymerase gene has been shown to be the best target for consensus PCR testing.[30]

More recently, a novel paramyxovirus was found during an investigation of an outbreak of neurorespiratory disease in a collection of Australian pythons.[59] Snakes infected with sunshine virus had hindbrain white matter spongiosis and gliosis, with extension to the surrounding gray matter and neuronal necrosis evident in severe cases. Sixty-three percent of infected snakes also had mild bronchointerstitial pneumonia.[59] Phylogenetic analyses supported the clustering of this virus within the family Paramyxoviridae but outside both of the current subfamilies.[59]

BACTERIAL DISEASE
Devriesea agamarum

Devriesea agamarum, a newly discovered species of bacteria, is a gram-positive, short rod in the phylum Actinobacteria that has been associated with severe hyperkeratotic dermatitis, cheilitis, and potential septicemia in Uromastyx species and agamid species.[60] Approximately 1 to 2 mm in length, the organisms are non–spore-forming, nonmotile, non–acid-fast rods that occur singly, in pairs, or in short chains. Hellebuyck and colleagues[61] have evaluated the significance of the organism as a new normal flora isolate or if it has truly emerged as a primary pathogen. In 1 report of a D agamarum infection causing dermatitis in a beaded dragon, D agamarum was identified as a normal oral flora isolate and classified as a facultative pathogen in Pogona vitticeps.[61] In this study, Koch's postulates were shown when the investigators inoculated abraded areas of the dragon's skin with D agamarum, caused the pathologic hyperkeratotic lesions, and reisolated the same bacteria from the lesions.

Although D agamarum is considered normal oral flora in asymptomatic Pogona species,[62] it has not been isolated as oral flora of Uromastyx species. Sixty-nine lizards, including Pogona (n = 21), Uromastyx (n = 31), Agama (n = 4), Crotaphytus (n = 8), Laudakia (n = 4), and Eublepharis (n = 1) species, were sampled for D agamarum in a study performed at Ghent University in Belgium.[62] The phylogenetic analysis of isolates obtained from asymptomatic bearded dragons and clinical Uromastyx species revealed 8 different genotypes of D agamarum. Two genotypes were exclusively associated with diseased Uromastyx lizards, suggesting that these strains are primary pathogens for the species.

D agamarum has been shown to exist for over 5 months in humid sand and distilled water, and was detected in dermal crusts removed from affected animals for up to 57 days.[62] Environmental control of the pathogen can be obtained by using the following common agents to disinfect hard surfaces with a minimum contact time of 5 minutes: sodium hypochlorite (0.05%–0.5%), chlorhexidine (0.05%–0.5%), boric acid (0.01%), and ethanol (70%). In addition, it has been shown that initial debridement and intramuscular administration of cetiofur at 5 mg/kg every 24 hours for an average of 18 days in Pogona vitticeps and 12 days in Uromastyx sp serves as an effective treatment. Enrofloxacin did not eliminate the bacteria.[63]

FUNGAL DISEASE
Chrysosporium

As members of the Opisthokonta group, fungi are amongst the closest relatives of metazoan animals.[64] Historically, mycotic infections in reptiles have likely remained underdiagnosed.[26] Most recognize fungal infections as secondary infections resulting primarily from poor husbandry and underlying chronic comorbidities. The global impact of primary fungal pathogens such as Batrachochytrium dendobatidis in amphibians and Geomyces destructans in bats has rapidly changed the generalized perception of mycotic infections as secondary invaders. Although opportunistic infections can occur in reptiles, Chrysosporium, ascomycetous teleomorphic fungi in the order Onygenales, has provided evidence to support that they are contagious primary pathogens of squamates. The order Onygenales contains most of the most serious fungal pathogens of vertebrates, including Blastomyces dermatitidis, Histoplasma capsulatum, Coccidioides immitis, Microsporum, Trichophyton, Lacazia loboi,

Paracoccidioides brasiliensis, and *Chrysosporium.* The Onygenales have been shown to have reduced numbers of plant cell wall–degrading enzymes, and tend to have increased numbers of proteases, especially keratinases, which may be adaptations for living on animal hosts.[65]

The nomenclature used to classify fungi is inconsistent with the rest of biology. There are separate genus and species names for asexual anamorph stages and sexual teleomorph stages of the same organism, resulting in multiple species names and paraphyletic taxa. The anamorph species *Blastomyces dermatitidis* and *Histoplasma capsulatum* are in different genera, but the identical teleomorphs *Ajellomyces dermatitidis* and *Ajellomyces capsulatus* are congeneric. The anamorph genus *Chrysosporium* contains organisms identical to those in several teleomorph genera, including *Amaurascopsis, Amauroascus, Aphanoascus, Arthroderma, Bettsia, Ctenomyces, Neogymnomyces, Pectinotrichum, Renispora, Uncinocarpus,* and *Nannizziopsis.*[66]

An understanding of *Chrysosporium* sp in reptiles is still being developed. Although there are numerous reports in the literature of the *Chrysosporium* anamorph of *Nannizziopsis vriesii* causing disease, these identifications are morphologic, and there are no sequence data in GenBank supporting these identifications, *Chrysosporium* sp are paraphyletic and widely distributed across the Onygenales. Although sequenced reptile isolates form a well-supported clade with *Nannizziopsis vriesii*, there are no reptile isolate sequences in GenBank that would support identification as *Chrysosporium* anamorph of *Nannizziopsis vriesii* (CANV). The closest related available sequence, from a bearded dragon, shares 90% identity with *Nannizziopsis vriesii* over the ITS2 region. For comparison, *Blastomyces dermatitidis* shares 90% identity with *Histoplasma capsulatum* over this region. We have yet to see a reptile isolate with sequence that would support identification as *Nannizziopsis vriesii* (Wellehan, unpublished, 2013). There are limitations to morphologic identification of microbes with limited identifying characteristics, and cryptic speciation is common. We strongly encourage sequence-based identification of future reptile *Chrysosporium* isolates.

A CANV-related species, *Chrysosporium guarroi,* has been reported as an emerging pathogen of captive iguanas in Spain[67,68] and South Korea.[69] The cause of an ulcerative dermatomycosis reported in 2 captive green iguanas, this CANV-related species shared 81% genetic homology with CANV[67] and 91% homology to 3 cases reported in captive iguanas in South Korea.[69] In the case of the isolates from Spain, the isolate grew at 35°C. On histology, the hyphae residing in the coalescing granulomas were identified on periodic acid-Schiff reaction or Grocott methenamine silver stain. Antifungal medications were chosen based on culture inhibition of the isolate. Oral ketoconazole (20 mg/kg every 24 hours by mouth), in combination with topical 2% chlorhexidine and terbinafine, led to a clinical resolution for both patients.[67]

An unnamed *Chrysosporium* sp, related to but distinct from CANV, has been identified in inland bearded dragons.[70] *Chrysosporium* seems to be a common problem in the species and is commonly known amongst hobbyists as yellow fungus disease.

Chrysosporium ophiodiicola has been identified as an emerging primary pathogen of wild timber rattlesnakes[71] and the endangered eastern massasauga rattlesnake.[72,73] *Chrysosporium ophiodiicola* do not cluster near the *Chrysosporium guarroi/Nannizziopsis vriesii* clade. It was first reported in association with a mycotic granuloma in a black rat snake,[74] and has emerged as a suspected cause of facial disfiguration syndrome in free-ranging snakes in the eastern United States.[73] The keratophilic fungus causes a granulomatous dermatitis and osteomyelitis, resulting in close to 100% mortality of eastern massasaugas. A recent survey of 14 wild timber rattlesnakes in New England revealed *Chrysosporium ophiodiicola* as the cause of an emerging fungal dermatitis that has been witnessed in routine biological surveys since 2009.[71] *Chrysosporium ophiodiicola* has also been identified with systemic mycosis in a cottonmouth in Florida (Wellehan, unpublished data, 2013).

PARASITIC DISEASES

Although several parasites have eluded previous classification, new molecular and genetic advances have provided species identification. This section overviews emerging primary pathogens that have caused significant disease in reptiles and reviews the prevalence of *Pentastomids* and *Isospora amphiboluri*.

Cryptosporidium

Cryptosporidium, a genus of coccidian parasites that infect many orders of vertebrates, is a significant concern in squamates. Identified in at least 57 reptile species,[75] although reliable morphologic species identification is not possible, *Cryptosporidium* species have been characterized using DNA sequence-based techniques. Phylogenetic analyses have revealed 2 major clades of *Cryptosporidium*; one with tropism for the intestine, and the other with tropism for the stomach. In most cases, *Cryptosporidium* sp cause gastrointestinal disease, but extraintestinal infections including aural polyp–associated infections[76] and pharyngeal infections[77] have been reported in green iguanas.

Cryptosporidium serpentis has a tropism for the stomach. It causes hypertrophic gastritis, regurgitation, and chronic wasting in squamate species.[26] Experimental infections have shown that this agent causes gastric hypertrophy with focal necrosis and petechiation in snakes.[78] Clinically, regurgitation and midbody swelling are typical antemortem signs.

Commonly isolated from squamate species, *Cryptosporidium varanii* has often been mistakenly referred to in the literature as *Cryptosporidium saurophilum*.[79] Historically, the intestinal parasite *Cryptosporidium varanii* (*Cryptosporidium saurophilum*) has been shown to cause chronic wasting disease in lizard species and has been well studied in leopard geckos.[3] Coinfections with other enteric pathogens such as adenoviruses may exacerbate disease.[4]

Beyond the named species using squamate hosts, additional distinct clades of *Cryptosporidium* have been identified using sequence-based methodologies. A *Cryptosporidium* species was identified in a fecal sample from a viper boa (*Candoia asper*) and found to be distinct from other known reptile *Cryptosporidium*.[80] An identical organism was later found in 57 of 223 wild Japanese grass snakes (*Rhabdophis tigris*), and was associated with mucosal edema, goblet cell loss, and scattered necrosis in the small intestine.[81] Another *Cryptosporidium* has been found in the feces of a boa constrictor that is probably distinct at a species level.[80] *Cryptosporidium muris* and *Cryptosporidium parvum* have also been seen in reptiles, but were likely just passing through from ingested prey.[80]

Cryptosporidium has been identified in green iguanas,[82] with molecular and genetic characterization showing 100% sequence identity with a *Cryptosporidium* genotype isolated from cockatiels.[83] This isolate caused clinical cloacitis and cystitis in green iguanas and was shown to be contagious. The investigators note that there was a recurrence of clinical signs despite treatment with paromomycin.

One report[84] analyzed 171 fecal samples of 18 squamate species, and found *Cryptosporidium parvum* in 1 leopard gecko, raising the possibility of reptiles serving as a host to this zoonotic pathogen. However, the possibility of contamination and error for this single result must be considered. A previous experimental study conducted by Graczyk and Cranfield[36] provided evidence that *Cryptosporidium parvum* oocysts were not infectious to reptiles.

Richter and colleagues[85] have recently reported the prevalence of cryptosporidium in snakes and lizards in Austria. Among 672 fecal, gastric wash, or regurgitation samples, 16% of corn snake samples and 7% of leopard gecko samples were positive for *Cryptosporidium varanii*. *Cryptosporidium serpentis* was found in 2% of leopard gecko samples and in none of the snake samples. Unidentified isolates were discovered as well, and among the python samples, *Cryptosporidium muris*, *Cryptosporidium parvum*, and *Cryptosporidium baileyi* were noted, in addition to 3 unidentified isolates. This report contradicts previous findings, recognizing *Cryptosporidium serpentis* to infect predominantly snakes. These findings highlight the need for further investigation on regional prevalences and host ranges of reptile-associated *Cryptosporidium*.

Pentastomids

Pentastomids are large wormlike parasites that parasitize the upper respiratory tract of vertebrates, with 90% of extant species serving as parasites to reptiles.[26] Also known as tongue worms, these large arthropodlike worms can range from 0.5 to 12 cm long. Pentastomids reside in the upper respiratory tract, where they lay eggs, which are coughed and released into the sputum, swallowed, and passed through the feces. Intermediate hosts (IHs), usually small mammals, invertebrates and arthropods, ingest the eggs, which hatch and encyst in the IH body. Ingestion of the IH by a reptile species completes the life cycle of the parasite. The genus *Armillifer* can infect humans. Histologically, these parasites rarely cause severe pathologic reactions in their definitive hosts. However, antigenic stimulation may result when the adult worms molt. The disease potential of pentastomids in IHs is not insignificant; *Porocephalus crotali* has been shown to cause massive visceral pentastomiasis in dogs.[86] Identification of species is crucial to assessing disease risk; the order Porocephalida is more strongly associated with disease in mammalian IHs.[87] DNA sequence-based identification is available and may be especially useful for identification of eggs and larvae.[87]

Pentastomids are an understudied clade of parasites, but have been identified in all orders of reptiles, including testudines, squamates, crocodilians, and birds.[88] In Brazil, several pentastomid prevalence studies have been reported for several species of wild reptiles.[3] Almeida and colleagues[89] reported a prevalence of 55.5% (n = 9) in *Amphisbaena alba* species and 50% (n = 12) in *Amphisbaena vermicularis*. In addition, a new species of Pentastomida has been characterized in the lizard *Tropidururus hispidus*. In another study evaluating the prevalence of pentastomids in several reptile species originating from Pakistan, the countries of the European Union, Mali, Slovenia, Canary Islands, El Salvador, Lebanon, and Solomon isolates, the investigators obtained samples from 949 reptile necropsies, including tortoises, and reported a 6.9% prevalence in 331 non-snake lizard samples and a 11.1% prevalence in 55 snake samples.[90] Pharmaceutical therapy for pentastomids is generally unsuccessful. Endoscopic removal of adults from the lungs of definitive hosts is the treatment of choice.[87]

Isospora amphiboluri

Isospora amphiboluri is an important coccidial disease of captive bearded dragons. Studies that have evaluated prevalence, detection in feces, pathogenesis, and treatment have been recently presented. A 2008 cross-sectional study found that more than 23% of captive bearded dragons in a breeding colony were shedding *I amphiboluri* in their feces as diagnosed on single fecal samples, which likely represents an underestimate of the true prevalence.[91] Walden and colleagues[92] have also characterized the pathogenesis of *I amphiboluri* in bearded dragons. In their study, these investigators reported a prepatent period of 15 to 22 days. Initially, infective oocysts colonize the duodenum, and by day 4, merogony can be seen on histology in the proximal intestine. By day 8, meronts and gametes are noted; by day 12, late gametes are noted; and by day 16, unsporulated oocysts are seen in the intestine.[92] Oocysts are shed in the feces by day 22. No extraintestinal forms were noted, and histopathologic evidence showed that initial infections began in the duodenum and progressed to the colon.

Walden and Mitchell[93] have characterized the specificity and sensitivity of fecal flotation and direct smear evaluations for detecting coccidia oocysts. Direct smears revealed 76% sensitivity and 100% specificity when detecting oocysts, whereas fecal flotation was 100% specific and 93% specific. A recent clinical trial showed that sulfadimethoxine at 50 mg/kg by mouth every 24 hours for 21 days significantly reduced fecal shedding of *Isospora*.[93] Daily removal of feces from the cages of the treatment group and disinfection of the cages every 2 weeks may also have contributed to reduced exposure to the parasite and limited reinfection. In our subjective experience, ponazuril may have greater efficacy than sulfadimethoxine. At this time, it is not known if coccidial infections in bearded dragons are self-limiting or have cyclic shedding cycles, as seen with *Toxoplasma* in other species.[93]

SUMMARY

Several infectious diseases of reptiles are emerging, and further studies are needed to characterize the epidemiology of these agents. There is evidence to support host and class switching among invertebrate and reptile species in emergent viral diseases. Novel gram-positive bacteria are contributing to significant, species-specific disease in captive reptiles. Mycotic infections are causing fatal disease as primary pathogens. Novel species and host adaptation has been shown in zoonotic parasites. Although there have been major advances in identifying novel pathogens, controlled studies evaluating pathogenesis, environmental stability, and treatment are lacking. Further studies are warranted to help guide control and treatment recommendations.

REFERENCES

1. Fry BG, Vidal N, Norman JA, et al. Early evolution of the venom system in lizards and snakes. Nature 2005;439(7076):584–8.
2. Johnson AJ, Wellehan JF. Amphibian virology. Vet Clin North Am Exot Anim Pract 2005;8(1):53.
3. el Masri M, Saad AH, Mansour MH, et al. Seasonal distribution and hormonal modulation of reptilian T cells. Immunobiology 1995;193:15–41.
4. Wellehan JF, Johnson AJ, Harrach B, et al. Detection and analysis of six lizard adenoviruses by consensus primer PCR provides further evidence of a reptilian origin for the atadenoviruses. J Virol 2004;78(23):13366–9.
5. Jacobson EA. Viruses and viral associated diseases of reptiles. Acta Zool Pathol Antverp 1986;79:73–90.
6. Moormann S, Seehusen F, Reckling D, et al. Systemic adenovirus infection in bearded dragons (*Pogona vitticeps*): histological, ultrastructural and molecular findings. J Comp Pathol 2009;141(1):78–83.
7. Papp T, Fledelius B, Schmidt V, et al. PCR-sequence characterization of new adenoviruses found in reptiles and the first successful isolation of a lizard adenovirus. Vet Microbiol 2009;134(3):233–40.

8. Julian AF, Durham PJ. Adenoviral hepatitis in a female bearded dragon (*Amphibolurus barbatus*). N Z Vet J 1982;30(5):59–60.

9. Kim DY, Mitchell MA, Bauer RW, et al. An outbreak of adenoviral infection in inland bearded dragons (*Pogona vitticeps*) coinfected with dependovirus and coccidial protozoa (*Isospora* sp.). J Vet Diagn Invest 2002;14(4):332–4.

10. Jacobson ER, Kopit W, Kennedy FA, et al. Coinfection of a bearded dragon, *Pogona vitticeps*, with adenovirus- and dependovirus-like viruses. Vet Pathol 1996;33(3):343–6.

11. Parkin DB, Archer LL, Childress AL, et al. Genotype differentiation of agamid adenovirus 1 in bearded dragons (*Pogona vitticeps*) in the USA by hexon gene sequence. Infect Genet Evol 2009;9(4):501–6.

12. Ball I, Marschang RE. Establishment of an agamid cell line and first isolation of an adenovirus from a bearded dragon (*Pogona vitticeps*). Presented at Association of Reptilian and Amphibian Veterinarians. Oakland, October 23–26, 2012.

13. Hyndman T, Shilton CM. Molecular detection of two adenoviruses associated with disease in Australian lizards. Aust Vet J 2011;89(6):232–5.

14. Wellehan JF Jr, Schneider R, Childress AL. Identification of helodermatid adeovirus 2 in a captive central bearded dragon (*Pogona vitticeps*) in the United States. Presented at Association of Reptilian and Amphibian Veterinarians. Oakland, October 23–26, 2012.

15. Garner MM, Wellehan JF, Pearson M, et al. Characterization of enteric infections associated with two novel atadenoviruses in colubrid snakes. J Herpetol Med Surg 2008;18:86–94.

16. Perkins LE, Campagnoli RP, Harmon BG, et al. Detection and confirmation of reptilian adenovirus infection by in situ hybridization. J Vet Diagn Invest 2001; 13(4):365–8.

17. Schumacher J, Jacobson ER, Burns R, et al. Adenovirus-like infection in two rosy boas (*Lichanura trivirgata*). J Zoo Wildl Med 1994;25(3):461–5.

18. Raymond JT, Lamm M, Nordhausen R, et al. Degenerative encephalopathy in a coastal mountain kingsnake (*Lampropeltis zonata multifasciata*) due to adenoviral-like infection. J Wildl Dis 2003;39(2):431–6.

19. Pees M, Schmidt V, Marschang RE, et al. Prevalence of viral infections in captive collections of boid snakes in Germany. Vet Rec 2010;166(14):422–5.

20. Ogawa M, Ahne W, Essbauer S. Reptilian viruses: adenovirus like agent isolated from royal python (*Python regius*). Zentralbl Veterinarmed B 1992;39(1–10): 732–6.

21. Slomka-McFarland E. Disinfectants for the vivarium. In: Mader DR, editor. Reptile medicine and surgery, vol. 2. St Louis (MO): Saunders Elsevier; 2006. p. 1085–7.

22. Wellehan JF, Johnson AJ. Reptile virology. Vet Clin North Am Exot Anim Pract 2005;8(1):27.

23. Causey OR, Shope RE, Bensabath G. Marco, Timbo, and Chaco, newly recognized Arboviruses from lizards of Brazil. Am J Trop Med Hyg 1966;15: 239–43.

24. Monath TP, Cropp CB, Frazier CL, et al. Viruses isolated from reptiles: identification of three new members of the family Rhabdoviridae. Arch Virol 1979;60(1): 1–12.

25. Wellehan JF, Pessier AP, Archer LL, et al. Initial sequence characterization of the rhabdoviruses of squamate reptiles, including a novel rhabdovirus from a caiman lizard (*Dracaena guianensis*). Vet Microbiol 2012;158(3–4):274–9.

26. Jacobson E. Infectious diseases and pathology of reptiles: color atlas and text. Boca Raton (FL): CRC Press; 2007.
27. Marschang RE. Viruses infecting reptiles. Viruses 2011;3(11):2087–126.
28. Abbas MD, Marschang RE, Schmidt V, et al. A unique novel reptilian paramyxovirus, four atadenovirus types and a reovirus identified in a concurrent infection of a corn snake (*Pantherophis guttatus*) collection in Germany. Vet Microbiol 2011; 150(1):70–9.
29. Landolfi JA, Terio KA, Kinsel MJ, et al. Orthoreovirus infection and concurrent cryptosporidiosis in rough green snakes (*Opheodrys aestivus*): pathology and identification of a novel orthoreovirus strain via polymerase chain reaction and sequencing. J Vet Diagn Invest 2010;22(1):37–43.
30. Marschang RE, Papp T, Frost JW. Comparison of paramyxovirus isolates from snakes, lizards and a tortoise. Virus Res 2009;144(1):272–9.
31. Garner MM, Farina LL, Wellehan JF Jr, et al. Reovirus-associated syncytial cell enteropathy and hepatopathy in leopard geckos (*Eublepharis macularius*). Presented at Association of Reptilian and Amphibian Veterinarians. Milwaukee, Wisconsin, August 8–15, 2009.
32. Marschang RE, Donahoe S, Manvell R, et al. Paramyxovirus and reovirus infections in wild-caught Mexican lizards (*Xenosaurus* and *Abronia* spp). J Zoo Wildl Med 2002;33(4):317–21.
33. Raynaud A, Adrian M. [Cutaneous lesions with papillomatous structure associated with viruses in the green lizard (*Lacerta viridis* Laur.).] C R Acad Sci Hebd Seances Acad Sci D 1976;283(7):845 [in French].
34. Lamirande EW, Nichols DK, Owens JW, et al. Isolation and experimental transmission of a reovirus pathogenic in ratsnakes (*Elaphe* species). Virus Res 1999;63(1): 135–41.
35. Gravendyck M, Ammermann P, Marschang RE, et al. Paramyxoviral and reoviral infections of iguanas on Honduran Islands. J Wildl Dis 1998;34(1):33–8.
36. Graczyk TK, Cranfield MR. Experimental transmission of *Cryptosporidium* oocyst isolates from mammals, birds and reptiles to captive snakes. Vet Res 1998;29(2): 187–96.
37. Drury SE, Gough RE, Calvert I. Detection and isolation of an iridovirus from chameleons (*Chamaeleo quadricornis* and *Chamaeleo hoehnelli*) in the United Kingdom. Vet Rec 2002;150(14):451–2.
38. Vieler E, Baumgärtner W, Herbst W, et al. Characterization of a reovirus isolate from a rattle snake, *Crotalus viridis*, with neurological dysfunction. Arch Virol 1994;138(3):341–4.
39. Wellehan JF, Childress AL, Marschang RE, et al. Consensus nested PCR amplification and sequencing of diverse reptilian, avian, and mammalian orthoreoviruses. Vet Microbiol 2009;133(1):34–42.
40. Blahak S, Goebel T. A case reported of a reovirus infection in an emerald tree boa (Corallus caninus). In: Proceedings of the 4th International Colloquium on the Pathology of Reptiles and Amphibians. Giessen (Germany): Deutsche Veterinaermedizinische Gesellschaft; 1991. p. 13–6.
41. Blahak S, Ott I, Vieler E. Comparison of 6 different reoviruses of various reptiles. Vet Res 1995;26(5–6):470–6.
42. Jacobson ER, Kollias GV. Adenovirus-like infection in a savannah monitor. J Zoo Anim Med 1986;17(4):149–51.
43. Ahne W, Thomsen I, Winton J. Isolation of a reovirus from the snake, *Python regius*. Arch Virol 1987;94(1):135–9.

44. King AM, Lefkowitz E, Adams MJ, et al. Virus taxonomy: ninth report of the International Committee on Taxonomy of Viruses. London: Elsevier; 2011.

45. Jancovich JK, Bremont M, Touchman JW, et al. Evidence for multiple recent host species shifts among the ranaviruses (family Iridoviridae). J Virol 2010;84(6): 2636–47.

46. Mao J, Hedrick RP, Chinchar VG. Molecular characterization, sequence analysis, and taxonomic position of newly isolated fish iridoviruses. Virology 1997;229(1):212–20.

47. Wellehan JF, Strik NI, Stacy BA, et al. Characterization of an erythrocytic virus in the family Iridoviridae from a peninsula ribbon snake (*Thamnophis sauritus sackenii*). Vet Microbiol 2008;131(1):115–22.

48. Alves de Matos AP, da Silva Trabucho Caeiro MF, Papp T, et al. New viruses from *Lacerta monticola* (Serra da Estrela, Portugal): further evidence for a new group of nucleo-cytoplasmic large deoxyriboviruses. Microsc Microanal 2011;17(01):101 8.

49. Chatton E, Blanc G. Sur un hématozoaire nouveau, *Pirhemocyton tarentolae*, du Gecko, *Tarentola mauritanica*, et sur les altérations globulaires qu'il détermine. Comptes Rendus des Séances de la Société de Biologie et de ses Filiales 1914;11:496–8 [in French].

50. Marschang RE, Braun S, Becher P. Isolation of a ranavirus from a gecko (*Uroplatus fimbriatus*). J Zoo Wildl Med 2005;36(2):295–300.

51. Hyatt AD, Williamson M, Coupar BE, et al. First identification of a ranavirus from green pythons (*Chondropython viridis*). J Wildl Dis 2002;38(2):239–52.

52. Alves de Matos AP, Paperna I, Crespo E. Experimental infection of lacertids with lizard erythrocytic viruses. Intervirology 2002;45(3):150–9.

53. Just F, Essbauer S, Ahne W, et al. Occurrence of an invertebrate iridescent like virus (Iridoviridae) in reptiles. J Vet Med B Infect Dis Vet Public Health 2001; 48(9):685–94.

54. Weinmann N, Papp T, de Matos AP, et al. Experimental infection of crickets (*Gryllus bimaculatus*) with an invertebrate iridovirus isolated from a high-casqued chameleon (*Chamaeleo hoehnelii*). J Vet Diagn Invest 2007;19(6): 674–9.

55. Jay MT, Glaser C, Fulhorst CF. The arenaviruses. J Am Vet Med Assoc 2005; 227(6):904–15.

56. Stenglein MD, Sanders C, Kistler AL, et al. Identification, characterization, and in vitro culture of highly divergent arenaviruses from boa constrictors and annulated tree boas: candidate etiological agents for snake inclusion body disease. MBio 2012;3(4):e00180–12.

57. Foelsch DW, Leloup P. Fatale edemische Infektion in einem Serpentarium. Tierarztl Prax 1976;4:527–36 [in German].

58. Jacobson ER, Origgi F, Pessier AP, et al. Paramyxovirus infection in caiman lizards (*Draecona guianensis*). J Vet Diagn Invest 2001;13(2):143–51.

59. Hyndman TH, Marschang RE, Wellehan JF, et al. Isolation and molecular identification of sunshine virus, a novel paramyxovirus found in Australian snakes. Infect Genet Evol 2012;12(7):1436–46.

60. Martel A, Pasmans F, Hellebuyck T, et al. *Devriesea agamarum* gen. nov., sp. nov., a novel actinobacterium associated with dermatitis and septicaemia in agamid lizards. Int J Syst Evol Microbiol 2008;58(9):2206–9.

61. Hellebuyck T, Martel A, Chiers K, et al. *Devriesea agamarum* causes dermatitis in bearded dragons (*Pogona vitticeps*). Vet Microbiol 2009;134(3):267–71.

62. Hellebuyck T, Pasmans F, Blooi M, et al. Prolonged environmental persistence requires efficient disinfection procedures to control *Devriesea agamarum* associated disease in lizards. Lett Appl Microbiol 2011;52(1):28–32.

63. Hellebuyck T, Pasmans F, Haesebrouck F, et al. Designing a successful antimicrobial treatment against *Devriesea agamarum* infections in lizards. Vet Microbiol 2009;139(1):189–92.
64. Steenkamp ET, Wright J, Baldauf SL. The protistan origins of animals and fungi. Mol Biol Evol 2006;23(1):93–106.
65. Sharpton TJ, Stajich JE, Rounsley SD, et al. Comparative genomic analyses of the human fungal pathogens Coccidioides and their relatives. Genome Res 2009; 19(10):1722–31.
66. Hoog GS, Guarro J, Gené J, et al. Atlas of clinical fungi. Baarn (The Netherlands): Centraalbureau voor Schimmelcultures (CBS); 2000.
67. Abarca ML, Martorell J, Castella G, et al. Cutaneous hyalohyphomycosis caused by a *Chrysosporium* species related to *Nannizziopsis vriesii* in two green iguanas (*Iguana iguana*). Med Mycol 2008;46(4):349–54.
68. Abarca ML, Castellá G, Martorell J, et al. *Chrysosporium guarroi* sp. nov. a new emerging pathogen of pet green iguanas (*Iguana iguana*). Med Mycol 2010; 48(2):365–72.
69. Han JI, Lee SJ, Na KJ. Necrotizing dermatomycosis caused by *Chrysosporium* spp. in three captive green iguanas (*Iguana iguana*) in South Korea. J Exot Pet Med 2010;19(3):240–4.
70. Abarca ML, Martorell J, Castellá G, et al. Dermatomycosis in a pet inland bearded dragon (*Pogona vitticeps*) caused by a *Chrysosporium* species related to *Nannizziopsis vriesii*. Vet Dermatol 2009;20(4):295–9.
71. McBride M, Murray M, Wojick KB, et al. *Chryosoporium ophidiicola* isolated from skin lesions in wild timber rattlesnakes (*Crotalus horridus*). Presented at Association of Reptilian and Amphibian Veterinarians. Oakland, October 23–26, 2012.
72. Allender MC, Dreslik M, Wylie S, et al. *Chrysosporium* sp. infection in eastern massasauga rattlesnakes. Emerg Infect Dis 2011;17(12):2383.
73. Allender M, Dreslik MJ, Philips CA, et al. Facial disfiguration syndrome in free-ranging snakes throughout the eastern United States: an emerging pathogen associated with *Chrysosporium*. Presented at Association of Reptilian and Amphibian Veterinarians. Oakland, October 23–26, 2012.
74. Rajeev S, Sutton DA, Wickes BL, et al. Isolation and characterization of a new fungal species, *Chrysosporium ophiodiicola*, from a mycotic granuloma of a black rat snake (*Elaphe obsoleta obsoleta*). J Clin Microbiol 2009;47(4):1264.
75. O'Donoghue PJ. Cryptosporidium and cryptosporidiosis in man and animals. Int J Parasitol 1995;25(2):139.
76. Fitzgerald SD, Moisan PG, Bennett R. Aural polyp associated with cryptosporidiosis in an iguana (*Iguana iguana*). J Vet Diagn Invest 1998;10(2):179–80.
77. Uul EW, Jacobson E, Bartick TE, et al. Aural-pharyngeal polyps associated with *Cryptosporidium* infection in three iguanas (*Iguana iguana*). Vet Pathol 2001; 38(2):239–42.
78. Graczyk TK, Cranfield MR, Fayer R. A comparative assessment of direct fluorescence antibody, modified acid-fast stain, and sucrose flotation techniques for detection of *Cryptosporidium serpentis* oocysts in snake fecal specimens. J Zoo Wildl Med 1995;26(3):396–402.
79. Pavlasek I, Ryan U. *Cryptosporidium varanii* takes precedence over *C. saurophilum*. Exp Parasitol 2008;118(3):434–7.
80. Xiao L, Ryan UM, Graczyk TK, et al. Genetic diversity of *Cryptosporidium* spp. in captive reptiles. Appl Environ Microbiol 2004;70(2):891–9.
81. Kuroki T, Izumiyama S, Yagita K, et al. Occurrence of *Cryptosporidium* sp. in snakes in Japan. Parasitol Res 2008;103(4):801–5.

82. Kik MJ, van Asten AJ, Lenstra JA, et al. Cloaca prolapse and cystitis in green iguana (*Iguana iguana*) caused by a novel *Cryptosporidium* species. Vet Parasitol 2011;175(1):165–7.

83. Abe N, Makino I. Multilocus genotypic analysis of *Cryptosporidium* isolates from cockatiels, Japan. Parasitol Res 2010;106(6):1491–7.

84. Pedraza-Díaz S, Ortega-Mora LM, Carrión BA, et al. Molecular characterisation of *Cryptosporidium* isolates from pet reptiles. Vet Parasitol 2009;160(3):204–10.

85. Richter B, Nedorost N, Maderner A, et al. Detection of *Cryptosporidium* species in feces or gastric contents from snakes and lizards as determined by polymerase chain reaction analysis and partial sequencing of the 18S ribosomal RNA gene. J Vet Diagn Invest 2011;23(3):430–5.

86. Brookins MD, Wellehan JF Jr, Roberts JF, et al. Massive visceral pentastomiasis caused by *Porocephalus crotali* in a dog. Vet Pathol 2009;46(3):460–3.

87. Brock AP, Gallagher AE, Walden HD, et al. *Kiricephalus coarctatus* in an eastern indigo snake (*Drymarchon couperi*); endoscopic removal, identification, and phylogeny. Vet Q 2012;32(2):107–12.

88. Paré JA. An overview of pentastomiasis in reptiles and other vertebrates. J Exot Pet Med 2008;17(4):285–94.

89. Almeida WO, Freire EM, Lopes SG. A new species of *Pentastomida* infecting *Tropidurus hispidus* (Squamata: Tropiduridae) from Caatinga in Northeastern Brazil. Braz J Biol 2008;68(1):199–203.

90. Rataj AV, Lindtner-Knific R, Vlahović K, et al. Parasites in pet reptiles. Acta Vet Scand 2011;53(1):1–21.

91. Walden MR. The epidemiology of coccidia in bearded dragons (*Pogona vitticeps*). Baton Rouge (LA): Louisiana State University; 2008.

92. Walden M, Mitchell MA. Developing a better understanding of coccidia on bearded dragons (*Pogona vitticeps*). Presented at Association of Reptilian and Amphibian Veterinarians. Oakland, October 23–26, 2012.

93. Walden M, Mitchell MA. Evaluation of three treatment modalities against *Isospora amphiboluri* in inland bearded dragons (*Pogona vitticeps*). J Exot Pet Med 2012; 21(3):213–8.

94. Johnsrude JD, Raskin RE, Hoge AY, et al. Intraerythrocytic inclusions associated with iridoviral infection in a fer de lance (Bothrops moojeni) snake. Vet Path 1997; 34:235–8.

95. Marquardt WC, Yaeger RG. The Structure and Taxonomic Status of Toddia from the Cottonmouth Snake Agkistrodon piscivorus leucostoma. J Eukaryot Microbiol 1967;14(4):726–31.

96. Booker KA, Yongue WH Jr. Cytotoddia(= Toddia) infection of serpentes and its incidence in two geographical areas. Va J Sci 1982;33(2):11–21.

97. Smith TG, Desser SS, Hong H. Morphology, ultrastructure and taxonomic status of Toddia sp. in northern water snakes (Nerodia sipedon sipedon) from Ontario, Canada. J Wildl Dis 1994;30(2):169–75.

Avian Bornavirus and Proventricular Dilatation Disease
Diagnostics, Pathology, Prevalence, and Control

Sharman M. Hoppes, DVM, DABVP-avian[a],*,
Ian Tizard, BVMs, BSc, PhD, DACVM[b],
H.L. Shivaprasad, BVSc, MS, PhD, DACPV[c]

KEYWORDS

- Avian bornavirus • Proventricular dilatation disease • Parrot • Diagnosis
- Pathogenesis • Epidemiology

KEY POINTS

- Avian bornavirus (ABV) is the etiologic agent of proventricular dilatation disease (PDD).
- Birds intermittently shed the virus in their droppings, making diagnosis challenging, requiring multiple negative polymerase chain reaction (PCR) tests prior to determining that a bird is negative.
- Birds positive for ABV may or may not ever develop clinical disease.
- Different genotypes of ABV may be more or less virulent depending on species of bird infected. Having exposure to one strain does not provide immunity to another strain.
- Apparently healthy birds that are positive for ABV should not be euthanized.

INTRODUCTION

ABV is the only known etiologic agent of PDD, an infectious disease of birds (**Fig. 1**). PDD has been reported to occur in more than 80 species of psittacines. It has also been reported in toucans, honeycreepers, weaver finches, waterfowl, raptors, and passerines.[1] PDD is a fatal neurologic disease that uniquely affects the enteric nervous system. The disease was first recognized in the early 1970s in macaws exported to Europe and North America from Bolivia.[1] The infection has spread to Australia, Latin America, Japan, the Middle East, and Africa. Its name is derived from the predominant

[a] Department of Veterinary Small Animal Clinical Sciences, College of Veterinary Medicine and Biomedical Sciences, Texas A&M University, 4474 TAMU, College Station, TX 77843-4474, USA; [b] Department of Veterinary Pathobiology, College of Veterinary Medicine and Biomedical Sciences, Texas A&M University, 4467 TAMU, College Station, TX 77843-4467, USA; [c] California Animal Health and Food Safety Laboratory System - Tulare Branch, University of California, Davis. 18830, Road 112, Tulare, CA 93274, USA
* Corresponding author.
E-mail address: SHoppes@cvm.tamu.edu

Vet Clin Exot Anim 16 (2013) 339–355
http://dx.doi.org/10.1016/j.cvex.2013.01.004
1094-9194/13/$ – see front matter © 2013 Elsevier Inc. All rights reserved.

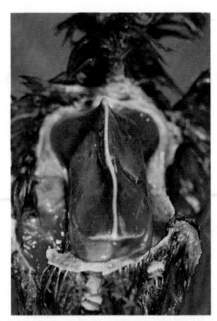

Fig. 1. Severe atrophy of pectoral muscles in a military macaw (Ara militaris) due to PDD.

clinical feature of the disease in parrots, namely, dilation of the proventriculus by accumulated food secondary to defects in intestinal motility (**Fig. 2**). The intestinal dysfunction is probably due to virus-induced immune damage to the autonomic nerves affecting the upper and middle gastrointestinal tract. The disease also is associated with significant central nervous system damage. Clinical signs range from weight loss, crop stasis, proventricular and intestinal dilatation, regurgitation, and maldigestion to eventually starvation and death. Signs involving the central nervous system may also be present, such as tremors, ataxia, seizures, and blindness. Affected birds may show both neurologic and gastrointestinal signs.[1]

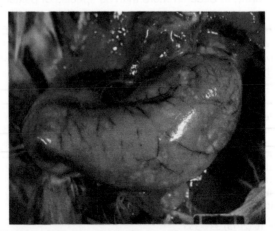

Fig. 2. Severely dilated and thin proventriculus in a Blue-throated macaw (Ara glaucogularis) due to PDD.

PDD was long considered an infectious disease based on its spread through aviaries. Nevertheless, the etiologic agent of PDD proved elusive. It was only in 2008 that pyroseqencing of complementary DNA from the brains of parrots with PDD and subsequent searching for viral sequences identified the presence of a novel bornavirus. Honkovuori and colleagues[2] detected this virus in the brain, proventriculus, and adrenal gland of 3 birds with PDD. It was absent in 4 unaffected birds. At the same time, a separate study by Kistler and colleagues[3] used a microarray approach to identify a bornavirus hybridization signature in 5 of 8 PDD birds and none in 8 controls. Using high-throughput pyrosequencing in combination with conventional PCR cloning and sequencing, a complete viral genome sequence was recovered and the agent shown to be a bornavirus. In this same time period, Villanueva and colleagues[4] detected ABV Nucleoprotein (N-protein) in the brains of birds with PDD.

Bornaviruses

Bornaviruses are negative-encoded, single-stranded, nonsegmented RNA viruses of the order Mononegavirales. Their most unique characteristic is that they undergo transcription inside the nucleus. These viruses also undergo alternative splicing and use different initiation and termination signals from other viruses. Before ABV was discovered the only known species in this family was Borna disease virus (BDV). BDV causes encephalitis in sheep, horses, and other domestic mammals in central Europe.[1] Although predominantly a disease of mammals, BDV has been detected in wild mallards and corvids in Scandinavia, and a neurologic disease has been associated with BDV infection in ostriches in Israel.[5,6] Experimental infections of chickens have been reported by Ludwig and colleagues,[7] who showed that 1-day old chicks inoculated intracerebrally with brain homogenates from rabbits with Borna disease developed paralysis of legs and wings. ABV, although sharing some features in common with BDV, has many significant differences.[8,9]

Etiology

In the 2 studies that first identified ABVs in parrots, 5 genotypes (ABV1–5) were recognized on the basis of nucleotide and amino acid sequence identity.[2,3] Two additional psittacine bornavirus genotypes (ABV6 and ABV7) have subsequently been identified.[10,11] Among these 7 genotypes, ABV4 and ABV2 are the most common genotypes in captive parrots worldwide.[10,12] Birds may also be infected with 2 genotypes simultaneously.[13]

Two additional ABV genotypes have been recently identified. One was recovered from a canary (*Serinus canaria*) and is identified as ABV-canary.[14] The second nonpsittacine ABV genotype was recovered from a wild Canada goose (*Branta canadensis*) and was named ABV-CG.[15] This was the first ABV identified in wild birds. ABV-CG is common across North America and has also been isolated from trumpeter swans (*Cygnus buccinator*) and mute swans (*Cygnus olor*).[15,16] Thus, to date, 9 ABV genotypes have been identified.

The causal association between experimental ABV infection of psittacine birds and the development of PDD has been demonstrated multiple times. Gancz and colleagues[17] were the first to demonstrate that PDD could be transmitted to healthy birds by the use of infected brain tissue. They inoculated cockatiels with a brain homogenate from an ABV4-positive bird or from a PDD/ABV− negative control bird. The birds inoculated with healthy brain homogenate remained healthy whereas all 3 birds inoculated with brain from ABV-infected birds developed both gross and microscopic lesions typical of PDD. Two infected birds exhibited clinical signs. These investigators went on to demonstrate the presence of ABV, with a sequence nearly identical to the challenge strain, in the brains of the challenged birds. High throughput pyrosequencing of the inoculum suggested, however, that other viruses may have been present in these brains although they were not identified in the challenged birds. Although persuasive, these results were, by themselves, insufficient to prove that ABV alone was responsible for PDD.[17]

Gray and colleagues[18] subsequently isolated ABV in cultured duck embryo fibroblasts (DEFs). After 6 passages, these infected cells were injected intramuscularly into 2 Patagonian conures (*Cyanoliseus patagonis*). Clinical signs of PDD developed within 66 days postinfection in both challenged birds. The presence of lesions typical of PDD was demonstrated on necropsy and histopathology. Reverse transcriptase - polymerase chain reaction (RT-PCR) demonstrated the presence of the inoculated strain in the brains of the challenged birds. A third, uninoculated control bird remained healthy. These conures, although apparently healthy, had previously been shown to be carriers of psittacine herpesvirus and, as a result, some uncertainty continued to persist regarding the cause of PDD.

In a subsequent experiment, 4 apparently healthy cockatiels from a flock known to be shedding ABV4 were challenged with a known virulent strain of ABV4 (strain M24). The challenged birds either died or were euthanized for humane reasons between days 92 and 110. Typical PDD was apparent on necropsy and the microscopic lesions were unusually severe. Control birds inoculated with uninfected cells remained healthy until euthanized on day 150, and no evidence of PDD was found at necropsy.[19]

Recently, Piepenbring and colleagues[20] inoculated 18 cockatiels by both the intracerebral and intravenous routes with an isolate of ABV4 cultured for 6 passages in a quail cell line (CEC-32). All challenged birds became persistently infected. Five birds developed clinical signs of PDD whereas 7 of the 18 had a dilated proventriculus on necropsy. All infected birds had histopathology characteristic of PDD.

Mirhosseini and colleagues[21] isolated ABV2 from an infected cockatiel and used infected DEFs to inoculate 2 adult cockatiels by the oral and intramuscular routes. One bird developed clinical signs on day 33, the second on day 41. Although both challenged birds had slightly enlarged proventriculi, histopathology showed typical PDD lesions in many organs. An uninoculated control cockatiel was apparently healthy when euthanized on day 50, and at necropsy, no gross abnormalities were observed. Lierz and colleagues[22] have subsequently conducted a similar challenge study using ABV2 and suggested that this genotype is more pathogenic in cockatiels than genotype 4.

The results of these experiments provide overwhelming support for the proposition that ABV is the sole cause of PDD in psittacines. That is not to say that PDD inevitably develops in every ABV-infected parrot. Many apparently healthy psittacines carry ABV for prolonged periods. Although theoretically, other as-yet unknown viruses may cause PDD or PDD-like disease, in the absence of any evidence for their existence, ABV should be considered the primary etiologic agent of PDD.

Transmission

PDD is contagious. The spread of ABV and PDD has been well reported by Kistler and colleagues,[23] who detailed the spread of disease through an aviary after introduction of an adult bird with fatal PDD. As a consequence, 10 additional birds (adults and unweaned birds) became sick and died. ABV2 was recovered from their tissues. In addition, 12 of 46 healthy exposed birds were also found to be shedding ABV2 by RT-PCR. Secondary spread was also documented because 3 chicks being temporarily boarded at this aviary developed PDD and carried ABV2. They subsequently transmitted it to 5 of 8 chicks in their home aviary. It was also clear from this study that ABV infection precedes development of PDD and provides additional confirmation that ABV is the causal agent of PDD.

This outbreak also provided evidence to suggest that the age of the host affected the disease outcome. Very young birds (as young as 5 weeks of age) developed central nervous system signs within 24 hours of first refusing food and death occurred within 3 days. This outbreak is also of significance because it documents the shortest recorded incubation period of PDD. Unweaned chicks developed clinical disease within 2 to 4 weeks of exposure to PDD.[23]

Because ABV can be detected in droppings—and if these droppings are consumed they infect naïve birds—the fecal-oral route of transmission is considered the most significant.[1,24] Heatley and Villalobos[25] demonstrated that urine of ABV-positive birds was also strongly positive with RT-PCR and immunohistochemical staining demonstrated viral N-protein and Phosphoprotein (P-protein) of ABV within the renal tubules. Heatley and Villalobos developed a nonsurgical method of collecting urine from parrots with little to no fecal contamination present and found that RT-PCR assays performed on samples from 5 infected birds were positive in all 5 urine samples. One urine sample was positive whereas the feces were negative, suggesting that in some cases urine could be even more infectious than feces.

High-volume air sampling has demonstrated the presence of ABV RNA in the air of an infected aviary. Likewise, ABV has been demonstrated within the lung tissue of infected birds. Thus, it is possible, but not proved, that ABV may also be transmitted by the respiratory route.[1] The presence of bornavirus in feather calami has also been demonstrated.[26] It is possible that this may provide a source of airborne virus in feather dust and explain positive RT-PCR results obtained from surface swabs of feathers.[1]

Vertical transmission of BDV has been observed in mice, horses, and humans. Monaco and colleagues[27] detected ABV in 10 of 61 eggs obtained from 2 confirmed ABV-positive aviaries. These eggs ranged from apparently nonviable to those that contained developing embryos. ABV RNA was also detected in the brain tissue of 2 embryos. As discussed later, ABV has also been detected in the brain tissue of embryos in commercial duck eggs. Similar evidence for the presence of ABV in eggs has been obtained by Lierz and colleagues[28] (**Fig. 3**). Kerski and colleagues[29]

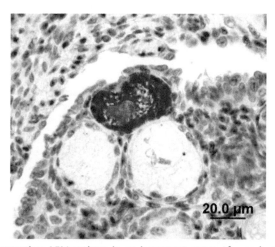

Fig. 3. IHC demonstrating ABV antigen in an immature ovum of a cockatiel.

obtained eggs, embryos, and hatchlings from 4 pairs of sun conures (*Aratinga solstitialis*) naturally infected with ABV2. ABV RNA was detected in early embryos of all 4 pairs. ABV RNA was also detected in multiple organs of late stage embryos and a 2-week-old hatching of 1 pair. This by itself does not confirm vertical transmission because, unless the eggs are incubator hatched and hand raised, infection may come from the parent post-hatch.

Collectively, these findings have important implications for transmission, diagnosis, and immunopathology. Thus, birds infected in ovo may be immunologically tolerant of ABV. If, as is believed, disease develops as a result of T-cell responses to the virus, this tolerance may ensure that ABV infection is inapparent in many birds.

PATHOGENESIS

PDD is characterized by the presence of lymphoplasmacytic infiltrates in the brain and nerves of affected birds. Lymphocytes are especially evident in the enteric ganglia and the enteric nerve plexuses in the anterior gastrointestinal tract and are readily found in the brachial, vagus, and sciatic nerves.[30] There is destruction of ganglia in the gastric plexus and, to a lesser extent, the duodenal myenteric plexus (**Fig. 4**).[31] It is assumed, therefore, that this destruction leads to interference with the motility of the affected gut segments. Such a failure leads to local atony and results in blockage of the passage of digesta. The loss of target neurons may result from direct damage to the nerve cells or, alternatively, destruction of their support cells as a result of ABV infection. Thus, in the cerebellum of infected birds, a significant loss of Purkinje cells is common. Immunohistochemistry (IHC), however, consistently fails to demonstrate that Purkinje cells themselves are infected. Nearby Bergmann glia cells are, however, heavily infected and it is likely that these cells are required to support Purkinje cell function and viability.[32] A major problem with the suggestion that ABV directly damages nerve cells is that ABV is noncytopathic. ABV can infect cells in tissue culture and not affect their viability to any significant extent. ABV associates with nuclear protein in such a way that it remains with daughter cells as they divide.[33] Thus direct viral cytopathic effects are unlikely to be significant in this infection.

It is more likely that the neuronal damage observed in PDD is secondary to the activities of cytopathic T cells. Evidence for this is based exclusively on studies on BDV in laboratory rodents.[34,35] Thus, in susceptible Lewis rats, BDV can induce severe neurologic disease. Immunization or selective removal of T cells with antiserum or immunosuppressive drugs, such as cyclosporine, significantly enhances rat survival.[36] It is hypothesized that cytotoxic T cells attack and destroy target cells expressing BDV

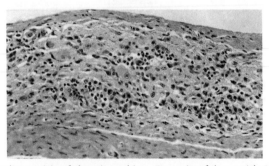

Fig. 4. Severe ganglioneuritis of the gizzard in a Peregrine falcon with PDD.

antigens. If this pathway also operates in birds infected with ABV, then it is anticipated that immunosuppressive protocols, especially selective T-cell elimination by drugs, such as cyclosporine, may be of therapeutic benefit.[36]

Under some circumstances, the immune system can cause neurologic disease by producing autoreactive antiganglioside antibodies. These antibodies are triggered by some viral infections and cause Guillain-Barré syndrome, a rare autoimmune disease sometimes seen in humans postvaccination. Rossi and colleagues[37] have proposed that the pathogenesis of PDD may involve a similar process. There is no doubt that birds with PDD may develop antibodies to brain tissues. For example, the authors have encountered ABV-infected birds with antimyelin antibodies (Villa-nueva I, PhD, unpublished data, 2008). It is, however, unclear just how significant these antibodies are, whether they develop secondary to tissue damage, and how they contribute to the disease process. They could be of use as diagnostic or prognostic indicators. It is relevant to point out that plasma cells are prominent among the lymphocytes within brain and nerve lesions and it may be assumed that they are making immunoglobulins against something. Stitz and colleagues,[36] however, showed that although T cells contributed significantly to the pathogenesis of BDV-induced disease in rats, antibodies seemed to play no significant role in this process.

It has been suggested that ABV-induced nerve damage might trigger local irritation and feather picking. The authors have never observed any association between ABV infection as determined by RT-PCR and feather-picking behavior. There is no evidence that ABV may cause feather-picking disorders. The authors have never observed feather picking in experimentally challenged birds. The occurrence of feather picking in a single ABV-positive bird is of no significance.[38]

DIAGNOSIS

PDD is a complex disease syndrome and affected birds may present with diverse clinical signs. In the classical form of the disease, the signs pertain to the slow emptying or total blockage of the movement of digesta through the proventriculus. As a result, the proventriculus dilates and birds begin to regurgitate ingested foods and ultimately die of starvation. Alternatively or additionally birds may exhibit neurologic signs, especially reflected as an inability to fly or perch or as loss of vision. A clinician who suspects PDD ideally likes to determine if the bird is actually infected with ABV. A reverse transcriptase–PCR is an efficient method of determining the presence of ABV RNA. Studies in the authors' laboratory have demonstrated, however, that selection of tissues or urofeces for PCR testing is critical to obtaining a meaningful result.

Urofecal PCR

Reverse transcriptase–PCR testing of urofeces has been extensively studied in the authors' laboratory. The greatest amount of virus is excreted in the urine.[25] Shedding, however, is intermittent. The great majority of healthy infected birds shed ABV infrequently and some confirmed cases of PDD have been encountered where the authors have failed to detect urofecal ABV even after multiple tests. Alternatively, some birds, especially those developing clinical disease, may shed the virus on a continuous basis. As a result of this variation, the testing of a single dropping from a single bird is of limited usefulness. Multiple droppings from a single bird may be pooled over a period of at least a week or, alternatively, samples from multiple birds in an aviary may also be sampled. Because of intermittent shedding, however, the test has limited sensitivity. It must also be pointed out that many healthy birds may shed ABV for years and the development of clinical PDD is not inevitable. There is no apparent difference in results between collecting fresh droppings or swabbing the cloaca.[1,39]

Feather PCR

de Kloet and colleagues[26] have suggested that RT-PCR performed on a feather sample is a reliable testing procedure. They reported that RT-PCR of the calami of plucked contour feathers detected sufficient ABV RNA and was more reliable than RT-PCR testing of cloacal swabs. They found this true even when the feathers were stored at room temperature for up to 4 weeks. The authors have had limited success using the RT-PCR assay on feather calami.

Blood PCR

Dalhausen and Orosz[40] have suggested that the use of real-time PCR on the whole blood of birds is a sensitive diagnostic test. The authors have limited experience with this test and, given that viremia does not seem to be a common feature of BDV or ABV infections, do not currently use this diagnostic method.

RT-PCR on Necropsy

ABV is readily detected in the tissues of birds that die as a result of PDD. In many cases, the birds' major organs contain detectable virus. In other cases, the virus is largely restricted to nervous tissue, such as the brain, spinal cord, and peripheral nerves. In the authors' experience, the vitreous of the eye is among the most consistent sources of the virus. Apparently healthy carrier birds that die of other causes may have detectable virus restricted to the adrenals and the vitreous. Lierz and colleagues[39] studied the anatomic distribution of ABV in a parrot with clinical PDD. They used a quantitative reverse transcriptase real-time–PCR assay and found virus in all tissues tested as well as a viremia. They also conducted a similar study in a healthy exposed bird and found ABV restricted to nervous tissue. Raghav and colleagues[41], Wunschmann and colleagues[42] examined the distribution of tissue antigen in psittacines suffering from clinical PDD and infected with ABV1. They found, consistent with the authors' experience with genotype 4, that antigen was largely restricted to neurons, astroglia, and ependymal cells in the central nervous system; neurons of the peripheral nervous system; and adrenal cells. In some birds, however, the virus was more widely distributed and detected in intestinal and urinary epithelial cells, retina, heart skeletal muscle, and skin. This widespread distribution further differentiates ABV from BDV because the latter is essentially restricted to nervous tissue.

Immunohistochemistry

Ouyang and colleagues[32] were able to detect the presence of ABV in 24 stored avian brain samples from birds previously diagnosed as suffering from PDD. These investigators used antiserum directed against the N antigen and detected this antigen in the cerebrum, cerebellum, peripheral nerves, enteric ganglia, and spinal cord. They also examined the brains of 11 birds not diagnosed with PDD; 10 were negative and 1 was apparently suffering from an unrecognized case of PDD **Fig. 5**.

Raghav and colleagues[42] also performed IHC using antinucleoprotein antibodies on birds with PDD. They consistently detected this antigen in brain, spinal cord, adrenal, pancreas, and kidney. It was also detected in multiple other organs, including the anterior gastrointestinal tract (crop, proventriculus, ventriculus, and duodenum) as well as heart, testes, ovary, and thyroid. Using histopathologic diagnosis as the gold standard, they found the sensitivity and specificity of IHC 100% for both. They

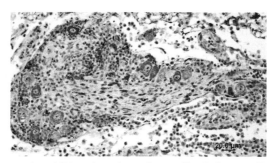

Fig. 5. IHC demonstrating ABV antigen in various cells of the ganglion of the heart of a canary.

also found, however, that many more tissues were positive for ABV by RT-PCR than by IHC, implying that there was inapparent infection in many tissues.

Viral Isolation

ABV is not, in the authors' experience, difficult to grow. The authors have generally used primary DEFs but, given the possibility of domestic duck eggs being already infected (discussed later), all DEF cultures must be screened by RT-PCR prior to use. Infection may be detected by immunofluorescence, IHC, or a Western blot.[8,43,44] Rubbenstroth and colleagues[10] have reported that ABV grows readily in the quail CEC-32 cell line. Isolation works best on freshly obtained tissues. It is not practical to attempt this on feces or cloacal swabs.

Serology

The assessment of ABV infection and the diagnosis of PDD are rendered difficult because, although ABV infection is common, the development of clinical PDD is more rare. Thus, tests that simply detect the presence of ABV may not be especially useful for the antemortem diagnosis of PDD. This issue is further complicated by some ABV-infected birds not seeming to develop a detectable antibody response,[44] although, conversely, there seems to be a positive correlation between the level of antibodies produced and the development of disease. In practice, the sensitivity and specificity of a serologic test can be based on the presence or absence of ABV or the presence or absence of disease and the results of these tests may not correlate well. Heffels-Redmann and colleagues[45] followed the natural course of infection in parrots by both serology (indirect immunofluorescence) and RT-PCR performed at 2-month to 6-month intervals. They found, in general, that birds with a high ABV load in their crop and cloaca combined with the presence of high levels of antibodies had the highest risk of developing disease. This, incidentally, confirmed the authors' experience that antibodies or prior ABV infection did not protect against disease.[19] This also tends to provide an explanation for the authors' observation that sudden seroconversion may immediately precede the onset of clinical disease (Villanueva I, PhD, Unpublished Data, 2008). The prognostic significance of low or inconsistent antibody levels and low PCR responses thus remains unclear.

Western Blot

The initial finding of ABV in the authors' laboratory was based on a Western blot assay.[4] Blood from PDD cases consistently produced antibodies that bound to a 40-kDa antigen in infected brain tissue or a lysate from infected embryonic duck fibroblasts; 27 of 30 PDD cases had detectable antibodies to this protein.

However, 13 of 87 apparently healthy birds also possessed these antibodies. There was no evidence from this study that the presence of antibodies was associated with a poor prognosis. Subsequent amino acid sequencing showed that the p40 antigen was ABV N-protein. Some birds made detectable antibodies to other viral antigens but N-protein was clearly immunodominant. Villanueva and colleagues,[4] therefore, detected antibodies to N-protein on the basis of a Western blot diagnostic test.

Immunofluorescence

Herzog and colleagues[44] used an indirect immunofluorescent assay to measure antibodies against ABV. The target antigen consisted of acetone-fixed Madin-Darby canine kidney cells infected with a horse strain of BDV. They compared this with ABV-infected quail CEC-32 cells and had comparable results. They validated the assay on serum from 77 psittacines taken from flocks where PDD was present; 45% of these birds had ABV-specific antibodies with titers ranging from 1:10 to 1:40,960; 64% of PCR-positive birds and 34% of PCR-negative birds had ABV-specific antibodies. Given these results, they recommended a combination of serology and PCR for PDD diagnosis.

ELISA

de Kloet and colleagues[26] used ELISA to detect antibodies to ABV nucleoprotein (also called p40) and reported that it could detect many infected birds. They found this assay more consistent than ELISA testing for the ABV phosphoprotein (p24) or the matrix protein (p16). This is consistent with the Western blot results (described previously). The authors have also tested ELISA assay for antibodies against the N-protein in PDD cases but found it to have a low sensitivity and specificity (75% sensitivity and 75% specificity) compared with fecal PCR. One of the major difficulties in developing a serologic assay, such as ELISA, is in determining the nature of the standard of comparison. There is poor correlation between the presence of antibodies, fecal shedding of ABV, and clinical disease. Clinically affected birds may or may not have detectable antibodies or fecal PCR positivity. A combination of fecal/feather RT-PCR with a serologic assay may offer the best combination to determine infection.

Antiganglioside Antibodies

Rossi and colleagues[37] have suggested that PDD results from the production of antiganglioside autoantibodies. They have, therefore, compared the level of antiganglioside antibodies with antibodies to ABV. There seemed little correlation between the two. Thus, of 57 blue-throated macaw sera tested, 3 had anti-ABV antibodies and 2 had antiganglioside antibodies but the 2 tests did not seem to overlap. It is unclear from the literature just how sensitive and specific antiganglioside antibody testing might be.

Treatment protocols

Practicing veterinarians are confronted with clinical PDD cases on a daily basis and are faced with the need to treat these birds. Based on the observed histopathologic lesions, it has generally been believed that the neurologic lesions are inflammatory in nature. As a result, it made sense to seek to inhibit or reduce this inflammation. Thus, nonsteroidal anti-inflammatory drugs are widely used to treat this disease. Many veterinarians believe that this treatment is beneficial. Effectiveness is difficult to measure, however, in uncontrolled studies. For example, the effectiveness of this treatment may depend critically on the time of onset of treatment and the stage of the disease when treatment is initiated. It could also be argued that the pathologic lesions of PDD are immunologically mediated, especially if a result of cytotoxic T-cell activity, and that prostanoids are not central to this process. Reuter and colleagues[46] demonstrated that ABV was able to evade the host immune response by failing to activate the pathogen receptor RIG-1 and, as a result, does nor induce production of type I interferons. It is possible that a similar mechanism may prevent overproduction of phospholipases and prostanoids.

Celecoxib

Dalhausen and colleagues[47,48] administered celecoxib at 10 mg/kg orally once daily to treat birds with clinically diagnosed PDD, They treated birds for 6 to 12 weeks and the birds were reported to show a marked clinical improvement. Based on these data, currently it is the standard of treatment. Unfortunately, no untreated control groups were provided so the significance of this report is unclear.

Meloxicam

Preliminary studies performed at the authors' facility (Sharman Hoppes, DVM, unpublished data, 2012) did not demonstrate efficacy of treatment with meloxicam in cockatiels experimentally challenged with ABV strain M24. In evaluating the utility of meloxicam, the birds treated with meloxicam that were challenged with ABV-M24 did not survive. Birds challenged with ABV-M24, however, that did not receive meloxicam and the birds that were unchallenged but did receive meloxicam all survived to the 150-day study endpoint. Only 1 bird in the challenge and untreated group had lesions consistent with PDD on necropsy. Additional studies need to be performed to evaluate both the safety of meloxicam in birds with ABV and the efficacy of meloxicam in the treatment of PDD. Given that these are preliminary studies, the sample sizes were small.

Cyclosporine

Cyclosporine is a calcineurin inhibitor that selectively suppresses T-cell function. As discussed previously, studies on BDV infection in laboratory rodents have indicated that disease is mediated by cytotoxic T cells and the onset of disease can be prevented by appropriate treatment with the immunosuppressive drug cyclosporine.[35-37] In preliminary studies performed at the authors' facility (unpublished data) evaluating the utility of cyclosporine in ABV-challenged cockatiels, there was no significant difference in the development of lesions between the control and treated groups, although on necropsy the treated birds had more organs that were RT-PCR positive for the presence of ABV. Additional studies need to be performed to evaluate the efficacy of cyclosporine in the treatment of PDD.

Ribavirin

The antiviral drug ribavirin readily kills ABV in tissue culture (Musser J and colleagues, unpublished data). In preliminary studies on ABV-infected birds it had no measurable effect on viral shedding. Preliminary data on the pharmacokinetics of ribavirin in birds does show that it is rapidly excreted and that doses appropriate to mammals are insufficient to reach and maintain therapeutic levels in birds. Studies on the use of higher and more frequent dosing with ribavirin are ongoing.

Control

In the absence of effective treatments, control must be sought by other methods. There is no available vaccine and should this disease prove immunologically mediated, it is possible that a vaccine may be ineffective. Certainly infection with one genotype does not seem to confer protection with a different genotype. Studies are ongoing.

The control of ABV in aviaries, therefore, requires a multimodal approach. Although there are still no data on survival of ABV in the environment or sensitivity to disinfectants, it may be assumed that it has much the same stability as other enveloped RNA viruses of similar size and structure. For practical purposes, it can be assumed that ABV has similar sensitivities to disinfectants and cleaners as Newcastle disease virus. Control, therefore, includes isolation of all new, sick, or ABV-positive birds, separation of birds from a flock when they are PCR positive, control of traffic, and good sanitation and thorough cleaning of all areas should be implemented. Existing birds and newly presenting birds should all be tested using both serology and multiple (up to 3) PCR tests, and birds should be separated and/or isolated based on the results of this testing. With the determination of vertical transmission, this makes the issue more difficult, requiring chicks from infected birds to be hand raised, preferably separated from other noninfected birds and monitored for development of disease. Due to the intermittent shedding and inconclusive serology testing, testing and separating birds may require years to obtain ABV-negative aviaries. The authors' studies on shedding patterns suggest, however, that a small number of infected birds are high-level persistent shedders. If such birds are detected, they should be promptly removed from a flock.

ORIGIN AND EPIDEMIOLOGY

PDD was first described in the late 1970s in birds imported from the Santa Cruz area of Bolivia. Given its great lethality to macaws and other large psittacines, it seems to be a completely new disease in these species. Presumably it originated in species other than macaws. Thus, attempts have been made to determine its presence in other species.

ABV in Other Avian Species

Diseases that look like PDD have been observed from time to time in many different bird species (Shivaprasad, unpublished data). After the discovery of ABV, only a few additional species have been shown infected with this virus. Most have been waterfowl.

ABV in Waterfowl

In 1991, Daoust and colleagues[49] described 2 cases of a PDD-like disease in Canada geese. Archived tissues from these birds were subsequently found positive for ABV.[15] Smith and colleagues[50] were the first to detect ABV in Canada geese (*Branta canadensis*) and trumpeter swans (*Cygnus buccinator*). They investigated birds suffering from a neurologic disease of unknown origin. ABV was identified in 11 of 12 goose brains and 2 of 2 swan brains by IHC. The PCR gene products confirmed the presence of a unique new genotype of ABV (ABV-CG).[15,50] In subsequent studies, they collected cloacal swabs from 200 wild Canada geese and 7 were PCR positive.[51] Payne and colleagues[52] tested cloacal swabs from Canada geese by RT-PCR directed against the ABV M genes; 24 of 409 were positive. Twelve of these PCR products were subsequently sequenced and shown to be ABV-CG. Canada geese brains were also tested and 11 of 25 were PCR positive. Positive results have also been obtained on brains from snow geese (*Chen caerulescens*), and Ross's geese (*Chen rossii*).

Delnatte and colleagues,[15] found ABV in 6 of 8 trumpeter swans with uncharacterized neurologic disease. Guo and colleagues[16] tested combined oropharyngeal and cloacal swabs from 219 mute swans (*Cygnus olor*) and 14 were PCR positive. Four positive samples were sequenced and confirmed ABV-CG.[51] Guo and colleagues[16] also tested brains from 197 mute swan and 45 (23%) were positive. Two of these isolates were cultured and found ABV-CG. ABV-associated neuropathology in a mute swan has been reported by Delnatte and colleagues.[51] The differences between apparent viral prevalence in mute swan cloacal swabs (6%) and brains (23%) reflect the intermittent nature of viral shedding in the urofeces.

Payne and colleagues[53] tested 212 brain samples for the ABV M gene from hunter-killed ducks in Texas. ABV was detected in 6.5% of northern pintails (*Anas acuta*), 24% of gadwalls (*Anas strepera*), 10% of mallards (*Anas platyrhynchos*) (10%), 33% of American widgeons (*Anas americana*), and 8% of redheads (*Aythya americana*) (8.3%). Overall, approximately 10% of Texas ducks tested were ABV positive. Two of 72 eggs purchased from commercial duck producers were found ABV positive by RT-PCR. Both viruses belonged to the ABV-CG genotype.[54] This also suggests that ABV may be vertically transmitted in Pekin ducks.

Brains from several species of gull have also been tested for the ABV M gene.[54] Three of 26 herring gulls (*Larus argentatus*), 1 of 5 ring-billed gulls (*L delawarensis*), and 3 of 13 laughing gulls (*L atricilla*) were positive.

Canaries

ABV has been detected in canaries (*Serinus canaria*). Weissenbock and colleagues[55] described a canary that had died after a few days of apathy. On necropsy, the bird had a severely dilated proventriculus. On histopathology, the bird had a nonsuppurative encephalitis and ganglioneuritis in the proventriculus and ventriculus. ABV antigen was detected in multiple tissues and confirmed by RT-PCR. Sequencing demonstrated that this was a new genotype of ABV (ABV-canary). Subsequently, Rinder and colleagues[14] described 2 additional canaries with neurologic disease associated with the presence of ABV. One bird showed apathy and sudden death; the other showed prolonged depression, neurologic disease (head tilting and inability to fly), and blindness due to chorioretinitis. Necropsy showed a dilated proventriculus with ganglioneuritis and nonsuppurative encephalitis. Sequencing identified variants of the previously reported ABV-canary genotype.

Raptors

A bald eagle (*Haliaeetus leucocephalus*) that was found unable to fly was submitted to an avian rehabilitator in Texas and subsequently died. Necropsy showed the presence of an acute encephalitis and ABV-CG strain was detected in its brain by RT-PCR. Bald eagles are known to predate on goose flocks in Texas. Thus transmission of ABV from geese to eagles is not unexpected. Shivaprasad[56] has observed PDD in a peregrine falcon *(Falco peregrinus)*—another waterfowl predator. Shivaprasad has also observed PDD lesions in a red-tailed hawk and a golden eagle but both birds were negative for ABV by PCR using conventional primers.

Mammals

ABV has not been grown in mammalian cells and the authors have never detected it in a mammal.[10,14] The authors continue to test waterside rodents, such as muskrat, and nutria, as well as waterfowl predators, such as mink and raccoon, but have yet to detect an ABV-positive animal. The authors have challenged both rats and mice with ABV4 with no apparent effects. At the present time, therefore, there is no evidence that ABV infects or causes disease in mammals.

SUMMARY

Throughout the years since this disease first appeared, observations on PDD cases have suggested sporadic infections and a relative lack of outbreaks. This led many investigators to believe that the agent was slowly or inefficiently transmitted. Because the etiologic agent is now identified and its presence reliably tested, it has become apparent that ABV infection is common and widespread throughout captive psittacines. It is present at a high level in North America and Europe and has also been detected in Latin America, the Middle East, Japan, Africa, and Australia. Healthy and subclinical carriers of many different species have been documented. There is an urgent need for efficient tests that diagnose clinical PDD with accuracy. There is an urgent need for effective and safe treatments. There is a need for a logical, scientifically sustainable method of stopping the spread of this virus and establishing ABV clean flocks. None of this will be easy but large, valuable endangered birds deserve no less.

REFERENCES

1. Hoppes S, Gray PL, Payne S, et al. The isolation, pathogenesis, diagnosis, transmission, and control of avian bornavirus and proventricular dilatation disease. Veterinary Clin North Am Exot Anim Pract 2010;13(3):495–508.
2. Honkavuori KS, Shivaprasad HL, Williams BL, et al. Novel borna virus in psittacine birds with proventricular dilatation disease. Emerg Infect Dis 2008;14: 1883–6.
3. Kistler AL, Gancz A, Clubb S, et al. Recovery of divergent avian bornaviruses from cases of proventricular dilatation disease: identification of a candidate etiologic agent. Virol J 2008;5:e88.
4. Villanueva I, Gray P, Mirhosseini N, et al. The diagnosis of proventricular dilatation disease: use of a western blot assay to detect antibodies against avian borna virus. Vet Microbiol 2010;143:196–201.
5. Berg M, Johansson M, Montell H, et al. Wild birds as a possible natural reservoir of Borna disease virus. Epidemiol Infect 2001;127:173–8.
6. Malkinson M, Weisman Y, Ashash E, et al. Borna disease in ostriches. Vet Rec 1993;133:304.
7. Ludwig H, Kraft W, Kao M, et al. Bornavirus infection (Borna disease) in naturally and experimentally infected animal: its significance for research and practice. Tierarztl Prax 1985;13:421–53.
8. Rinder M, Ackermann A, Kempf H, et al. Broad tissue and cell tropism of avian bornavirus in parrots with proventricular dilatation disease. J Virol 2009;83: 5401–9.
9. Staeheli P, Rinder M, Kaspers B. Avian bornavirus associated with fatal disease in psittacine birds. J Virol 2010;84:6269–75.
10. Rubbenstroth D, Rinder M, Kaspers B, et al. Efficient isolation of avian bornaviruses (ABV) from naturally infected psittacine birds and identification of a new ABV genotype from a salmon-crested cockatoo (Cacatua moluccensis). Vet Microbiol 2012;161(1–2):36–42.
11. Weissenbock H, Bakonyi T, Sekulin K, et al. Avian bornaviruses in psittacine birds from Europe and Australia with proventricular dilatation disease. Emerg Infect Dis 2009;15:1453–9.

12. Ogawa H, Sanada Y, Sanada N, et al. Proventricular dilatation disease associated with Avian Bornavirus infection in a Citron-crested cockatoo that was born and hand-reared in Japan. J Vet Med Sci 2011;73(6):837–40.

13. Nedorost N, Maderner CA, Kolodziejek J, et al. Identification of mixed infections with different genotypes of avian bornaviruses in psittacine birds with proventricular dilatation disease. Avian Dis 2012;56:414–7.

14. Rinder M, Kronthaler F, Hufen H, et al. Avian bornavirus infections in canaries (Serinus canaria). Proc Annu Conf Assoc Avian Vet 2012;331–2.

15. Delnatte P, Berkvens C, Kummrow M, et al. New genotype of avian bornavirus in wild geese and trumpeter swans in Canada. Vet Rec 2011;169:108.

16. Guo J, Covaleda L, Heatley JJ, et al. Widespread avian bornavirus infection in mute swans in the Northeast United States. Vet Med Res Rep 2012;3:49–52.

17. Gancz AY, Kistler AL, Greninger A, et al. Experimental induction of proventricular dilatation disease in cockatiels (Nymphicus hollandicus) inoculated with brain homogenate containing avian bornavirus 4. Virol J 2009;6:100.

18. Gray P, Hoppes S, Suchodolski P, et al. Use of avian bornavirus isolates to induce proventricular dilatation disease in conures. Emerg Infect Dis 2010;16:473–9.

19. Payne S, Shivaprasad HL, Mirhosseini N, et al. Unusual and severe lesions of proventricular dilatation disease in cockatiels (Nymphicus hollandicus) acting as healthy carriers of avian bornavirus (ABV) and subsequently infected with a virulent strain of ABV. Avian Pathol 2011;40:15–22.

20. Piepenbring AK, Enderlein D, Herzog S, et al. Pathogenesis of avian bornavirus in experimentally infected cockatiels. Emerg Infect Dis 2012;18:234–41.

21. Mirhosseini N, Gray PL, Hoppes S, et al. Proventricular dilatation disease in cockatiels (Nymphicus hollandicus) following infection with a genotype 2 avian bornavirus. J Avian Med Surg 2011;25:199–204.

22. Lierz M, Piepenbring A, Heffels-Redmann U, et al. Experimental infection of cockatiels with different avian bornavirus genotypes. Proc Annu Conf Assoc Avian Vet 2012;9–10.

23. Kistler AL, Smith JM, Greninger AL, et al. Analysis of naturally occurring avian bornavirus infection and transmission during an outbreak of proventricular dilatation disease among captive psittacine birds. J Virol 2010;84:2176–9.

24. de Kloet SR, Dorrestein GM. Presence of avian bornavirus RNA and anti-avian bornavirus antibodies in apparently healthy macaws. Avian Dis 2009;53:568–73.

25. Heatley JJ, Villalobos AR. Avian bornavirus in the urine of infected birds. Vet Med Res Rep 2012;3:19–23.

26. de Kloet AH, Kerski A, de Kloet SR. Diagnosis of avian bornavirus infection in Psittaciformes by serum antibody detection and reverse transcription polymerase chain reaction assay using feather calami. J Vet Diagn Invest 2011;23:421–9.

27. Monaco E, Hoppes S, Guo J, et al. The detection of avian bornavirus within psittacine eggs. J Avian Med Surg 2012;26:144–8.

28. Lierz M, Piepenbring A, Herden C, et al. Vertical transmission of avian bornavirus in psittacines. Emerg Infect Dis 2011;17:2390–1.

29. Kerski A, de Kloet AH, de Kloet SR. Vertical Transmission of Avian Bornavirus in Psittaciformes: avian bornavirus RNA and anti-avian bornavirus antibodies in eggs, embryos, and hatchlings obtained from infected sun conures (aratinga solstitialis). Avian Dis 2012;56:471–8.

30. Berhane Y, Smith DA, Newman S, et al. Peripheral neuritis in psittacine birds with periventricular dilatation disease. Avian Pathol 2001;30:563–70.

31. Manni A, Gerlach H, Leipold R. Neuropathic gastric dilatation in Psittaciformes. Avian Dis 1986;31:214–21.
32. Ouyang N, Storts R, Tian Y, et al. Histopathology and the detection of avian bornavirus in the nervous system of birds diagnosed with proventricular dilatation disease. Avian Pathol 2009;38:393–401.
33. Matsumoto Y, Hayashi Y, Omori H, et al. Bornavirus closely associates and segregates with host chromosomes to ensure persistent intranuclear infection. Cell Host Microbe 2012;11:492–503.
34. Rott R, Herzog S, Richt J, et al. Immune-mediated pathogenesis of Borna disease. Zentralbl Bakteriol Mikrobiol Hyg A 1988;270:295–301.
35. Hallensleben W, Schwemmle M, Hausmann J, et al. Borna disease virus-induced neurological disorder in mice: infection of neonates results in immunopathology. J Virol 1998;72:4379–86.
36. Stitz L, Soeder D, Deschl U, et al. Inhibition of immune-mediated encephalitis in persistently Borna disease virus-infected rats. J Immunol 1989;143:4250–6.
37. Rossi G, Ceccherelli R, Crosta L, et al. Anti-ganglioside auto-antibodies in ganglia of PDD affected parrots. Proc European Assn Avian Vets 2011;198–9.
38. Horie M, Ueda K, Ueda A, et al. Detection of avian bornavirus 5 RNA in Eclectus roratus with feather picking disorder. Microbiol Immunol 2012;56(5):346–9.
39. Lierz M, Hafez HM, Honkavouri KS, et al. Anatomical distribution of avian bornavirus in parrots, its occurrence in clinically healthy birds and ABV- antibody detection. Avian Pathol 2009;38:491–6.
40. Dahlhausen R, Orosz S. Avian bornavirus infection rates in domestic psittacine birds. Proc Annu Conf Assoc Avian Vet 2010;13–6.
41. Wunschmann A, Honkavouri K, Briese T, et al. Antigen tissue distribution of avian bornavirus (ABV) in psittacine birds with natural proventricular dilatation disease and ABV genotype 1 infection. J Vet Diagn Invest 2011;23:716–26.
42. Raghav R, Taylor M, DeLay J, et al. Avian bornavirus is present in many tissues of psittacine birds with histopathologic evidence of proventricular dilatation disease. J Vet Diagn Invest 2010;22:495–508.
43. Gray PL, Suchodolski P, Wigle W, et al. Isolation and growth of avian bornavirus from psittacine birds with proventricular dilatation disease. Emerg Infect Dis 2010;16:473–9.
44. Herzog S, Enderlein D, Heffels-Redmann U, et al. Indirect immunofluorescence assay for Intra vitam diagnosis of avian bornavirus infection in psittacine birds. J Clin Microbiol 2010;48:2282–4.
45. Heffels-Redmann U, Enderlein D, Herzog S, et al. Follow-up investigations on different courses of natural avian bornavirus infections in Psittacines. Avian Dis 2012;56:153–9.
46. Reuter A, Ackermann A, Kothlow S, et al. Avian bornaviruses escape recognition by the innate immune system. Viruses 2010;2:927–38.
47. Dahlhausen R, Aldred S, Colaizzi E. Resolution of clinical proventricular dilatation disease by cyclooxygenase 2 inhibition. Proc Annu Conf Assoc Avian Vet 2002;9–12.
48. Perpiñan D, Fernandez-Bellon H, Lopez C, et al. Lymphocytic myenteric, subepicardial and pulmonary ganglioneuritis in four nonpsittacine birds. J Avian Med Surg 2007;21:210–4.
49. Daoust PY, Julian RJ, Yason CV, et al. Proventricular impaction associated with nonsuppurative encephalomyelitis and ganglioneuritis in 2 Canada geese. J Wildl Dis 1991;27:513–7.

50. Smith D, Berkvens C, Kummrow M, et al. Identification of avian bornavirus in the brains of Canada geese (Branta canadensis) and trumpeter swans (Cygnus buccinator) with non-suppurative encephalitis. Proc Wildlife Disease Assoc. Puerto Iguazu, May 30 - June 4, 2010.
51. Delnatte P, Ojkic D, DeLay J, et al. Pathology and diagnosis of avian bornavirus infection in wild Canada geese (Branta canadensis), trumpeter swans (Cygnus buccinator) and mute swans (Cygnus olor) in Canada: a retrospective study. Avian Pathol, in press.
52. Payne S, Covaleda L, Jianhua G, et al. Detection and characterization of a distinct bornavirus lineage from healthy canada geese (Branta canadensis). J Virol 2011; 85:12053–6.
53. Payne SL, Guo J, Tizard I. Bornaviruses. In: Hambrick J, Gammon LT, editors. North American Waterfowl. In Ducks: habitat, behavior and diseases. New York: Nova Scientific Publishers; 2012. p. 1–20.
54. Payne SL, Delnatte P, Guo J, et al. Birds and bornaviruses. Animal Health Reviews And Reports 2012;13(2):145–56.
55. Weissenbock H, Sekulin K, Bakonyi T, et al. Novel avian bornavirus in a nonpsittacine species (canary; Serinus canaria) with enteric ganglioneuritis and encephalitis. J Virol 2009;83:11367–71.
56. Shivaprasad HL. Proventricular dilatation disease in a Peregrine falcon (Falco peregrinus). Proc Annu Conf Assoc Avian Vet 2005;107–8.

Emerging and Reemerging Diseases of Avian Wildlife

Susan J. Pello, VMD, MS[a],*, Glenn H. Olsen, DVM, MS, PhD[b]

KEYWORDS

- Aspergillosis • Avian influenza • Emerging diseases • Inclusion body disease
- Poxvirus • Wellfleet Bay virus • West Nile virus

KEY POINTS

- Several new and emerging diseases such as inclusion body disease of cranes and Wellfleet Bay virus are documented only in one species or group of species.
- Some established diseases have taken a new focus as more is learned about genomics.
- Some established diseases found in other parts of the world have the potential for deadly spread to North American wildlife populations, such as occurred with West Nile virus, and could occur with inclusion body disease or Old-World strains of avian influenza.
- New techniques in genomics, treatment, reporting of wildlife disease, and wildlife tracking, such as miniature satellite transmitters, are increasing our knowledge of how these diseases act and spread.

ASPERGILLOSIS

Introduction

There are 4 fungal genera: *Aspergillus*, *Fusarium*, *Penicillium*, and *Claviceps*. Aspergillosis, as the name implies, is caused by fungi in the genus *Aspergillus*. *A flavus* and *A fumigatus* commonly affect avian species, specifically raptors, and have been described in captive and wild bird species.[1] Mycotoxins are poisonous secondary metabolites produced by fungi including species of *Aspergillus* and *Fusarium* (**Fig. 1**). Aflatoxins, produced by *A flavus*, are a group of compounds that act as biosynthetic inhibitors, which can cause liver impairment.[2]

Etiology

Aspergillus fungi are ubiquitous and found in the soil, whereas the fungal organisms causing aflatoxicosis are often linked to corn, cereal, oil seeds, feeds, grains, peanuts, and decomposing vegetables.[2–4] Common species of this genus that cause aspergillosis are *A fumigatus*, *A niger*, *A glaucus*, *A nidulans*, and *A flavus*.[5,6] *A fumigatus* is the

[a] Animal & Bird Health Care Center, Cherry Hill, NJ 08003, USA; [b] USGS Patuxent Wildlife Research Center, 12302 Beech Forest Road, Laurel, MD 20708, USA
* Corresponding author.
E-mail address: PelloVMD@gmail.com

Vet Clin Exot Anim 16 (2013) 357–381
http://dx.doi.org/10.1016/j.cvex.2013.02.001
1094-9194/13/$ – see front matter

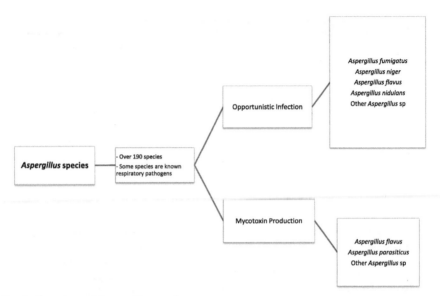

Fig. 1. Overview of *Aspergillus* species.

most pathogenic species to affect wild birds and poultry, which may be attributed to the fact that the spores, also known as conidia, are much smaller than other species of aspergillosis.[5] *A fumigatus* conidia are 2 to 3 μm in diameter, which is small enough to reach the air capillaries of even a songbird (3 μm).[7] Aspergillosis is primarily an infection of the respiratory tract caused by inhalation of spores. However, aspergillosis has also been isolated from the skin, gastrointestinal tract, central nervous system (CNS), bone, and eye.[2,8]

A fumigatus, a saprophytic fungus, has an essential role in recycling carbon and nitrogen in the soil, specifically organic debris.[8] Culture identification of *A fumigatus* is based on conidia and conidiophore morphology (**Fig. 2**). The organism is characterized by septate hyphae and asexual fruiting structures that are produced on conidiophores. The conidiophore is produced from the vegetative mycelium and consists of hyphal branches originating from a foot cell. The asexual reproductive units, conidia, arise on flask-shaped phialides on the vesicle of the hyphal foot cell and are produced in chains basipetally.[9] These conidia may be greenish in color or white, and can measure 6 to 8 by 2 to 3 μm in size.[8] The color of *Aspergillus*, depending on the species, varies from blue-green, brown, black, to yellow. *A fumigatus* grows within 5 days on Sabouraud dextrose agar, and is velvety or granular with bluish-green color and narrow white peripheries. *A flavus* colonies have a fluffy texture and are yellowish-green in color.[10]

Predilection

Factors that may predispose a bird to mycosis infection include immunosuppression, recent vaccination, concurrent viral infection, parasitisim, babesiosis,[11] lymphoproliferative disorders, starvation, hypovitaminosis A, and overcrowding. Some factors that may increase spore concentration in the environment include poor environmental ventilation, poor sanitation, elevated humidity and temperature, and long-term storage of feed.[5]

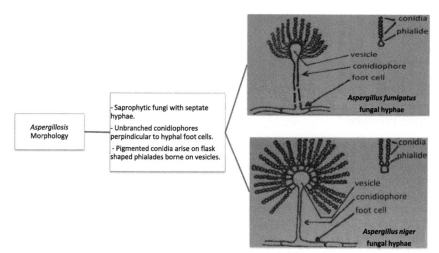

Fig. 2. Overview of *Aspergillus* morphology.

Clinical Correlation

Aspergillosis and candidiasis are the most common fungal infections in birds. Wild noncaptive birds are typically negative for *Aspergillus*, but once placed in a captive environment may become infected owing to stress or other factors.[3] Inhalation is the main route of infection for aspergillosis. *A fumigatus*, which has conidia measuring 2 to 3 μm in size, disperse easily through the air, allowing them to be inhaled. Once they reach the lower respiratory tract, the conidia attach to the mucosa and produce the vegetative form that makes up the visible plaques. The plaques are commonly noted in the dorsal air sacs or in the syrinx. Tracheal endoscopy, coelomoscopy, radiography, and computed tomography (CT) may be used for diagnosis in conjunction with clinical findings, polymerase chain reaction (PCR) of lesions or blood, and serum antibody and antigen levels. Coelomoscopy/endoscopy to identify and biopsy fungal plaques is the gold standard for diagnosis,[12] followed by fungal culture and microscopic examination.

There are 2 forms of aspergillosis infection, acute and chronic. Acute infection commonly affects the young, whereas chronic infections are more common in adult birds.[1–3] *A fumigatus* infection in newly hatched chicks (brooder pneumonia) causes somnolence, inappetance, and death. In adult birds, clinical signs of aspergillosis include inappetance, emaciation or weight loss, change of voice, respiratory distress, and exercise intolerance. On physical examination the bird may be fluffed and unkempt. On necropsy or endoscopy, yellow nodules may be found in the syrinx, air sacs, lungs, and other organs. The air sacs may appear thickened and opaque. Histopathologic examination and culture of the affected tissues would be necessary for diagnosis. A complete blood count may show a severe leukocytosis (white blood cell count >40,000), possibly characterized by a monocytosis and a toxic heterophilia.[12] In some cases, hepatomegaly and elevated liver values occur. These cases with liver involvement may indicate *A flavus* as the culprit, because it produces an aflatoxin.

Acute toxicity of aflatoxin B1, produced by *A flavus*, causes death with few gross lesions other than hepatomegaly and pallor.[2] Acute aflatoxicosis in ducklings results in stunted growth, inappetance, ataxia, and death. In very young birds slight hepatomegaly and renomegaly may be noted, with pallor of the liver and kidneys. Petechiation of the kidneys and pancreas may also be found.[2] Hepatic fibrosis, nodular hyperplasia, hydropericardium, and coelomic effusion have been reported in older ducks. Hemorrhages may be found in the pancreas, kidney, feet, and webbing. Other histologic lesions that have been noted include hepatocellular degeneration or necrosis with biliary proliferation.[2] Chronic aflatoxin intake results in hepatic carcinomas, immunosuppression, and subsequent susceptibility to bacterial and parasitic infections.[2]

Treatment

Aspergillosis is a common disease that affects both captive and wild raptors. Treatment options include endoscopic removal of fungal lesions, oral antifungal therapy (**Table 1**), and supportive care.[3,13–15] Other therapies include nebulization with antifungal agents, such as amphotericin B or clotrimazole, which can also be administered intratracheally and parentally. Anti-inflammatories and antibiotics to cover secondary infections should also be considered. Further research into the use of tumor necrosis factor in birds may prove useful.[14]

Newer antifungal options include voriconazole (VRC), which can be administered orally or intravenously, and terbinafine, which can be administered orally or via nebulization. VRC has been used successfully in both wild and captive avian species, and has been shown to be effective in humans.[12,13,17,18,22–24] It is a broad-spectrum second-generation triazole antifungal agent, which functions by enzymatic inhibition to block synthesis of ergosterol. VRC is a synthetic derivative of fluconazole[24] and is metabolized in the liver by cytochrome P450. It has excellent oral bioavailability, with wide tissue distribution and CNS penetration in humans.[24] VRC is effective against Aspergillus, Candida, and Cryptococcus species.[18] The most common side effect noted with VRC treatment is polyuria in birds.[17,23] However, this may be an adverse effect of the treatment and/or may be stress related because of handling and medication administration.[17] VRC has been used successfully in the treatment of aspergillosis and has shown stability when compounded.

Of note, cases of A fumigatus resistance to VRC and other triazole antifungals in humans and avian species have been reported.[19,25] The most reported cause of VRC resistance is due to a mutation in the A fumigatus cyp51A gene, and several mutations in this gene have been associated with triazole resistance.[19] For those cases of VRC-resistant A fumigatus infections in humans, posaconazole is used. Use of posaconazole, a second-generation triazole,[19] has not been documented in avian species.

Summary

Aspergillosis is an important disease of avian wildlife, specifically captive raptors. During rehabilitation and captivity, raptors are at risk for A fumigatus infection, which is a significant cause of morbidity and mortality despite medical advances and the development of new antifungal agents.[13] Avian aspergillosis commonly involves lesions developing in the air sacs and lungs. The new current standard of treatment is endoscopic removal of florid lesions and topical antifungal treatment, followed by systemic antifungal and nebulization therapy. VRC has been used successfully in the treatment of aspergillosis and has shown stability when compounded, in comparison with itraconazole. VRC may become the new standard of care in the treatment of fungal infections in birds, both wild and captive species. This new standard for treatment offers much improved outcomes over previous therapies and is easier to administer to avian patients than such therapies as amphotericin B.

Table 1
Antifungals available for aspergillosis treatment

Drug	Route of Administration	Oral Bioavailability	Site Metabolized	Mechanism of Action	Miscellaneous Notes
Macrocyclic Polyketides					
Amphotericin B	Nebulization Intravenous Topical	Poor	Renal	Binds sterols causing transmembrane channels	Nephrotoxicity[16] Poorly soluble in water
Imidazoles					
Clotrimazole	Nebulization Topical	Poor	Hepatic	Blocks synthesis of ergosterol Causes lysis of fungal membrane[16]	Must be compounded Water soluble
Enilconazole (Imazalil 13.8%)	Nebulization Topical	Poor	Liver	Blocks synthesis of ergosterol	Used to treat environment Renal excretion
Ketoconazole	Oral	Yes	Hepatic CYP450	Blocks synthesis of ergosterol	Low stomach pH required for absorption Hepatotoxicity risk
Triazoles					
Fluconazole	Oral Intravenous	Yes	Hepatic CYP450	Blocks synthesis of ergosterol	Fungistatic Caution with impaired renal function due to renal excretion[17] Water soluble Absorption not influenced by food Hepatotoxicity risk

(continued on next page)

Table 1
(continued)

Drug	Route of Administration	Oral Bioavailability	Site Metabolized	Mechanism of Action	Miscellaneous Notes
Itraconazole	Oral Intravenous	Variable 50% on empty stomach 100% on full stomach	Hepatic CYP450	Blocks synthesis of ergosterol	Broad spectrum (more than fluconazole) Use with caution in African gray parrots Drug accumulation
Voriconazole (VRC)	Oral (poor in chickens[18]) Intravenous	Yes	Hepatic CYP450	Blocks synthesis of ergosterol	Broad spectrum (more than itraconazole) Highly active against *Aspergillus* spp and *Candida* spp[17]
Posaconazole	Oral	Yes	Hepatic CYP450	Blocks synthesis of ergosterol	Superior activity to VRC in reducing lung fungal burden in mice with VRC mutation of *A fumigatus*[19] Water insoluble[20] Closely related to Itraconazole Fungicidal and fungistatic Excreted in urine and feces
Allylamine					
Terbinafine	Oral Nebulization	Yes	<5% of hepatic CYP450	Inhibits synthesis of ergosterol	Fungicidal and fungistatic antifungal[21]

WEST NILE VIRUS
Introduction

West Nile virus (WNV), a flavivirus, is an arthropod-borne single-stranded RNA virus.[26] Within the genus *Flavivirus*, family Flaviviridae, there are 70 viruses. The main antigens of flaviviruses are contained in 3 structural proteins, which cause the high degree of cross-reactivity in serologic testing and high similarity among viruses in this genus.[6] WNV is a member of the Japanese encephalitis serocomplex, and was first isolated in humans from the West Nile region of Uganda in 1937.[6,26] From Uganda the virus spread across Africa and the Middle East, and into Europe. In 1999, WNV emerged on the east coast of the United States and has migrated west. WNV is now found throughout the United States, 7 Canadian provinces, Jamaica, Guadeloupe, Mexico, Puerto Rico, and El Salvador. Two distinct lineages of WNV exist. Lineage 1 viruses have been isolated from northeastern United States, Europe, Israel, Africa, India, and Russia. Lineage 2 viruses have been isolated from sub-Saharan Africa and Madagascar.[27] The strain in the western hemisphere is most similar to that of one isolated from Israel.[6,28] The strain introduced in New York in 1999 was especially virulent to some native North American avian species that caused high mortality. The route by which WNV entered the western hemisphere is still unknown.[6]

The disease, even though a decade old in North America, is still recurring and spreading to previously undocumented locations, especially in 2012.[29] Indeed, 5290 human cases of WNV were documented in 2012 across the entire United States by the Centers for Disease Control and Prevention (CDC), but especially in the Northeast, southern Arizona, Central Valley of California, and the Red and Missouri River Valleys of the Midwest.[29] There have been more than 200 human deaths in 2012.[30] To date, 326 avian species have been found carrying the virus[29] and more than 43 mosquito species are considered vectors of WNV.[31] Surveillance reports show WNV infection increasing in companion avian species. Psittaciformes that have been reported with WNV include budgerigars (*Melopsittacus undulatus*), Pacific parrotlets (*Forpus coelestis*), canary-winged parakeets (*Brotogeris versicolorus*), cockatiels (*Nymphicus hollandicus*), rosellas (*Platycercus* spp), lories and lorikeets (*Eos, Lorius pseudeos*, and *Trichoglossus* spp), cockatoos (*Cacatua* spp), macaws (*Ara* spp), amazons (*Amazona* spp), African grays (*Psittacus* spp) Meyer's (*Poichephalus* spp), and blue-crowned conure (*Thectocercus acuticaudata*).[32]

Etiology

Domestic and wild avian species are the primary amplifying host of WNV, and more than 300 avian species have shown susceptibility.[26] WNV also infects more than 30 vertebrate species including marine mammals, squirrels, chipmunks, bats, horses, hoofstock, camelids, canids, felids, and some reptiles, particularly alligators.[6,27,33] The most common form of transmission is mosquito borne (*Culex* spp in western hemisphere); however, louse flies (*Icosta americana*), ticks (*Carios capensis*), and tabanid flies (family Hippoboscidae, *Pseudolynchia*) have been implicated. Other routes of infection include horizontal transmission among corvids, ingestion of WNV-infected prey or blood contamination of wounds.

Birds are the natural reservoir host of WNV; however, species susceptibility, morbidity, and mortality vary. Species that have shown extremely high titers and mortality following infection include corvids, magpies *(Pica pica)*, common grackle (*Quiscalus quiscula*, house finch, house sparrow, ring-billed gull (*Larus delawarensis*), and loggerhead shrikes (*Lanius ludovicianus migrans*). Passeriformes and *Charadriiformes* species have very high viremias without clinical disease, and therefore are a more competent viral reservoir than species of other orders.[6] Northern breeding species that have shown 100% mortality include the snowy owl (*Bubo scandiaca*), northern hawk owl (*Surnia ulula*), northern saw-whet owl (*Aegolius acadicus*), boreal owl (*Aegolius funereus*), and great gray owl (*Strix nebulosa*). An intermediate mortality is seen in species with a pan–North American breeding range, such as the short-eared owl (*Asio flammeus*), long-eared owl (*Asio otus*) and great horned owl (*Bubo virginianus*). Very little mortality is noted in southern breeding species such as the barn owl (*Tyto alba*), eastern screech owl (*Megascops asio*), and burrowing owl (*Athene cunicularia*). Low susceptibility is also noted in the northern goshawk (*Accipiter gentilis*) and the peregrine falcon (*Falco peregrines*).

Antemortem Detection

Viremia is often detectable 1 day after infection and is cleared by days 6 to 8.[26] Shedding (cloacal, oral) occurs during viremia, 1 to 4 days after infection, and may continue for 14 days or longer. When determining which diagnostic test should be used, it is important to deduce which period of infection the patient is in (**Tables 2** and **3**). Reverse transcription (RT)-PCR of blood, feces, and/or a crop/cloacal swab to detect viral RNA can be used during the 1- to 8-day postinfection period. From days 5 to 7 postinfection, antibodies are produced by the body, and therefore serology and a plaque-reduction neutralization test (PRNT) may be used for detection.[36,37] If the virus has already been cleared and the active viremia is missed, running a PRNT

Table 2
West Nile virus: diagnostic testing based on sample

Sample for Submission	Optimal Time Period for Sample Collection	Important Diagnostic Details	Diagnostic Test
Cloacal and oral shedding	Viremia 1–4 d, up to 14 d or longer	A bird must have sufficient viremia for the virus to be shed in mucosal secretions of oropharynx and cloaca, because this period is brief in avian species and false negatives are likely[34]	RT-PCR
Blood	1–8+ d	Good during viremia; however, the viremic phase usually precedes clinical signs, which appear 10–12 d postinfection[35,36]	PRNT ELISA RT-PCR
Tissue biopsy	5–45+ d		PRNT ELISA IHC RT-PCR
Insect/mosquito carcass CSF/ blood/tissues		Requires infectious virus in sample Should be used when testing carcasses, for screening critical patients, or surveillance of mosquitoes or other insects	PRNT RT-PCR Antigen detection IHC Culture VecTest

Abbreviations: CSF, cerebrospinal fluid; ELISA, enzyme-linked immunosorbent assay; IHC, immunohistochemistry; PRNT, plaque-reduction neutralization test; RT-PCR, reverse transcription–polymerase chain reaction.

Table 3
Explanation of diagnostic testing for WNV

Diagnostic Test	Sample to Submit	Optimal Time Period for Sample Collection	Detection	Results	Laboratory
Real-time TaqMan RT-PCR	Whole blood, fecal, crop/cloacal swab, brain, heart, kidney, bone marrow, oropharyngeal swab, CSF, spinal cord, feather pulp	1–8 d postinfection or during active infection	Viral RNA[36]	Negative once virus cleared	Veterinary Molecular Diagnostics, Inc (VMD Labs) Cornell Avian Biotech State labs
Nucleic acid sequence based amplification (NASBA reactions)	Brain, CSF, cloacal/crop swab, whole blood	Best used in first 1–8 d postinfection	Viral RNA	Negative once virus cleared	Avian Biotech
PRNT **GOLD STANDARD**	Whole blood, serum, plasma, or CSF	From day 5+	WNV-specific NABs	Fourfold increase indicates WNV-positive infection	Cornell
Viral neutralization	Whole blood, serum, plasma, or CSF	From day 5+	WNV-specific NABs	Fourfold increase indicates WNV-positive infection	Michigan State University Diagnostic Center for Population and Animal Health
IgG (indirect ELISA)	Serum or CSF Paired titers 2–4 wk apart	5–45 d postinfection	IgG (antispecies conjugates are not available for every host)	Positives must be confirmed by PRNT Cannot discriminate WNV from other flaviviruses More cross-reactions than MAC-ELISA Variable sensitivity and specificity, depending on test manufactured	State labs

(continued on next page)

Table 3
(continued)

Diagnostic Test	Sample to Submit	Optimal Time Period for Sample Collection	Detection	Results	Laboratory
MAC-ELISA (IgM antibody capture)	Serum or CSF Paired titers 2–4 wk apart	5–45 d postinfection	IgG IgM (antispecies conjugates are not available for every host)	Fourfold increase is a positive result Positives must be confirmed by PRNT Cannot discriminate WNV from other flaviviruses Sensitivity 91.7%, specificity 99.2% (equine Sera)[36]	State labs
IFA	Blood	5–45 d postinfection	IgM	Discriminates flavivirus specific IgM-associated antibodies	
Histopathology	Feather pulp, heart, kidney, liver, CNS, spleen, lung, pancreas, proventriculus, intestine, adrenal glands, integument, gonads, eye	Best used in first 1–8 d postinfection	Inflammatory lesions associated with WNV (lymphoplasmocytic and histiocytic inflammation)	Evaluation of target tissues for signs of inflammatory damage	Private labs that perform histopathology
IHC	CNS, spleen, kidney, heart, lung, pancreas, proventriculus, intestine, adrenal glands, integument, gonads, tissue macrophages, endothelial cells, vascular feather pulp	From day 5+	WNV antigen	Antigen distribution can vary as infection progresses[37]	Private labs that perform IHC

Virus isolation	Brain, heart, kidney, bone marrow, crop/cloacal swab, CSF, spinal cord	Best used in first 1–8 d postinfection	Virus	Negative once virus cleared	Cornell
VecTest antigen-capture assay	Mosquito Insects Tissue samples Blood CSF Saliva	During viremia	Antibodies against WNV	Sensitivity and specificity variable depending on species and site tested[38] Sensitivity 83.3%, specificity 95.8% of oral swabs in crows[39] Not affected by freezing tissue	Louisiana State University State labs

Abbreviations: CNS, central nervous system; IFA, immunofluorescent antibody; IgG, immunoglobulin G; IgM, immunoglobulin M; NABs, neutralizing antibodies; WNV, West Nile virus.

(the gold standard) is appropriate. WNV affects multiple organ systems and is cleared in 1 to 2 weeks, but may be present up to 27 days after infection, depending on the immune status and age of the bird.[26] If the period of infection cannot be determined, running a PCR and paired PRNT would be recommended. Once the virus is cleared clinical signs can remain, owing to inflammatory damage to organ systems such as the brain.

Sample collection for WNV detection in live patients includes blood and oral/cloacal swabs, as well as feather, organ, and skin biopsies. PRNT and serology are useful, especially when paired titers are run 2 to 4 weeks apart.[26] The occurrence of a 4-fold antibody titer increase indicates acute or recent WNV infection. There are several methods to detect WNV in avian species. The gold standard is PRNT. Other tests (see **Table 3**) include enzyme-linked immunosorbent assay, RT-PCR, histopathology, immunohistochemistry, and feather-pulp testing (vascular vs nonvascular) (see **Table 3**). A recent study of WNV distribution in North American owls (Strigidae family) and select psittacine species found that the kidney is the most reliable location for the detection of WNV.[32,40] Another study of experimentally infected hamsters found persistent WNV infection in the brain and kidneys.[31]

Postmortem Detection

Appropriate samples to collect in determining if an avian carcass is WNV positive include brain, heart, kidney, blood, and skin, as well as oropharyngeal and cloacal swabs.[41,42] WNV detection has been well demonstrated in vascular feather pulp of corvid carcasses.[42] A VecTest WNV antigen assay can be used when performing mosquito surveillance, and is used to test mosquitoes and avian carcasses for WNV infection.[26,38,39] In acute infections, postmortem virus isolation of homogenized tissue via RT-PCR may be useful.[26] However, chronic infections (≥2–3 weeks postinfection) are more difficult to diagnose because the birds may have cleared the virus. These birds may succumb to chronic inflammatory sequelae of WNV,[40] and in these cases it would be difficult to detect WNV infection by most means. Immunohistochemistry, viral isolation, and histopathology of organ tissue should be submitted. Histopathology of the brain may reveal perivascular cuffing of mononuclear inflammatory cells, and perivascular lymphocytic and plasmacytic infiltrates. Histopathology of the eyes may reveal mild to marked retinal necrosis, retinal atrophy, and lymphoplasmacytic and histiocytic uveitis; pectinitis, papillitis, segmental multifocal choroiditis, and iriocyclitis may be noted in birds with antemortem pectinitis and chorioretinitis.[43] In chronic infections ocular, CNS, renal, and feather samples have yielded positive results.[26,34,42]

Clinical Correlation

Clinical signs of WNV in avian species appear 10 to 12 days after infection,[35] and in some avian species viremia remains for only 0 to 4 days after infection.[34] On initial physical examination, poor body condition, lethargy, and head tilt may be noted. Common clinical findings with WNV are due to encephalitis. Primarily neurologic signs will be noted including head tilt, tremors, ataxia, disorientation, inability to perch, missing perches, and visual impairment. Other findings include anterior uveitis and chorioretinitis. Blood work may reveal a moderate leukocytosis characterized by a heterophilia and lymphocytosis with reactive heterophils.[44] Additional findings include atypical feather morphology (pinched-off feathers), myocarditis, myalgias, arthralgias, rashes, pancreatitis, hepatitis, and inflammation of the pectin and choroid.[43,45–48]

In humans, clinical signs and complications can persist for more than a year after infection and release from hospital. Complications included fatigue, difficulty ambulating, memory difficulties, weakness, confusion, and recent onset of depression.[31] Studies on Rhesus monkeys support persistent WNV infection in humans. It was even noted that WNV phenotypic characteristics changed over the course of infection in clinical and nonclinical Rhesus monkeys and hamsters.[31] This finding supports the notion that WNV infection can persist in humans and other mammals, which may also occur in avian species showing persistent clinical signs. One study found that relapses of neurologic signs occurred in educational raptors for more than 4 years after initial infection.[45]

Treatment

At present, specific antiviral therapy does not exist and the only approved therapy in humans is supportive care.[31] Treatment of WNV infected avian patients includes supportive care (intravenous/intraosseous fluid therapy, gavage feedings, heat support) and anti-inflammatory medications[44] because of the severe inflammatory sequelae caused by WNV in the body. It is important to stress prevention, including vaccination and mosquito control, to zoologic and raptor facilities. Treatment and prevention among noncaptive populations of wild birds is not feasible.

Prevention

Because of the high morality of WNV in birds, avian practitioners, veterinarians, and zoologic parks are searching for a way to protect their patients. Despite the lack of research on vaccine efficacy in birds, veterinarians began using the equine WNV vaccination in an off-label manner. Two vaccines are commonly used, the Fort Dodge killed vaccine and the Merial Recombitec canarypox vectored vaccine. Both vaccines are used off-label and may not produce seroconversion in every patient, but the lack of seroconversion may indicate tissue-mediated immunity and does not necessarily correlate with lack of protection.[28] Both vaccines have been used successfully in avian species,[28,36,49] and in some cases have shown antibody development. One study in sandhill cranes (*Grus canadensis*) showed reduced viremia and shedding following vaccination with a killed vaccine, despite a lack of detectable antibody titer.[28,42] This result shows that high antibody production following vaccination does not correlate with protection.[28] A recent article presented the use of vectored WNV vaccines in the domestic goose as a model for WNV vaccine efficacy using a fowlpox virus vector for delivery of WNV genes that provided protection.[50] Further development and research of similar vaccines may lead to the production of an avian labeled WNV vaccine, the first of its kind.

The CDC promotes educating the public on the 5 'Ds' for WNV,[31] some of which can be translated into protecting outdoor captive wildlife. It is recommended to remain indoors between dusk and dawn. Although this is not feasible for much of our wildlife, it can be instituted for at-risk companion psittacines. The use of mosquito nets placed around outdoor enclosures from dusk to dawn can reduce mosquito access. Mosquito breeding sites can be eliminated and reduced by draining standing water. These measures will also help to reduce the threat to the surrounding human population.

Summary

WNV is the most important infectious disease of raptors and is very common in passerines and charadriiform species, which serve as critical vectors owing to their high viral load. Captive psittacines who are housed in WNV-endemic regions with large mosquito-vector areas are at high risk for exposure. WNV has been well documented in wildlife and noncaptive avian species; however, it has become an emerging issue in captive psittacines.[34] It is important that research is continued on the pathogenesis of WNV and vaccine development in avian species.

POXVIRUS

Introduction

Avipoxvirus is the genus of poxviruses in birds. Avian poxviruses affect many avian species, including more than 230 species of free-ranging and domestic birds.[51–53] Many forms of poxviruses exist; however, 16 have been defined[54] and are named mainly after the species they infect. A few that have been defined include canarypox (canaries and canary hybrids), psittacinepox (South American parrots), mynahpox (mynahs), starlingpox (starlings and mynahs), fowlpox (gallinaceous birds, ostrich chicks in the United States), and penguinpox (African penguin). Avipoxvirus will typically be seen in canaries, chickens, pigeons, turkeys, and vultures housed outdoors and in free-ranging flocks, but has also been found in jungle crows, Hawaiian crows, jungle mynahs, rough-legged hawks, short-toed larks, peafowl, eagles, partridges, falcons, African penguins, and stone curlews.[53,55–57] Many reports of avipoxviruses are in passerines, but some report infections in raptorial species.[56]

In free-ranging birds, infection with an avipoxvirus would have implications in endangered or threatened species. These viruses are not fatal to all avian species, but may reduce the viability of a species[2] and are a threat to isolated native avifauna of the Hawaiian, Galapagos, and Canary Islands.[54,58,59] In India, where avipoxviruses are reemerging, phylogenic analysis was performed, and showed that virus isolates from wild and domestic birds were identical.[60] This finding indicates that avipoxviruses are not host specific and can infect any avian species, be they wild, domestic, or endangered.[60] Avifauna of the Hawaiian Islands are at risk for extinction because of complex infections with avipoxvirus, *Plasmodium* blood parasites, and arthropod vectors.[58] The history of avipoxvirus, which dates back to 1899 in wild bird populations on the Galapagos, may reveal a possible contribution to the population decline of avifauna.[58] Recently, avipoxvirus has been reported in kiwis (*Apteryx mantelli*) in New Zealand,[54] although the virulence in this species is unknown.

Etiology

The route of transmission for avipoxviruses occurs mechanically by bloodsucking or biting vectors, such as mosquitoes and mites.[61–65] Other forms of transmission include direct contact with aerosols, contaminated food, water, or fomite. However, poxviruses cannot penetrate the epithelium unless compromised by trauma,[51,66] owing to the large size of the virus. Outbreaks are seen in all age groups during summer and fall, in relation to the vector life cycle. However, young birds (older than 3 weeks) are especially susceptible.[2]

Clinical Correlation

There are 3 forms of infection: cutaneous or external form, internal diphtheroid form, and septicemic form.[2] Finches usually develop the cutaneous form, whereas canaries develop the internal diphtheroid or septicemic form, which causes high mortality.[51,66] Severity and duration of disease is dependent on the strain of virus, species infected, and route of infection.[51]

The cutaneous (dry form) is localized to unfeathered regions such as limbs, periocular region, nares, bill, and under the wings. Lesions typically develop from raised smooth to nodular 2- to 4-mm papules and may progress to vesicles that ulcerate, dry out, and crust. Secondary bacterial or fungal infections of the ulcerated lesions can occur. Periocular lesions can progress and affect the palpebrae, causing a secondary conjunctivitis and keratitis. Severe ocular infections may impair vision. Mutilation of lesions and mechanical trauma can result in hemorrhage, and further compromise of tissue vascularization may cause loss of digits or nails.[51] The mortality rate is low for the cutaneous form of avipoxvirus infection. In this form lesions occur rapidly, but resolve slowly over 3 to 6 weeks.[66]

The diphtheroid form (wet form or mucosal pox) affects mainly the upper respiratory and gastrointestinal tracts.[51] This form is found in canaries, mynahs, and some psittacines, such as lovebirds and Amazons. Typical findings with mucosal pox include conjunctivitis, chemosis, blepharitis, and ocular discharge causing bleophoredema. Diphtheric lesions occur in the oropharynx and on the lingual surface. Lesions are fibrinous gray brown and caseous.[51,66] As the lesions progress they can cause obstruction of the airway and esophagus, resulting in respiratory distress and dysphagia. Some patients may survive with aggressive treatment, but may have persistent ocular lesions. Wet pox may accompany dry pox.[51]

The most severe form is septicemic or systemic poxvirus. This form has a high mortality rate of 90% to 100% and is the predominant form noted in canaries.[51] Acute-onset presents with severe respiratory distress and cyanosis. Other clinical signs include chemosis, depression, and anorexia. Death typically occurs quickly, and necropsy findings include air sacculitis and pneumonia. Cutaneous lesions may persist in patients that survive.[51]

Diagnosis

Biopsy and light microscopic examination of avipoxvirus lesions reveal characteristic large eosinophilic intracytoplasmic inclusions (Bollinger bodies).[51] Cytology and impression smears of lesions reveal Bollinger bodies within epithelial cells. A recent study in Hawaiian birds infected with avipoxvirus used RT-PCR for genetic characterization and confirmation of suspected pox infections.[59] Histopathology, RT-PCR, electron microscopy, virus isolation, cell culture, and serology are other methods used to determine avipoxvirus infection.[51,66] Gross necropsy reveals hepatic hemorrhage and splenomegaly.[66]

Treatment

There is no treatment for avipoxvirus infections; however, supportive care and prevention are important. Lesions should be treated locally with dilute iodine and topical silver sulfadiazine. Ulcerated lesions may require wound management and antibiotics for secondary bacterial infections. Supplementation with vitamins A and C may be indicated to support epithelial healing.[51] Surgical removal of pox lesions is not recommended.[66]

To prevent avipoxvirus infections, reported methods include administration of an attenuated live vaccine in the wing web every 6 months, before the mosquito season. Successful vaccination is indicated by a whitish swelling or crust at the injection site 8 to 10 days after vaccination. This vaccine can be used in birds as young as 4 weeks of age.[51] There has been more interest in avipoxvirus vaccination recently because of the success of the avipoxvirus vaccination in commercial flocks,[55] which may translate into the production of other successful vaccines for birds.

Summary

Avipoxvirus is an important disease of wildlife and affects many avian species. It is important to understand the disease process and methods of prevention in protecting captive wildlife. Avipoxvirus threatens Galapagos and Canary Island avian species, and has already caused extensive morbidity and mortality in native Hawaiian species.[59] As described in a collection of captive stone curlews,[57] the avipoxvirus can spread quickly through a flock and can cause varying levels of disease. It is important to understand avipoxvirus and the effect it can have on avifauna.

WELLFLEET BAY VIRUS

The common eider (*Somateria mollissima*) is a large sea duck that breeds from Maine north to Labrador and winters as far south as the mouth of the Chesapeake Bay.[67] Other subspecies of common eider live and breed in the Hudson Bay area of Canada, and along the United States and Canadian Pacific and Arctic coasts. The species is circumpolar, occurring in Europe and Asia as well as North America. Starting in 1998, 11 mortality events have occurred in wintering common eiders around Cape Cod, Massachusetts (USA),[68] resulting in the deaths of thousands of these birds. The cause of death identified on necropsy was anemia and emaciation.[68] In 2010 samples were collected and submitted to the United States Geological Survey (USGS) National Wildlife Health Center and to the University of Georgia's Southeastern Cooperative Wildlife Disease Study. A new orthomyxovirus, tentatively called Wellfleet Bay virus (WFBV), with the species name *Quarjarvirus*, has been associated with these deaths.[69]

Some of the dead and recovered common eider were originally banded in eastern Quebec, Nova Scotia, Newfoundland, and eastern Maine.[69] During any single mortality event, often the great majority of birds will be from only one sex, but the sex varies from one mortality incident to another.[69] This information would make one suspect that exposure to the virus is during periods when eider segregate by sex, such as nesting or molting.

The orthomyxoviruses are RNA-type viruses and are associated with the avian influenza group. The avian influenza viruses are normally involved with aerosol transmission, although other routes have been documented (mostly gastrointestinal routes involving feces).[70] The mode of transmission of WFBV is unknown, but may possibly involve arthropod vectors on the breeding grounds.

Deaths have occurred only in the Cape Cod area, but a study conducted by the USGS Patuxent Wildlife Research Center, US Fish and Wildlife Service, Rhode Island Department of Environmental Management, and University of Rhode Island and Wildlife Services (US Department of Agriculture) during November and December, 2011 detected titers to WFBV. Common eider wintering in Naragansett Bay and Block Island Sound, Rhode Island were tested, and of 66 common eider tested, 3 male eider were found with titers to the WFBV.[71] None of the eider with positive titers had clinical signs of the disease, and all 3 had results of complete blood count and serum chemistry within the normal ranges for the other common eider found in this area.

The orthomyxoviruses are RNA viruses and are divided into 5 genera. The influenza A group infects humans, other mammals, and birds. At present the WFBV has not been completely characterized, but is thought to be in the orthomyxovirus group.[72]

The etiology of WFBV is still unknown, but it is possible that the common eider are contracting disease somewhere other than wintering areas, thus explaining the positive eider found in Rhode Island. It is also possible that there are interactions between the common eider populations of Rhode Island and Cape Cod. However, further analysis of data is needed to identify the amount of interaction between eider wintering in the different areas and to assess the potential linkages to their breeding and molting areas. Thus far, the virus has only been confirmed in common eider, but further testing of other waterfowl associating with common eider needs to be conducted. The disease currently is not considered a threat to domestic poultry nor is it considered a zoonotic disease.

AVIAN INFLUENZA

The emergence and spread of the highly pathogenic H5N1 form of avian influenza across Asia, Europe, and parts of Africa in the past 17 years has increased interest in this group of viral diseases of birds and other species.

Influenza viruses are in the family Orthomyxoviridae. From a viral descriptive view they are considered enveloped, segmented, negative-stranded RNA viruses with 2 surface glycoproteins.[73] Influenza viruses are subdivided into 3 types (A, B, and C) based on M and nucleocapsid proteins.[74] Influenza A virus is the only form recovered from avian species, whereas types B and C are primarily human forms of the virus.[70]

Influenza A viruses are grouped into subtypes based on differences in hemagglutinin (H) and neuraminidase (N), which are the surface nucleocapsid proteins. Sixteen H proteins and 9 N proteins have been identified[74] for a total of 144 subtype combinations such as H1N1 or H5N1, H7N3, and so forth. During viral replication there can be changes or mutations in the proteins, especially the H proteins, leading to newly emerging forms of avian influenza.

Avian influenza viruses are further classified based on their pathogenicity to domestic chickens. There are 2 forms, high pathogenic avian influenza (HPAI) and low pathogenic avian influenza (LPAI). A form that is highly pathogenic in chickens may cause little or no illness in some other bird species, especially waterfowl. All the HPAI viruses identified to date have been H5 or H7, with H5N1, H5N2, H7N3, and H7N7 being some of the causes of recent epizootics of avian influenza in poultry.[73]

Avian influenza viruses are widespread in wild bird populations, and have been isolated from more than 100 species of birds and 13 genera. Waterfowl (order Anseriformes: ducks, geese, and swans) and shorebirds (Charadriidae and Scolopacidae) are considered common reservoir hosts of the low pathogenic forms of avian influenza.[75] Transmission generally occurs by a fecal-oral transmission route[76]; however, some strains of the highly pathogenic H5N1 have evolved to transmit via aerosol.[77]

Influenza has a 1- to 5-day incubation period in most avian species. In poultry the LPAI form produces no or mild clinical signs, such as mild respiratory signs of coughing, sneezing, or nasal discharge, decreased appetite, and decreased egg production. For LPAI, spread can be by direct contact with feces or respiratory secretions, or by contact with contaminated water, equipment, or clothing on farm personnel. HPAI can be manifested as lethargy, facial edema, discoloration of areas such as swollen eyelids, cob, and wattle, swollen hocks or legs, decreased egg production, diarrhea, incoordination, and death.[73]

The influenza viruses are always changing and use mutation, reassortment, insertion, deletion, and recombination to create new viral forms.[78] Reassortment has been detected in influenza viruses found in wild birds.[79] Insertion, deletion, and recombination have been found in influenza viruses in poultry and mammals, but not in wild birds. Insertion occurs in the H5 and H7 viruses and is associated with the creation of the high-pathogenicity forms that occur in poultry.[80]

Timing of peak viral load and the spread of the influenza viruses differs among avian species.[78] For ducks in North America, the peak period for isolation of influenza viruses occurs during the staging period just before fall migration, a time when there are many naïve juveniles in the population. For shorebirds, the peak influenza period is during the spring migration.[78] Migrating shorebirds feed in large mixed flocks on the eggs of abundant horseshoe crabs (*Limulus polyphemus*) on the shores of Delaware Bay (USA). Ruddy turnstones (*Arenaria interpres*) may be a key agent in spreading influenza viruses.[78] It is also considered possible that the influenza viruses overwinter in the frozen earth of the high Arctic in both North America and Eurasia.[81,82] Until the 2005 outbreak of the H5N1 influenza virus in bar-headed geese (*Anser indicus*) and other species,[83] wild waterfowl were considered to be natural reservoir hosts, although the influenza viruses caused no disease signs in these wild birds.

There are geographic variations in the incidence of the influenza viruses. All influenza A subtypes, H1 to H16, have been isolated from Eurasian waterfowl, but H14, H15, and H16 have not been isolated from birds in the Americas.[78] This finding would indicate some separation of the viruses into 2 different clades by geography. After the pathogenic outbreak of H5N1 avian influenza virus in bar-headed geese in the Qinghai Lake region of China,[83] wild-bird sampling for avian influenza viruses became an increasingly important subject of research and monitoring. Many of these surveillance programs involved one or more combinations of (1) recovery and testing of dead birds, (2) target sampling of live birds, or (3) opportunistic sampling of live birds.[84] There have been extensive surveys for avian influenza in Eurasia and more recently in the Americas, including the United States,[85,86] Argentina,[87,88] Barbados,[89] Bolivia,[90] Brazil,[91] Chile,[92] and Peru.[93] To date, no cases of wild birds carrying or transmitting HPAI H5N1 avian influenza have been documented in the Americas, unlike Eurasia and Africa, where multiple separate or connected epizootics of H5N1 avian influenza have occurred in the last 6 years.

These findings lend strength to the theory that there are two clades or superfamilies of avian influenza viruses, one in the Americas and one in Eurasia.[78] Migratory pathways of wild waterfowl are generally north-south or latitudinal, with overlapping breeding areas between some Old-World and New-World species occurring in northeastern Siberia/Alaska, and to a lesser extent Greenland, Baffin Island, and Labrador (Greenland-Labrador Straits). A greater appreciation of migratory flyways has been developed in the past decade with the advent of satellite radio transmitters capable of being carried by migrating waterfowl. No overlapping migratory waterfowl pathways are found in the southern hemisphere.

Summary

Continued monitoring for HPAI H5N1 and other forms of avian influenza should continue in both the active and passive (opportunistic) monitoring modes. Regular and repeated active monitoring is important where New-World and Old-World migratory pathways overlap. Passive monitoring programs such as sampling birds in rehabilitation situations, bird banding sites, and bird mortality events constitute a useful tool, are far less expensive to implement than an active monitoring program, and should continue.

INCLUSION BODY DISEASE OF CRANES
Introduction

Inclusion body disease of cranes (IBDC) is a viral herpes infection that caused the death of 17 of 51 cranes of 4 species at the International Crane Foundation, Baraboo, Wisconsin in 1978.[94] Species that died included sandhill cranes (*Grus canadensis*), blue cranes (*Anthropoides paradisea*), red-crowned cranes (*Grus japonensis*), and hooded cranes (*Grus monacha*). The onset was sudden and all cranes died over a 15-day period. This outbreak of this disease has been the only one known in North America. However, there have been epizootics of similar herpesvirus infections in several locations in Europe. In 1973, 12 gray-crowned cranes (*Balearica regulorum*) and 7 demoiselle cranes (*Anthropoides virgo*) died at a zoo in Austria, also during a 15-day period.[95] Another similar outbreak of a herpesvirus infection in cranes occurred at a zoo in France in 1982.[96]

Clinical Correlation

Clinical signs include depression, anorexia, diarrhea, inability or reluctance to stand,[70] lethargy, weakness, and dyspnea.[97] Often infected cranes died within 2 days of the onset of clinical signs, with mortality ranging from 35% to 100%. One experimental study indicated unequal susceptibility among crane species.[98] Eurasian cranes (*Grus grus*), red-crowned cranes, and sandhill cranes exposed by conjunctival, intra-tracheal, intracloacal, intranasal, oral, or intramuscular routes died within 6 to 12 days. A white-naped crane (*Grus vipio*) experimentally infected in a similar fashion showed no clinical signs and developed a 1:16 titer 14 days after exposure[98] after 5 doses of the virus, ranging from 500 to 50,000,000 plaque-forming units and given by intra-nasal, intratracheal, intracloacal, and conjunctival routes.[98] Indeed, the researchers suspect that the later inoculations may have functioned more to vaccinate the crane than to challenge it.

Dead cranes had enlarged and turgid livers and spleens. There were off-white colored, 1- to 2-mm diameter foci throughout the surface and parenchyma of these 2 organs. On histopathology, focal areas of coagulative necrosis were found in the liver, spleen, bursa, and thymus.[98]

Other lesions reported included the formation of diphtheritic membranes of the oral, esophageal, and intestinal mucosa.[94] A tan to white discoloration of the liver was also reported.[99] Intranuclear inclusion bodies were found in the liver and also in other tissues including intestines, spleen, thymus, and bursa.[94,99,100]

Prevention

The International Crane Foundation monitored individual crane neutralizing antibody titers to IBDC for up to 27 months for the gray-crowned crane (n = 1), demoiselle crane (n = 1), sandhill crane (n = 1), Sarus crane (n = 2) (*Grus antigone*), Eurasian crane (n = 9), hooded crane (n = 8), and red-crowned crane (n = 2). Titers varied from 1:8 to 1:128. By the 27th month, 8 of the cranes tested still had persistent titers, but 7 were negative.[98] The fact that the titers of some individual cranes remained elevated for months while other titers waned is a typical herpesvirus response.[101] The trigeminal ganglion is thought to be a possible site of latent infection. When inoc-ulated with IBDC virus experimentally by the intranasal route, increasing amounts of shed virus are found in the cloaca, especially near death.[70] Thus, fecal passage of the virus is the probable source of infection for cranes. The shedding pattern in experimental infections was intermittent.[98] No vertical transmission via eggs from infected cranes was found.

Treatment

No treatment is effective for IBDC. Because of the high mortality associated with IBDC and the potential to spread the disease in either captive or wild flocks, and the poten-tial for carrier states to develop, euthanasia of infected cranes or complete isolation from other cranes in recommended. The fact that IBDC virus may persist in a dormant state makes detection by virus isolation difficult. Only one laboratory (USGS National Wildlife Heath Center, Madison, WI) offers IBDC antibody testing (virus neutralization test) for samples submitted in the United States.

Summary

IBDC is not found in wild North American cranes at present. In the wild, the disease has been found only in common cranes from southwestern Russia.[102] The great danger is that this is an important disease with high mortality among several crane species. It may yet again occur in a zoo or in a wild flock of cranes.

OVERALL SUMMARY

It is important when working with avian wildlife to recall that many of the diseases are zoonotic and can have an impact on humans, such as avian influenza. Some diseases in avian wildlife, such as WNV, are important in disease surveillance. Reporting WNV-positive cases to the state aids in mapping the progression of the virus, which is important for the human population and captive wildlife at risk. Other diseases that are a concern for avian wildlife are less studied and emerging, such as Wellfleet Bay virus, or established but not well known in North America, such as IBDC. Another established important disease of wildlife, aspergillosis, is important because of its impact on raptors and other captive wildlife. The current treatment for aspergillosis is considered emerging, owing to the advent of new and more effective treatments such as VRC. Avipoxvirus genomics have shed light on the progression of the avipoxvirus and its relation to infection across avian species. Moreover, the study of avipoxvirus vaccination may lead to the development of an effective WNV avian labeled vaccine. Of course, this list is not exhaustive; indeed, there are many important avian wildlife diseases. This article is intended as an introduction to and refresher course in some of the diseases that are important in wild avian species.

REFERENCES

1. Cacciuttolo E, Rossi G, Nardoni S. Anatomopathological aspects of avian aspergillosis. Vet Res Commun 2009;33:521–7.
2. Wobeser G. Diseases of wild waterfowl. 2nd edition. New York (NY): Plenum Press; 1997. p. 327.
3. Orosz SE. Overview of aspergillosis: pathogenesis and treatment options. Semin Avian Exot Pet 2000;9(2):59–65.
4. Joseph V. Aspergillosis in raptors. Semin Avian Exot Pet 2000;9(2):1–9.
5. Beernaert L, Pamans F, Waeyenberghe L, et al. *Aspergillus* infections in birds: a review. Avian Pathol 2010;39(5):325–31.
6. Thomas NJ, Hunter DB, Atkinson CT. Infectious diseases of wild birds. Ames, Iowa: Blackwell Publishing; 2007:1–490.
7. King AS, McLelland J. Birds: their structure and function. 2nd edition. London (UK): Bailliere Tindall; 1984. p. 334.
8. Latgé J. *Aspergillus fumigatus* and aspergillosis. Clin Microbiol Rev 1999;12(2): 1–42.
9. Hirsh DC, MacLachlan NJ, Walker RL. Veterinary microbiology. Ames, Iowa: Wiley-Blackwell; 2004. p. 535.
10. Quinn PJ, Markey BK. Concise review of veterinary microbiology. Ames, Iowa: Wiley-Blackwell; 2003. p. 152.
11. Tarello W. Etiologic agents and diseases found associated with clinical aspergillosis in falcons. Int J Microbiol 2011;2011:1–6.
12. Scott DE. Successful treatment of aspergillosis with voriconazole in a red-tailed hawk (*Buteo jamaicensis*). Association of Avian Veterinarians 32nd Annual Conference. Seattle (WA), 2011. p. 53–7.

13. Di Somma A, Bailey T, Silvanose C, et al. The use of voriconazole for the treatment of aspergillosis in falcons (*Falco* species). J Avian Med Surg 2007;21(4):307–16.

14. Orosz SE, Frazier D. Antifungal agents: a review of their pharmacology and therapeutic indications. J Avian Med Surg 1995;9(1):1–12.

15. Orosz SE, Lichtenberger M. Avian respiratory distress: etiology, diagnosis, and treatment. Veterinary Clin North Am Exot Anim Pract 2011;14(2):241–55.

16. Hector R. An overview of antifungal drugs and their use for treatment of deep and superficial mycoses in animals. Clin Tech Small Anim Pract 2005;20(4):240–9.

17. Flammer K, Osborne JA, Webb DJ, et al. Pharmacokinetics of voriconazole after oral administration of single and multiple doses in African grey parrots (*Psittacus erithacus timneh*). Am J Vet Res 2008;69:1–8.

18. Burhenne J, Haefeli W, Hess M, et al. Pharmacokinetics, tissue concentrations, and safety of the antifungal agent voriconazole in chickens. J Avian Med Surg 2008;22(3):199–207.

19. Natesan S, Wu W, Cutright J, et al. In vitro–in vivo correlation of voriconazole resistance due to G448S mutation (cyp51A gene) in *Aspergillus fumigatus*. Diagn Microbiol Infect Dis 2012;74(3):272–7.

20. Nagappan V, Deresinski S, Nagappan V, et al. Posaconazole: a broad-spectrum triazole antifungal agent. Clin Infect Dis 2007;45(12):1610–7.

21. Emery LC, Cox SK, Souza MJ. Pharmacokinetics of nebulized terbinafine in Hispaniolan Amazon parrots (*Amazona ventralis*). J Avian Med Surg 2012; 26(3):161–6.

22. Tell L, Clemons K, Kline Y, et al. Efficacy of voriconazole in Japanese quail (*Coturnix japonica*) experimentally infected with *Aspergillus fumigatus*. Med Mycol 2010;48:1–11.

23. Guzman D, Flammer K, Papich M. Pharmacokinetics of voriconazole after oral administration of single and multiple doses in Hispaniolan Amazon parrots (*Amazona ventralis*). Am J Vet Res 2010;71(4):460–7.

24. Kline Y, Clemons K, Woods L, et al. Pharmacokinetics of voriconazole in adult mallard ducks (*Anas platyrhynchos*). Med Mycol 2011;49:1–13.

25. Beernaert L, Pasmans F, Waeyenberghe L, et al. Avian *Aspergillus fumigatus* strains resistant to both itraconazole and voriconazole. Antimicrobial Agents Chemother 2009;53(5):2199–201.

26. Miller RE, Fowler ME. Fowler's zoo and wild animal medicine current therapy, vol. 7. St Louis (MO): Elsevier Saunders; 2011.

27. van der Meulen KM, Pensaert MB, Nauwynck HJ. West Nile virus in the vertebrate world. Arch Virol 2005;150:637–57.

28. Olsen GH, Miller KJ, Docherty DE, et al. Pathogenicity of West Nile virus and response to vaccination in sandhill cranes (*Grus canadensis*) using a killed vaccine. J Zoo Wildl Med 2009;40(2):263–71.

29. CDC. West Nile virus: information and guidance for clinicians. CDC; 2012. p. 1–48. Available at: www.cdc.gov.

30. Ogunfiditimi F. Infectious diseases: West Nile virus on the rise. JAAPA 2013;1–4.

31. Murray K, Walker C, Goulde E. The virology, epidemiology, and clinical impact of West Nile virus: a decade of advancements in research since its introduction into the Western Hemisphere. Epidemiol Infect 2011;139(6):807–17.

32. Palmieri C, Franca M, Uzal F, et al. Pathology and immunohistochemical findings of West Nile virus infection in psittaciformes. Vet Pathol 2011;48(5):975–84.

33. Nevarez J, Mitchell M, Morgan T, et al. Association of West Nile virus with lymphohistiocytic proliferative cutaneous lesions in American alligators (*Alligator mississippiensis*) detected by RT-PCR. J Zoo Wildl Med 2008;39(4):562–6.

34. Carboni D, Nevarez J, Tully T, et al. West Nile virus infection in a sun conure (*Aratinga solstitialis*). J Avian Med Surg 2008;22(3):240–5.

35. Hinten S, Komar N, Langevin S, et al. Experimental infection of North American birds with the New York 1999 strain of West Nile virus. Emerg Infect Dis 2003; 9(3):311–22.

36. Dauphin G, Zientara S. West Nile virus: recent trends in diagnosis and vaccine development. Vaccine 2007;25(30):5563–76.

37. Busquets N, Bertran K, Costa T, et al. Experimental West Nile virus infection in gyr-saker hybrid falcons. Vector Borne Zoonotic Dis 2012;12(6):482–9.

38. Kramer E, Stone W, Okoniewski J, et al. VecTest as diagnostic and surveillance tool for West Nile virus in dead birds. Emerg Infect Dis 2004;10(12):2175–81.

39. Nayar G, Lindsay R, Barker I, et al. Rapid antigen-capture assay to detect West Nile virus in dead corvids. Emerg Infect Dis 2003;9(11):1406–10.

40. Gancz AY, Smith DA, Barker IK, et al. Pathology and tissue distribution of West Nile virus in North American owls (family: Strigidae). Avian Pathol 2012;35(1):17–29.

41. Godhardt JA, Beheler K, O'Connor MJ, et al. Evaluation of antigen-capture ELISA and immunohistochemical methods for avian surveillance of West Nile virus. J Vet Diagn Invest 2006;18:85–9.

42. Nemeth NM, Young GR, Burkhalter KL, et al. West Nile virus detection in nonvascular feathers from avian carcasses. J Vet Diagn Invest 2009;21(5):616–22.

43. Pauli A, Cruz-Martinez L, Ponder J. Ophthalmologic and oculopathologic findings in red-tailed hawks and Cooper's hawks with naturally acquired West Nile virus infection. J Am Vet Med Assoc 2007;231(8):1241–8.

44. Phalen DN, Dahlhausen B. West Nile virus. Semin Avian Exot Pet 2004;13(2): 67–78.

45. Nemeth NM, Kratz GF, Bates R, et al. Clinical evaluation and outcomes of naturally acquired WNV in raptors. J Zoo Wildl Med 2009;10(1):1–13.

46. Wunschmann A, Shivers J, Bender J, et al. Pathologic findings in red-tailed hawks (*Accipiter cooperi*) naturally infected with West Nile virus. Avian Dis 2004;48(3):570–80.

47. Willis AM, Wilkie DA. Avian ophthalmology, part 2: review of ophthalmic diseases. J Avian Med Surg 1999;13(4):245–51.

48. Fitzgerald SD, Patterson JS, Kiupel M, et al. Clinical and pathologic features of West Nile virus infection in native North American owls (family Strigidae). Avian Dis 2003;47(3):602–10.

49. Okeson D, Llizo S, Miller C, et al. Antibody response of five bird species after vaccination with a killed West Nile virus vaccine. J Zoo Wildl Med 2007;38(2): 240–4.

50. Silva M, Ellis A, Karaca K, et al. Domestic goose as a model for West Nile virus vaccine efficacy. Vaccine 2013;31(7):1045–50.

51. Harrison GJ, Lightfoot TL. Clinical Avian Medicine. Palm Beach (FL): Spix Publishing, Inc; 2006;2:1008.

52. Wobeser G, Docherty. A solitary case of duck plague in a wild mallard. J Wildl Dis 1987;23:479–82.

53. Joshi S, Mudasir M, Sharma D, et al. Histopathological study of cutaneous form of avipoxvirus infection in Jungle crow (*Corvus macrorhynchos*). Vet World 2012;5(10):1–3.

54. Ha H, Howe L, Alley M, et al. The phylogenetic analysis of avipoxvirus in New Zealand. Vet Microbiol 2011;150(1–2):80–7.

55. Carulei O, Douglass N, Williamson AL. Phylogenetic analysis of three genes of penguinpox virus corresponding to *Vaccinia* virus G8R(VLTF-1), A3L (P4b) and

H3L reveals that it is most closely related to turkeypox virus, ostrichpox virus and pigeonpox virus. Virol J 2009;6:52.

56. Tarello W, Perugia IS. Prevalence and clinical signs of avipoxvirus infection in falcons from the Middle East. Vet Dermatol 2008;19(2):101–4.

57. Lierz M, Bergmann V, Isa G, et al. Avipoxvirus infection in a collection of captive stone curlews (*Burhinus oedicnemus*). J Avian Med Surg 2007;21(1):50–5.

58. Parker P, Buckles E, Farrington H, et al. 110 years of avipoxvirus in the Galapagos Islands. PLoS One 2011;6(1):e15989.

59. Farias M, LaPointe D, Atkinson C, et al. Taqman real-time PCR detects avipoxvirus DNA in blood of Hawaii amakihi (*Hemignathus virens*). PLoS One 2010; 5(5):e10745.

60. Pawar R, Bhushan S, Poornachandar A, et al. Avian pox infection in different wild birds in India. Eur J Wildl Res 2011;57(4):785–93.

61. Forbes NA, Simpson GN. A review of viruses affecting raptors. Vet Rec 1997; 141(5):123–6.

62. Schoemaker N, Dorrestein G, Lumeij J. An avipoxvirus infection in a goshawk (*Accipiter gentilis*). Avian Pathol 1998;27(1):103–6.

63. Wikelski M, Foufopoulos J, Vargas H, et al. Galápagos birds and diseases: invasive pathogens as threats for island species. Ecol Soc 2004;9(1):1–10.

64. Rampin T, Pisoni G, Manarolla G, et al. Epornitic of avian pox in common buzzards (*Buteo buteo*): virus isolation and molecular biological characterization. Avian Pathol 2007;36(2):161–5.

65. Mikaelian I, Martineau D. Cutaneous avian pox in a house sparrow. Can Vet J 1996;37(7):434.

66. Adams CJ, Feldman SH, Sleeman JM. Phylogenetic analysis of avian poxviruses among free-ranging birds of Virginia. Avian Dis 2005;49(4):601–5.

67. Griggs JL. All the birds of North America. American Bird Conservancy, Harper Perennial. New York (NY); 1997. p. 180.

68. Ellis J, Courchesne S, Shearn-Bachsler V, et al. Cyclic mass mortality of common eiders at Cape Cod, MA: an ongoing puzzle. Pacific Seabird Group Annual Meeting. 2010. p. 17–8. 37.

69. Mickley R. Investigating the newly described Wellfleet Bay virus. The Carrier; 2012. p. 4.

70. Richie BW. Avian viruses, function and control. Lake Worth (Fl): Wingers Publishing, Inc; 1995. p. 525.

71. Olsen GH, Gibbs S, Beuth J, et al. Searching for Wellfleet Bay virus in common eiders in Rhode Island. Association of Avian Veterinarians 33rd Annual Conference, Louisville (KY), 2012. p. 355.

72. Allison A. Wellfleet Bay virus. in press.

73. Blackmore C, Rabinowitz PM. Influenza. In: Rabinowitz PM, Conte LA, editors. Human-animal medicine: clinical approaches to zoonosis, toxicants and other shared health risks. Maryland Heights (MO): Saunders; 2012. p. 177–86.

74. Knipe DM, Howley DM, editors. Fields virology. 5th edition. Philadelphia: Lippincott Williams & Wilkins; 2007.

75. Swayne DE, Suarey DL. Highly pathogenic avian influenza. Rev Sci Tech 2000; 19:463–82.

76. Brown JD, Berghaus RD, Costa TP, et al. Intestinal secretion of a wild bird-origin H3N8 low pathogenic avian influenza virus in mallards (*Anas platyrhynchos*). J Wildl Dis 2012;48(4):991–8.

77. Lebarbenchon C, Feare CJ, Renaud F, et al. Persistence of highly pathogenic avian influenza viruses in natural ecosystems. Emerg Infect Dis 2010;16(7):1057–62.

78. Webster RG, Krauss S, Hulse-Post D, et al. Evolution of influenza A viruses in wild birds. J Wildl Dis 2007;43(Suppl 3):S1–6.
79. Obenauer JC, Denson J, Mehta PK, et al. Large-scale sequence analysis of avian influenza isolates. Science 2006;311:1575–80.
80. Rott R. Genetic determinants for infectivity and pathogenicity of influenza viruses. Philos Trans R Soc Lond B Biol Sci 1980;288:393–9.
81. Ito T, Okazaki K, Kawaoka Y, et al. Perpetuation of influenza A viruses in Alaskan waterfowl reservoirs. Arch Virol 1995;140:1163–72.
82. Okazaki K, Takada A, Ito T, et al. Precursor genes of future pandemic influenza viruses are perpetuated in ducks nesting in Siberia. Arch Virol 2000;145:885–93.
83. Li Y, Shi J, Qi Q, et al. H5N1 avian influenza outbreak in wild birds in Western China in 2005. J Wildl Dis 2007;43(Suppl 3):S21.
84. Guberti V, Newman SH. Guidelines on wild bird surveillance for highly pathogenic avian influenza H5N1 virus. J Wildl Dis 2007;43(Suppl 3):S29–34.
85. DeLiberto TJ, Swafford SR, Nolte DL, et al. Surveillance for highly pathogenic avian influenza in wild birds in the USA. Integr Zool 2009;4:426–39.
86. Dusek RJ, Bortner JB, DeLiberto TJ, et al. Surveillance for high-pathogenicity avian influenza virus in wild birds in the Pacific Flyway of the United States, 2006-2007. Avian Dis 2009;53:222–30.
87. Pereda AJ, Uhart M, Perez AA, et al. Avian influenza virus isolated in wild waterfowl in Argentina: evidence of a potentially unique phylogenetic lineage in South America. Virology 2008;378:363–70.
88. Alvarez P, Mattiello R, Rivailler P, et al. First isolation of an H1N1 avian influenza virus from wild terrestrial non-migratory birds in Argentina. Virology 2010;396:76–84.
89. Douglas KO, Lavoie MC, Kim LM, et al. Isolation and genetic characterization of avian influenza viruses and a Newcastle Disease virus from wild birds in Barbados: 2003-2004. Avian Dis 2007;51:781–7.
90. Spackman E, McCracken KG, Winker K, et al. An avian influenza virus from waterfowl in South America contains genes from North American avian and equine lineages. Avian Dis 2007;51:273–4.
91. Senne DA. Avian influenza in North and South America, 2002-2005. Avian Dis 2007;51:167–73.
92. Suarez DL, Senne DA, Banks J, et al. Recombination resulting in virulence shift in avian influenza outbreak in Chile. Emerg Infect Dis 2004;10:693–9.
93. Williams R, Segovia-Hinostroza K, Ghersi BM, et al. Avian influenza infections in nonmigrant land birds in Andean Peru. J Wildl Dis 2012;48(4):910–7.
94. Docherty DE, Henning DJ. The isolation of a herpes virus from captive cranes with inclusion body disease. Avian Dis 1980;24:278–83.
95. Burtscher H, Grunberg W. Epizootic virus hepatitis in cranes (Balearica pavonia and Anthropoidea virgo). In: Proceeding Int. Symp. Ertankungen Zootiere. 1975. p. 277–9.
96. Foerster S, Chastek C, Kaleta EF. Crane hepatitis herpesviruses. J Vet Med 1989;36:433–41.
97. Carpenter JW. Infectious and parasitic diseases of cranes. In: Fowler ME, editor. Zoo and wild animal medicine, current therapy 3. Philadelphia: W.B. Saunders Company; 1993. p. 617, 229–37.
98. Schuh JC, Yuill TM. Persistence of inclusion body disease of cranes virus. J Wildl Dis 1985;21(2):111–9.
99. Schuh JC, Sileo L, Siegfried LM, et al. Inclusion body disease of cranes: comparison of pathologic finings in cranes with acquired versus experimentally induced disease. J Am Vet Med Assoc 1986;189:993–6.

100. Schuh JC, Yuill TM. Inclusion body disease of crane virus: a herpes virus of captive cranes. In: Proceedings American Association Zoo Veterinarians. New Orleans (LA): 1982. p. 19–20.
101. Openshaw HT, Sekizawa T, Mohlenberg C, et al. The role of immunity in latency and reactivation of herpes simplex virus. In: Nahmias AJ, Dowdle WR, Schianazi RF, editors. Human Herpesviruses. New York: Elsevier North Holland Inc; 1981. p. 292–3.
102. Olsen GH, Carpenter JW, Langenberg JA. Medicine and surgery. Chapter 8. In: Ellis DH, Gee GF, Mirande CM, editors. Cranes: their biology, husbandry, and conservation. Washington, DC: National Biological Service; 1996. p. 308, 137–74.

Update on Diseases of Chinchillas

Christoph Mans, med vet[a],*,

Thomas M. Donnelly, BVSc, Dipl ACLAM, Dipl ABVP (Exotic Companion Mammal)[b]

KEYWORDS

- *Chinchilla lanigera* • Pyometra • Periodontal disease • Caries
- *Pseudomonas aeruginosa* • Giardia • Urolithiasis • Cardiac disease

KEY POINTS

- In chinchillas, a membrane covers the vulva except during estrus and birth. The membrane is also absent in many cases of uterine disease.
- Urolithiasis is predominately a problem in male chinchillas. The underlying etiology remains unknown. High-calcium diets are unlikely to be the cause, as chinchillas excrete excess calcium in the feces and not in the urine.
- Bacterial middle ear infections in chinchillas are reported with increasing frequency. A minimally invasive transbullar middle ear sampling technique enables diagnostic sample collection.
- Periodontal disease and caries are common problems in chinchillas. The diagnosis is greatly facilitated by the use of oral endoscopy. Untreated periodontal disease and caries will lead to progressive tooth resorption.
- *Pseudomonas* infection attributable to exposure or ingestion of high infective doses, often in water bottles, or because of an impaired immune system is common. Conjunctivitis is a common initial sign of pseudomoniasis in chinchillas.
- Giardia are found in both healthy and sick chinchillas. Infection is self-limiting in healthy chinchillas. Treatment lessens the duration of clinical signs and prevents zoonotic transmission.

FEMALE REPRODUCTIVE TRACT DISORDERS

Chinchillas possess a uterus duplex, with 2 cervixes entering the vagina. The urethra ends outside the vagina on the cranially located urethral papilla (**Fig. 1**), therefore hemorrhagic discharge originating from the vulva, is never associated with a urinary tract disorder in chinchillas. A membrane covers the vulva in chinchillas, except during estrus and birth, when the vulva is visible as a horizontal slit between the urethral papilla and the anus (see **Fig. 1**). The membrane is also absent in many cases of

[a] Department of Medical Sciences, Special Species Health Service, School of Veterinary Medicine, University of Wisconsin, 2015 Linden Drive, Madison, WI 53706, USA; [b] The Kenneth S. Warren Institute, 712 Kitchawan Road, Ossining, NY 10562, USA
* Corresponding author.
E-mail address: cmans@vetmed.wisc.edu

Vet Clin Exot Anim 16 (2013) 383–406
http://dx.doi.org/10.1016/j.cvex.2013.01.007
1094-9194/13/$ – see front matter © 2013 Elsevier Inc. All rights reserved.

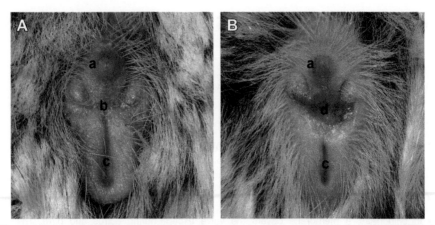

Fig. 1. (*A*) Normal female external genitalia in a chinchilla. The external urethral orifice is located on the urethral papilla (a). The vaginal orifice is sealed by a membrane (b) and located between the urethral papilla and the anus (c). (*B*) Normal female external genitalia in a chinchilla in estrus. Note the absence of the vaginal membrane and instead the open vaginal orifice (d). The vaginal closure membrane is also absent after birth and in most cases of underlying uterine disease.

uterine disease. During estrus, a mucoid vaginal discharge and a change in perianal color may be observed.

Chinchillas are seasonally polyestric and breeding season in the northern hemisphere is from approximately November to May.[1] Chinchillas are spontaneous ovulators with the estrus lasting 3 to 4 days and the entire estrus cycle about 28 to 35 days; the gestation period is 111 days on average and the typical litter size is 2.[2,3] The first estrus usually occurs by 3 to 4 months of age.[4]

Endometritis and Pyometra

Endometritis and pyometra and less commonly hydrometra or mucometra have been reported in farmed chinchillas and are increasingly reported in pet chinchillas.[3,5–8] Pyometra (purulent endometritis) is characterized by accumulation of purulent discharge within the uterine lumen, cystic endometrial hyperplasia, and secondary bacterial infections.[9,10] Prolonged high progesterone levels following initial estrogenic stimulation of the endometrium, result in endometrial hyperplasia, increased endometrial gland secretion, and cystic endometrial changes.[9] It is assumed that local immunity of the endometrium is reduced, due to progesterone, increasing the risk of secondary bacterial infections, caused often by physiologic vaginal flora.[9] The causes for endometritis and pyometras are frequently not revealed during diagnostic workups, but cases of stump pyometras secondary to incomplete ovariectomy have been reported in chinchillas.[6] Therefore, careful and complete resection of all ovarian tissue should be performed during ovariectomy or ovariohysterectomy.

Female chinchillas suffering from uterine disease may present with nonspecific mild signs, such as weight loss, lethargy, and reduced appetite, or can present severely depressed, dehydrated, and in poor body condition, because of severe or prolonged underlying uterine disease. The most consistent and common clinical finding is the absence of the vaginal membrane (see **Fig. 1**) and vaginal discharge, which can result in soiled perianal fur. Vaginal discharge can be mucoid, mucopurulent, purulent, or hemorrhagic, and may or may not be malodorous. Some mucoid discharge is normal during estrus in chinchillas, and should not be confused with pathologic vaginal discharge. Cytologic characterization of vaginal smears can be helpful for differentiation between physiologic and pathologic conditions causing vaginal discharge.[1] The predominant cells during estrus are partially to completely cornified superficial epithelial cells. Neutrophils are absent during estrus, but common during proestrus and metestrus.[1] Some chinchillas with uterine disease may not have an open vulva or vaginal discharge. Instead, these animals may present with severe uterine enlargement leading to abdominal distension. Abdominal palpation may induce vaginal discharge or detect uterine enlargement. Radiographs and, in particular, transabdominal ultrasonography are helpful for evaluation of the uterus. Vaginal cytology should be performed to differentiate pathologic vaginal discharge from physiologic vaginal discharge during estrus.[1] Ovariohysterectomy is the treatment of choice for endometritis and pyometra in chinchillas.[5] In cases of mild endometritis with vaginal discharge (open cervix), in which the animal is in good general condition, systemic antimicrobial therapy based on culture and susceptibility can be attempted.[11] As in other species, prognosis will depend on underlying and coexisting causes, such as hepatic lipidosis, ketosis, and possible complications in severe cases, such as sepsis.

Fetal Resorption, Mummification, Retention, and Abortion

Fetal death can be caused by any systemic disease process or trauma. In farmed chinchillas, primary infectious causes, such as *Listeria*, *Salmonella*, or *Pseudomonas* infections, have been associated with increases in abortion and high mortality.[4,12,13] In pet chinchillas, primary noninfectious causes are more likely to cause fetal death. Incompletely reabsorbed, retained, or mummified fetuses and retained placentas can remain in the uterus for extended periods and lead to sterility and endometritis (**Figs. 2** and **3**). In chinchillas presenting with hemorrhagic vaginal discharge, abortion or fetal or placental retention should be considered, especially if housed with a male conspecific (see **Figs. 2** and **3**). Diagnosis is made based on the history, ultrasonography and exploratory surgery. Ovariohysterectomy is the treatment of choice, unless the ability to breed needs to be maintained.

Neoplasia of the Female Reproductive Tract

Neoplasia of the female reproductive tract is rare. A review of 300 chinchilla biopsy and necropsy submissions revealed only 1 case of uterine neoplasia in a 13-year-old nulliparous chinchilla that was diagnosed as uterine leiomyosarcoma (Reavill DR, personal communication, 2012). In addition, a 5-year retrospective review (1991–1996) of

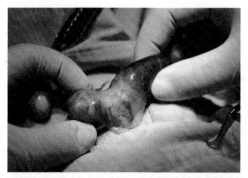

Fig. 2. Ventral midline laparotomy in a 7-year-old female chinchilla, which presented with acute onset of hemorrhagic vaginal discharge. Note the severely enlarged uteri. Placental retention, incomplete fetal resorption, and endometritis were the final histopathological diagnosis.

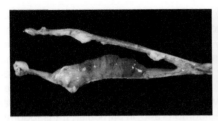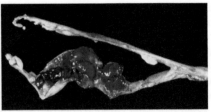

Fig. 3. Postmortem images of a uterus containing retained macerated fetal tissue. (*Courtesy of* Arno Wuenschmann, Dr med vet, Dipl. ACVP, St Paul, MN.)

chinchillas presented to the Animal Medical Center in New York revealed 1 case of uterine leiomyosarcoma.[14] In these 2 cases of leiomyosarcoma, there were no associated metastases. One case of uterine leiomyoma in a 2-year-old chinchilla has been reported in a retrospective study (1990–1999) of necropsy submissions to the University of Veterinary Medicine, Vienna, Austria. One additional case of uterine leiomyoma in a 15-year-old chinchilla was submitted to the College of Veterinary Medicine, University of Minnesota (Wuenschmann A, personal communication, 2012).

No reports of ovarian neoplasia in chinchillas exist. Neoplasia of the mammary glands has been reported, with 3 cases of 300 biopsy and necropsy submissions. Fibroadenoma, adenoma, and adenocarcinoma were the histopathological diagnosis in these 3 cases (Reavill DR, personal communication, 2012).

PENILE DISORDERS

The penis in chinchillas is sigmoid-shaped and in the flaccid state is directed posteriorly, ending caudal to the anus; it assumes a cranially oriented position during erection. A 1-cm-long os penis (baculum) is present in the distal penis.[15] As in other hystricomorph rodents (eg, guinea pigs, degus, porcupines) male chinchillas possess a structure termed variously as the "intromittent sac," "sacculus urethralis," or "penile pouch."[16] This structure is located just ventral to the urethra, and its orifice should not be confused with the external urethral opening during catheterization. The intromittent sac is lined with spurs and, like the membranous glans penis, becomes everted during tumescence, so that during erection the proximal portion of the penis is extruded outside the body, significantly adding to the length of the external penis.[17]

"Fur Rings"

Accumulation of fur at the base of the membranous glans penis, while still enclosed within the prepuce, is a common incidental finding during physical examination in chinchillas. In some cases the accumulated fur can predispose to balanoposthitis and paraphimosis, secondary to being a nidus for bacterial infections and/or leading to constriction of the glans penis, by forming a so-called "fur ring" (**Fig. 4**A). Accumulated fur that cannot be removed digitally may need to be carefully cut with small scissors with the chinchilla under sedation.

Balanoposthitis and Preputial Abscesses

Balanoposthitis is an inflammatory condition of the prepuce and glans penis usually secondary to infection. In all cases of balanoposthitis, excessive accumulation of smegma (see **Fig. 4**B) or fur should be removed, as it usually serves as a nidus for infection. If no underlying fur ring or smegma accumulation is found, then the balanoposthitis should be considered as part of a systemic or localized *Pseudomonas aeruginosa* infection (see **Fig. 4**C).[4,18] In cases of chronic balanoposthitis, preputial

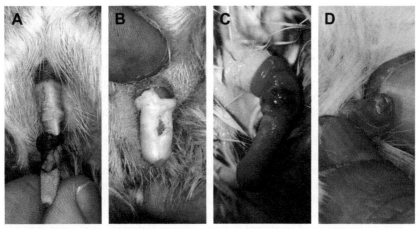

Fig. 4. Penile disorders of chinchillas. (*A*) "Fur ring." (*B*) Excessive smegma accumulation. (*C*) Paraphimosis secondary to acute balenoposthitis. Heavy and pure growth of *Pseudomonas aeruginosa* was cultured. (*D*) Phimosis secondary to formation of adhesions between the visceral layer of the prepuce and the glans penis, which prevented the extrusion of the glans penis from the prepuce. (*From* Mayer J, Donnelly TM. Clinical Veterinary Advisor: Birds and Exotic Pets. St Louis (MO): Saunders-Elsevier; 2013; with permission.)

abscesses can develop, becoming considerably large and leading to swelling of the prepuce, which prevents extrusion of the penis from the prepuce.

The glans penis should be completely extruded from the prepuce in any male chinchilla during physical examination and closely examined. Any accumulated fur or smegma should be removed with diluted chlorhexidine solution. Preputial abscesses should be aspirated, to reduce the tension within the prepuce, and then removed either by extrusion of the glans penis, or if necessary by surgical lancing through the prepuce.

Paraphimosis

Acute severe balanoposthitis or fur rings can lead to paraphimosis (see **Fig. 4**C), which is characterized by prolapse of the glans from the prepuce, and the inability to replace the glans back into the prepuce. In severe cases of paraphimosis, anuria may also develop due to inflammation, trauma, and self-mutilation of the prolapsed glans penis. If the glans and prepuce are viable, carefully clean the tissue with diluted chlorhexidine solution, and apply a lubricant gel or petroleum ointment (eg, Vaseline) to facilitate replacement of the glans penis in the prepuce. Do not attempt to reposition the glans penis if significant preputial swelling is present and substantial force is necessary. Instead, continue to apply ointments or hydrogels to the everted prepuce and glans penis to prevent drying of the exposed tissue. Topical treatment should be performed 3 to 4 times daily, until swelling has resolved. If self-mutilation or overgrooming occurs, an E-collar should be considered. Treat with systemic antibiotics if a bacterial balanoposthitis is present and provide pain relief and anti-inflammatory drugs. If the prolapsed glans penis is not viable, then penile amputation and perianal urethrostomy should be considered, but the prognosis of this procedure in chinchillas is unknown.[19]

Phimosis

Phimosis is defined by the inability to completely protrude the glans penis from the prepuce or entrapment of the penis within the prepuce.[20,21] Phimosis in chinchillas can occur secondary to preputial abscesses. Another cause is the formation of adhesions between the visceral layer of the prepuce and the glans penis (see **Fig. 4D**) or due to stricture formation of the preputial opening. The etiology of phimosis caused by adhesions in chinchillas is unknown. In other species, phimosis can be congenital or acquired (ie, secondary to chronic inflammation, trauma, or neoplasia).[21] An insufficiently small preputial opening may cause phimosis in other species, but this has not been described in chinchillas.[20,21] Phimosis can be subclinical, but may lead to the development of balanoposthitis because of secondary infections from the accumulation of smegma.[21] In cases of secondary balanoposthitis, purulent discharge is often present.

Treatment of phimosis is surgical resection of any adhesions between the visceral layer of the prepuce and the glans penis or resolution of the preputial abscesses. Adhesions should be removed under general anesthesia using magnification. On resolution of the adhesions, completely evert the glans from the prepuce and examine for any abnormalities. Following surgery, manually extrude the glans penis from the prepuce and apply a petroleum ointment (eg, Vaseline) once daily for 10 to 14 days. Then reduce frequency of treatment to once weekly. Reformation of adhesions often occurs, especially as the primary underlying cause is usually not apparent. If adhesions reoccur, consider partial resection of the distal prepuce, to prevent recurrence of phimosis and secondary balanoposthitis.

UROLITHIASIS

Male chinchillas are predominately diagnosed with urinary calculi.[22–24] Urolith analysis from 73 chinchillas (70 male, 1 female, 2 unknown sex) showed that in about 90% of the cases the stones were composed of calcium carbonate (Osborne CA and Lulich JP, personal communication, 2013).[25] A dietary cause for calcium carbonate urolithiasis in chinchillas is unlikely, because excessive dietary calcium is excreted to more than 80% in the feces of chinchillas. Even if high high-calcium diets are fed, urinary calcium excretion does not exceed 3%.[26] Therefore dietary calcium restriction is unlikely to affect the chance of development of uroliths in chinchillas or the recurrence after surgical removal. Chinchillas diagnosed with urolithiasis usually present for hematuria and/or stranguria. Radiographically most animals have a single uroliths located in either the urinary bladder or urethra. In some cases, uroliths are present in both locations (**Fig. 5**). Uroliths should be removed by cystostomy. Because of the unknown underlying etiology of urolithiasis in chinchillas, the risk for recurrence needs to be considered. Surgical removal appears to carry a good prognosis for cystic calculi. However, for urethral calculi, the prognosis is generally guarded, because

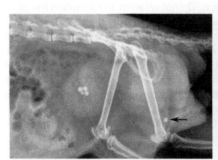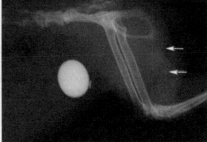

Fig. 5. Lateral abdominal radiographs of 2 male chinchillas diagnosed with urolithiasis. Note the presence of multiple uroliths in the bladder as well as in the urethra (*arrows*) of both animals.

uroliths might be unable to be dislodged and retropulsed in the bladder. Postsurgical treatment should include antimicrobials, and animals should be closely monitored for recurrence of urolithiasis.

MIDDLE EAR INFECTIONS

Natural-occurring otitis media is being increasingly seen in chinchillas, but the literature on the management and diagnosis remains limited.[13,14] Chinchillas have very large tympanic bullae (25 × 22 × 12 mm in adults with volume of 1.5–2 mL), large tympanic membranes, and a relatively short and simple external ear canal.[27] These anatomic features have made chinchillas the gold-standard animal model to study otitis media, a multifactorial and polymicrobial disease process in humans.[28]

Anatomy

The tympanic bullae in chinchillas are divided into a ventral and a dorsal bulla, which are separated by multiple bony septa.[17] The ventral bulla is larger, extends caudally, and reaches half the height of the skull (**Fig. 6**).[17,29] The dorsal bulla forms the roof the tympanic bulla and reaches to the inner side of the meatus. The Eustachian tube connects the oropharynx with the tympanic bulla, is about 4.5 mm long, and enters the ventral tympanic bulla about 7 mm from the bottom of the ventral bulla on its medial aspect.[30]

Clinical Presentation

Middle ear infections (otitis media) in chinchillas can be subclinical and may be diagnosed as an incidental finding in animals during physical examination or during diagnostic imaging of the skull. If the infection is clinical, animals may present with a discharge from the external ear canal and head shaking, or in severe cases may exhibit a head tilt, facial paresis, or severe neurologic deficits.[13] Otitis externa is often the result of a perforated tympanic membrane secondary to otitis media. Any discharge from the ear canal should prompt the clinician to rule out a middle ear infection (**Fig. 8**).

Etiology

Middle ear infections (**Fig. 7**) develop in most cases from bacterial translocation through the Eustachian tube.[13] Predisposing factors include dysfunction of the

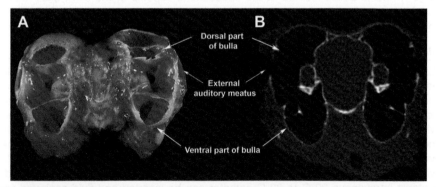

Fig. 6. (A) Caudal view of a chinchilla skull with the caudal walls of the tympanic bullae resected. (B) Computed tomography image at the level of the tympanic bullae. Note the large and multichambered tympanic bullae. ([A] Courtesy of Arno Wuenschmann, Dr med vet, Dipl. ACVP, St Paul, MN.)

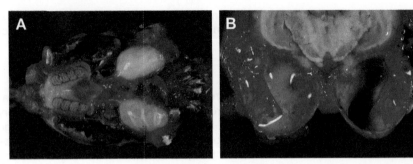

Fig. 7. Postmortem photographs of a chinchilla with bilateral otitis media. (*A*) Ventral view of the skull showing bilateral purulent effusion of both tympanic bullae. (*B*) Cross section through the ventral tympanic bullae showing bilateral purulent effusion. (*Courtesy of Arno Wuenschmann, Dr med vet, Dipl. ACVP, St Paul, MN.*)

Eustachian tube because of viral or bacterial infections, altered upper respiratory tract flora, insufficient immune response of the host, or concurrent disease. All these factors may predispose to ascending secondary bacterial infections with bacterial organisms from the upper respiratory tract via the Eustachian tube.

Diagnosis

The diagnosis of otitis media should be made based on a combination of physical examination findings, diagnostic imaging, and cytologic and microbiological evaluation of the middle ear effusion. Otoscopy will aid in the evaluation of the external ear canal and the integrity and appearance of the tympanic membrane. A normal ear canal in chinchillas is wide, free of any debris or purulent material, and visualization of the large tympanic membranes should be possible in every chinchilla (see **Fig. 8**A, B). The tympanic membrane should be avascular and semitransparent (see **Fig. 8**B). Any changes in vascularity, opacity, or bulging of the tympanic membrane signify inflammation of the middle ear and should prompt further investigation. Purulent discharge present in the external ear canal should prompt further investigation of the tympanic membrane and middle ear by means of diagnostic imaging, because primary otitis externa is rare in chinchillas, and most cases of otitis externa are a result of otitis media and a perforated tympanic membrane (see **Fig. 8**C, D). Because of the large tympanic bullae located at the caudolateral aspects of the skull, skull radiographs are easier to interpret compared with other rodents or rabbits. Computed tomography (CT) can provide additional detail and should be performed if available.

Middle Ear Sampling

A transbullar approach to the middle ear in chinchillas can be used to collect middle ear effusion samples for cytologic and bacteriologic testing (**Fig. 9**).[31] The technique requires general anesthesia but is minimally invasive and has a low risk of complications. Diagnostic samples collected by this method are of superior quality compared with samples collected via the external ear canal in cases of ruptured tympanic membranes. The technique consists of a skin incision over the dorsal aspect of the tympanic bulla, followed by perforation of the bone forming the dorsal tympanic bulla with an 18-G to 20-G needle. Once access to the middle ear has been established, a sterile intravenous 20-G to 22-G catheter can be inserted and fluid aspirated for diagnostic testing. After completion of the sample collection, careful lavage with sterile saline should be performed to remove pathogens.[31] Although closure of the skin incision is performed, closure of the perforated tympanic bone is not necessary.

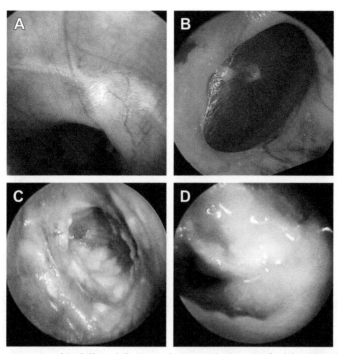

Fig. 8. Otoscopy in chinchillas. (*A*) Normal external ear canal. (*B*) Normal tympanic membrane. (*C* and *D*) Otitis externa secondary to otitis media. Note the purulent material in the external horizontal ear canal, partially covering the tympanic membrane which is abnormally opaque and vascularized (*C*) and perforated (*D*).

Therapy

In chinchillas, otitis media is often chronic at the time of diagnosis. Systemic antibiotic therapy should be initiated, owing to the difficulty of effective topical treatment and the risk of progression to otitis interna and meningoencephalitis. For effective antimicrobial therapy, it is critical to achieve sufficient drug concentrations within the middle ear, to reduce the chance of treatment failure or recurrence of disease.[32,33] Antimicrobial therapy should be based on culture and sensitivities of bacterial organisms isolated from effusions of the middle ear. Although penicillins achieve sufficient concentrations in middle ear fluid and have been successfully used in chinchillas, this medication must be given parentally, to avoid intestinal dysbacteriosis. Penicillins should be used in combination with a fluoroquinolone to improve the anaerobic and gram-positive coverage or following confirmed susceptibility of the isolated pathogen from the middle ear.

Ciprofloxacin, the active metabolite of enrofloxacin, penetrates the middle ear in chinchillas well and although concentrations in the middle ear fluid are lower than in plasma, the half-life is significantly longer (15.0 ± 11.8 hours), compared with the half-life in plasma (3.2 hours).[34]

Azithromycin (30 mg/kg orally every 24 hours for 10 days) and clarithromycin (15 mg/kg orally every 12 hours for 10 days) have been shown to be effective for sterilizing experimentally infected middle ears in chinchillas.[35–37]

Although several drugs have been shown to be effective in eliminating bacterial infections in the middle ears of chinchillas, effusion and inflammation often persist

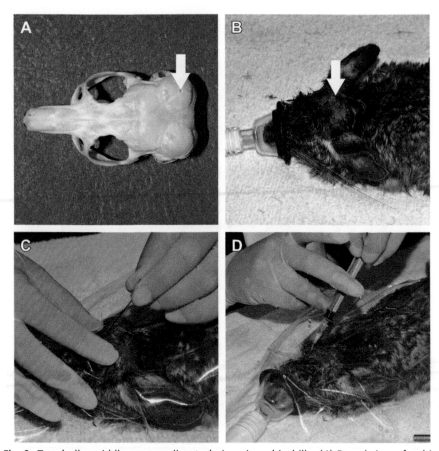

Fig. 9. Transbullar middle ear sampling technique in a chinchilla. (*A*) Dorsal view of a chinchilla skull. The access to the tympanic bulla is obtained through the dorsal aspect of the bulla (*arrow*). (*B*) An anesthetized chinchilla in ventral recumbency. The dorsal aspect of the caudal skull was clipped and aseptically prepared before performing the sampling (*arrow*). (*C*) Following a small skin incision, a 20-G hypodermic needle is used for perforation of the bone forming the roof of dorsal tympanic bulla. (*D*) Aspiration of middle ear effusion using a sterile 22-G catheter attached to a 3-mL syringe.

for weeks beyond sterilization of the middle ear.[38] Therefore, chronic clinical signs, such has persistent head tilt, often persist beyond the treatment period.

DENTAL AND PERIODONTAL DISEASE

Dental disease is one of the most common presenting disorders of pet chinchillas. Most chinchillas with dental disease present with weight loss, anorexia, and drooling. Historically, dental disease in chinchillas has been primarily described as malocclusion and elongation of the cheek teeth. However, periodontal disease, caries, and tooth resorption are disease processes that are common in chinchillas, but are frequently missed during intraoral examination, even if the examination is performed under general anesthesia. Endoscopy-assisted intraoral examination (stomatoscopy) (see **Figs. 10–12**) provides superior visibility and increases the chance for detection of dental lesions. Stomatoscopy also greatly simplifies intraoral procedures for

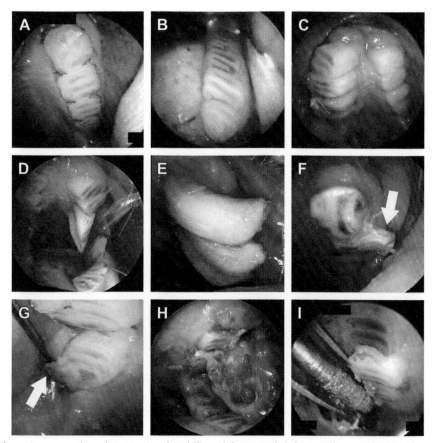

Fig. 10. Intraoral endoscopy in chinchillas. (*A*) Normal left maxillary and mandibular (*B*) dental arcades. Note the short clinical crowns of the cheek teeth (CT) and the lack of any interproximal spaces between the CT. (*C*) Elongation of the right maxillary CT. (*D*) Elongation and malocclusion of the left maxillary and mandibular CT. (*E*) Severe elongation of the left maxillary CT secondary to lack of attrition owing to previous extraction of the left mandibular CT. (*F*) Buccal spike formation of CT-2 (*arrow*) of the left maxillary arcade. (*G*) Buccal spur formation of CT-4 (*arrow*) of the right maxillary arcade. These buccal spurs on CT-3 or CT-4 are easily missed and therefore the buccal aspects of these teeth should be carefully examined in any chinchilla undergoing a dental examination. (*H*) Severe ulceration of the left cheek secondary to buccal spur formation of the left maxillary CT. (*I*) Removal of a buccal spur using a diamond burr in combination with a soft-tissue protector.

diagnostic and treatment purposes, as well as provides the opportunity for documentation of intraoral findings.[39] All cheek teeth should be carefully examined for evidence of crown elongation, malocclusion, mobility, and periodontal disease, as well as caries and resorptive lesions. Sharp dental spike formation might be easily overlooked, particularly if arising from the maxillary cheek teeth and directed buccally (see **Fig. 10**). These spikes frequently lead to ulceration of the buccal mucosa (see **Fig. 10**H). Other common intraoral findings involving the cheek teeth include coronal elongation, changes in the occlusal surface, and widened interproximal coronal spaces that facilitate impaction and promote development of periodontal disease (see **Fig. 11**).[40,41] Treatment of cheek teeth malocclusion and elongation includes

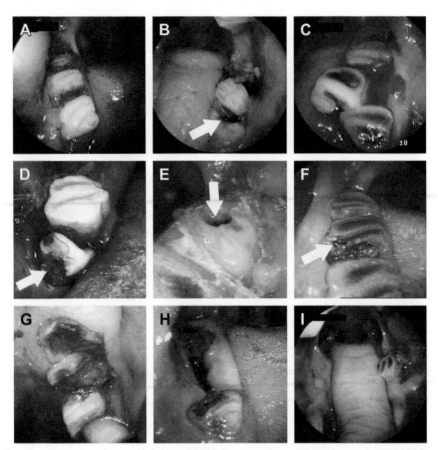

Fig. 11. Intraoral endoscopy of periodontal disease, caries and resorptive lesions in chinchillas. (*A*) Increased interproximal spaces between the right mandibular cheek teeth (CT) owing to absence of a CT. This has lead to impaction of food and debris in the interproximal spaces. (*B*) Increased interproximal spaces and periodontal disease of the left mandibular CT. Note the resorption of the distal aspect of the clinical crown of CT-2 (*arrow*). Tooth resorption is a common consequence of severe periodontal disease in chinchillas. (*C*) Severe periodontal disease of the left mandibular cheek teeth and lingual displacement of CT-2, which is commonly caused by periodontal abscessation. (*D*) Periodontal disease and tooth resorption (*arrow*) of the mesial aspect of CT-1. (*E*) Resorptive tooth lesion (*arrow*) of left mandibular CT-4. (*F*) Periodontal disease and carious lesion of right mandibular CT-3 (*arrow*). (*G*) Severe caries present on the occlusal surfaces of left maxillary CT-1 and -2. Note the severe gingival hyperplasia. (*H*) Subtotal resorption of the crowns of CT-2 and CT-3 of the right mandibular arcade. Note the discoloration and presence of carious lesion on the occlusal surfaces of CT-1 and -4. (*I*) Pseudo-oligodontia in a 15-year-old chinchilla secondary to tooth resorption. Note the absence of all right mandibular CT and of CT-1 and -2 of the left mandibular arcade.

reduction of coronal height and restoration of the horizontal occlusal surfaces. Any sharp spikes on the cheek teeth should be removed to promote healing of soft tissue. All corrections of the cheek teeth should be performed using a low-speed dental handpiece and a diamond burr (see **Fig. 10**I). The use of a soft-tissue protector will greatly reduce the risk of iatrogenic damage during the dental procedure. Resection of gingiva using monopolar electrosurgery may be indicated in cases of severe gingival hyperplasia, which prevent reduction of clinical crown height or removal of dental spikes.

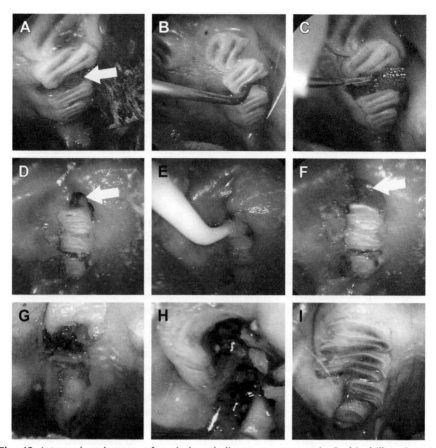

Fig. 12. Intraoral endoscopy of periodontal disease treatments in 3 chinchillas. Case 1: (*A*) Increased interproximal space between CT-2 and CT-3 of the left maxillary arcade leading to food entrapment and predisposition to periodontal disease (*arrow*). (*B*) Manual removal of the accumulated debris. (*C*) Administration of 2% hydrogen peroxide for lavage and disinfection of the periodontal pocket. Case 2: (*D*) Absence of the clinical crown of CT-1 of the right maxillary arcade, resulting in a deep periodontal pocket (*arrow*). (*E*) Subgingival instillation of a doxycycline containing sustained-release biodegradable liquid (Doxirobe) into the periodontal pocket. (*F*) Final appearance after successful instillation of Doxirobe. Note that the liquid has solidified and prevents impaction of the periodontal pocket with food and debris. Case 3: (*G*) Severe periodontal disease, partial tooth resorption, food impaction, and gingival hyperplasia of the right maxillary arcade. (*H*) Postextraction of severely mobile and diseased clinical crowns and lavage of the periodontal pockets with 2% hydrogen peroxide. (*I*) Four months after initiation of local and systemic treatment for periodontal disease. Note that the CT have regrown and no further signs of periodontal disease are present.

DENTAL CARIES

Dental caries (cavities, tooth decay) of the cheek teeth are common in chinchillas and are characterized by brown discoloration and loss of tooth substance along the occlusal and interproximal tooth surfaces (see **Fig. 11**).[40–43] In 52% of 181 skulls from captive chinchillas, dental caries were found on the occlusal and approximal surfaces of the cheek teeth.[41]

Dental caries can be defined as a bacterial infection that leads to demineralization and destruction of tooth substance. In chinchillas, a mixture of gram-positive and gram-negative bacteria has been reported to be associated with caries.[42] The reason why dental caries are more common in chinchillas, compared with other rodents or rabbits, remains unknown. Sugary treats in the diet and reduced abrasion of the teeth secondary to low-fiber diets may lead to increased bacterial plaque formation and reduced salivation, thus possibly predisposing chinchillas to the development of dental caries.[42] No treatment guidelines for dental caries in chinchillas have been established. Diseased tooth substance should be removed using a dental burr until healthy tooth substance is apparent. Periodontal disease is often associated with caries lesions and should be treated appropriately.

PERIODONTAL DISEASE AND TOOTH RESORPTION

Periodontal disease is a very common intraoral disease process in chinchillas. Evaluation of 181 skulls found signs of periodontal disease in 63%.[41] Although the primary cause for the development of periodontal disease in chinchillas remains to be identified, it is assumed that the same mechanisms are involved in periodontal disease as in other species, including dental disease, genetics, age, microflora, and diet.[44]

Resorptive processes can affect the tooth itself, but also the alveolar bone.[42] Odontoclastic resorption of teeth is believed to occur secondary to periodontal infection or trauma to the periodontal structures.[42] Tooth resorption was found in 18% of 181 examined chinchilla skulls in one study.[41] In chinchillas, resorptive tooth lesions are often found in direct association with periodontal disease and gingival pockets; resorption can result in occlusal surface defects or in absence of part or the entire clinical crown of a cheek tooth (see **Fig. 11**).[41]

Resorption of the clinical crowns of the cheek teeth often leads to food entrapment in the widened interproximal spaces. Periodontal disease is usually associated with tooth resorption. Careful and thorough removal of any retained food material in the oral cavity and assessment of every tooth for mobility and associated periodontal abnormalities is critical for detection of periodontal disease in chinchillas. Untreated periodontal disease can result in further bone and tooth resorption and chronic intraoral pain, leading to insufficient food intake and subsequent cachexia, ketoacidosis, and hepatic lipidosis.

Treatment of periodontal disease in chinchillas is challenging because of the small size of the oral cavity and the often-advanced stage of periodontal disease at the time of diagnosis. The goal of therapy is to reduce periodontal infection and intraoral pain to improve food intake. The treatment of periodontal disease in chinchillas consists of local and systemic therapy.

Local Periodontal Therapy

During a complete intraoral examination, all retained food should be removed, and any interproximal spaces cleaned and probed (see **Fig. 12**). If periodontal pockets or periodontal infection is identified, the lesions should be carefully lavaged with a disinfectant solution. The authors prefer the use of 2% hydrogen peroxide, because of its foaming action, which leads to superior retention at the site of application, and therefore minimizes the risk of aspiration (see **Fig. 12C**). Hydrogen peroxide has antimicrobial properties, particularly against anaerobic bacteria, which may help in reduction of periodontal infection and dental plaque formation.

The application of locally applied sustained-release antibiotics is a common practice in human and small animal dentistry for treatment of periodontal disease.[45,46]

Biodegradable antibiotic-containing or antiseptic-containing formulations are available, which are administered subgingivally in sufficiently deep gingival pockets, and provide high antimicrobial drug concentrations for prolonged periods.[45] Doxycycline is the most commonly used local antibiotic in veterinary dentistry and is available as a commercial product for veterinary use (Doxirobe; Pfizer Animal Health, New York, NY) (see **Fig. 12**D–F). This doxycycline-containing formulation is a biodegradable liquid that contains doxycycline and solidifies on contact with fluids. It also provides a physical barrier and therefore may help to prevent impaction with food material and reinvasion of bacteria in gingival pockets, while promoting healing of the pocket, through its antimicrobial action. Locally applied antimicrobial formulation should be instilled only into deep periodontal pockets to increase the chance for prolonged retention at the site of administration (see **Fig. 12**D–F).

Systemic Antimicrobial Therapy

Perio-odontopathogenic bacteria in rodents and lagomorphs are usually mixed aerobic-anaerobic populations.[47] Therefore, antimicrobials need to be chosen based on their effectiveness against anaerobic bacteria. Systemic antimicrobial therapy should be considered for any chinchilla with advanced periodontal disease to reduce the severity of periodontal infection and slow disease progression. Parenteral long-acting penicillin G benzathine (50,000 U/kg subcutaneously every 5 days) has been used extensively by the authors and has been shown to be effective and safe in chinchillas. Penicillin G provides excellent coverage against anaerobic bacteria.[47] The duration of treatment is dependent on the severity of periodontal disease. Other antibiotics that are effective against anaerobic bacteria and safe in chinchillas include chloramphenicol, metronidazole, and azithromycin. Trimethoprim-sulfonamide combinations and fluoroquinolones are poor choices for treatment of periodontal infections in any species, and should therefore not be used unless indicated by culture and sensitivity results and combined with antibiotics that are effective against anaerobic bacteria.

CARDIAC DISEASE

Limited information on cardiac diseases of chinchillas is available. Chinchillas that present with clinical signs consistent with cardiac disease, such as labored breathing, weakness, lethargy, and possible heart murmurs should be evaluated radiographically and echocardiographically. Echocardiographic abnormalities reported in chinchillas include mitral valve insufficiency, dynamic right ventricular outflow tract obstruction, tricuspid valve insufficiency, and left ventricular hypertrophy.[48,49] Reports about ventral septal defects and dilated cardiomyopathy also exist (Reavill DR, personal communication, 2012).[50]

A retrospective evaluation of 300 chinchilla necropsy and biopsy submissions over a 16-year period revealed 9 cases of left ventricular hypertrophy and 3 cases of dilated cardiomyopathy. Pathology of the heart valves was rare and found in only 1 chinchilla. Several chinchillas had evidence of myocarditis or suppurative epicarditis. Most cases of suppurative epicarditis were associated with bacterial pneumonia or pleuritis (Reavill DR, personal communication, 2012).

Heart murmurs are common in chinchillas and most heart murmurs in chinchillas are innocent (synonym: physiologic). In a recent multi-institutional study, the prevalence of heart murmurs in 260 chinchillas presented to veterinary teaching hospitals was 23% (59/260).[48] Of the 15 animals with heart murmurs that underwent echocardiography for further evaluation, 7 of 15 had no echocardiographic abnormalities (innocent murmur), and 8 of 15 had various echocardiographic abnormalities.[48]

Echocardiographic measurement for healthy chinchillas under manual restraint, as well as isoflurane anesthesia, has been reported (**Table 1**).[49] Isoflurane anesthesia has a significant effect on echocardiographic measurements, and therefore the type of chemical restraint needs to be considered, especially when comparing measurements obtained from clinical cases with published values.[49]

Reports on the successful clinical management of chinchillas with cardiac disease are currently lacking, and therefore therapy should be guided based on treatment recommendations in other animal species.

PSEUDOMONAS IN CHINCHILLAS

Pseudomonas aeruginosa infections and epizootic outbreaks in chinchillas have been reported frequently,[51–57] primarily in fur-farmed chinchillas. However, *Pseudomonas* infection can also be isolated from clinically healthy animals.[58–60] Chinchillas with intact host defenses are generally not at risk for serious infection with *P aeruginosa*, unless exposed to high infective doses, but those chinchillas with low neutrophil counts (eg, chronic stress, intercurrent disease) are at risk for invasive infection. Initially infections are often localized to one organ (see **Fig. 4C**).[53,61] Conjunctivitis is a common initial sign of pseudomoniasis in chinchillas. Anorexia, lethargy, and decreased fecal output often follow. Other organ-related signs include enteritis,[51,61,62] pneumonia,[63] otitis media and interna (see **Figs. 8** and **9**),[13] endometritis, and abortion.[13] The infection often progresses with development of neurologic manifestations, sepsis, and death.[13]

Epidemiology and Transmission

Although experimental models of *P aeruginosa* infection in chinchillas have been often described in recent years, there are only a few reports on the distribution and abundance of natural infection in chinchillas that are bred as laboratory animals or pets.

Table 1
Echocardiographic measurements (mean ± SD) obtained from a group of 17 clinical healthy chinchillas

Variable	Manual Restraint	Isoflurane Anesthesia
Heart rate, bpm	169 ± 32	170 ± 22
IVSd, cm	0.2 ± 0.03	0.18 ± 0.03
LVPWd, cm	0.24 ± 0.04	0.26 ± 0.02
LVID, cm	0.59 ± 0.08	0.64 ± 0.05
LVIS,[a] cm	0.29 ± 0.06	0.38 ± 0.05
FS, %	50 ± 8	40 ± 5
LA,[a] cm	0.53 ± 0.06	0.49 ± 0.06
Ao,[a] cm	0.41 ± 0.04	0.36 ± 0.05
LA/Ao ratio[a]	1.28 ± 0.13	1.38 ± 0.2

Echocardiography was performed with animals positioned in right lateral recumbency under manual restraint as well as under isoflurane anesthesia.

Abbreviations: Ao, aortic diameter; bpm, beats per minute; FS, fractional shortening; IVSd, interventricular septum in diastole; LA, left atrial diameter; LVID, left ventricular diastolic dimension; LVIS, left ventricular systolic dimension; LVPWd, left ventricular free wall in diastole.

[a] Anesthesia had a statistically significant effect on variable.

Data from Linde A, Summerfield NJ, Johnston M, et al. Echocardiography in the chinchilla. J Vet Intern Med 2004;18(5):772–4.

In one study, P aeruginosa was isolated from 30% of pet chinchillas and 48% of laboratory chinchillas.[64] In all, P aeruginosa was isolated from 42% of seemingly healthy chinchillas.

Two types of infection are known to occur. Autogenous infection occurs only in those animals whose colonization resistance has been perturbed (eg, bacteremia secondary to gastrointestinal colonization in immunocompromised hosts). However, most infections caused by P aeruginosa are probably acquired exogenously, such as conjunctivitis, otitis media, and osteochondritis. Ocular and deep-tissue infections are likely associated with penetrating injuries.

The occurrence of P aeruginosa infection in laboratory and fur-farmed chinchilla colonies was thought to be transmitted by equipment such as water and water bottles.[18] The detection rate of Pseudomonas from water bottles is generally higher than from the oral cavity or feces, and infections have been related with the presence of up to 10^4 colony-forming units per milliliter of Pseudomonas in the drinking water bottles.[61,64] In contrast, the risk of colonization from ingesting P aeruginosa in free-flowing drinking water is low.[65] In addition to these contaminations, transient infections may result in silent chronic infections from coprophagia.[66]

Pathology

Although Pseudomonas can be isolated from the upper respiratory and gastrointestinal tracts, and from areas of the intertriginous skin (eg, axilla of forelimb, anogenital region, nares, and between digits), the numbers of organisms are usually controlled by competition from normal bacterial flora. Inflammation or injury to these mucosal areas or chronic antibacterial therapy can lead to a proliferation of P aeruginosa.

P aeruginosa, which has few nutritional requirements, thrives in moist environments outside the host and creates microcolonies that allow it to grow on moist surfaces. Animals that are immunosuppressed and have implanted catheters or open wounds are particularly susceptible to contamination from these moist environments or surfaces.

P aeruginosa possesses intrinsic resistance to many antibiotic classes and has the ability to develop resistance by mutations. Susceptibility testing of this organism is difficult, especially for mucoid isolates, because of increasing resistance, lack of reproducibility of results, and lack of clinical correlation. In addition, biofilm-producing P aeruginosa isolates appear to be protected from killing by antibiotics.[67]

When P aeruginosa is recovered from a normally sterile body site, such as blood, pleural fluid, or joint space, it usually constitutes a true infection. The presence of small clusters of gram-negative organisms surrounded by amorphous material is indicative of biofilm formation compatible with a chronic infection. The presence of Pseudomonas organisms intracellularly in polymorphonuclear cells is a strong indication of a true infection; however, pseudoinfection should be considered when there is a cluster of infections with the same strain of Pseudomonas, especially when such infections had not been frequently seen previously, and the animals are neither severely ill nor at enhanced risk of such infection. A search for the source of the cluster should include culture of water bottles, feed, or in a hospital the antiseptic used for skin preparation for venipuncture or similar procedures.

Treatment and Prevention

Multidrug-resistant, reduced-antibiotic susceptibility, and highly virulent strains of P aeruginosa are widespread in chinchillas[64] Because affected animals are often in a critically compromised condition, empiric drug selection is necessary. Susceptibility to fluoroquinolones, third-generation cephalosporins, and aminoglycosides, such as amikacin, is usually high. Susceptibility to trimethoprim-sulfonamide combinations, chloramphenicol, or tetracyclines varies greatly and resistance is common. Use topical polymyxin B and gentamicin-containing formulations to treat ocular and other local infections because of the low prevalence of *P aeruginosa* isolates resistant against these drugs.

GIARDIA IN CHINCHILLAS

Historically, group-housed chinchillas in fur ranches and research colonies had a high prevalence of giardiasis.[68,69] However, the role of *Giardia* in causing disease in chinchillas is difficult to establish. *Giardia* are found rarely in fecal samples from wild chinchillas, but *Giardia* are found in both healthy and sick captive-bred animals.[70–72] A survey of 3 Italian chinchilla-breeding facilities found a 40% presence of *Giardia* cysts despite all animals appearing healthy and not showing any clinical signs.[72] The infection rate was similar to studies conducted in Brazil and Chile.[71,73] In a Belgian survey, 80 pet chinchillas from both pet owners and breeders were screened and 66% excreted *Giardia* cysts.[74] Why the infection rate was higher in Belgium breeding facilities despite the similar management conditions in which the animals were maintained and the similar consistence of the studied population is unknown.

Infection with *Giardia* occurs through fecal-oral transmission or the ingestion of cysts in contaminated food or water. However, experimental infection of healthy chinchillas with *Giardia* cysts has failed to induce clinical disease.[70,75] Predisposing factors, such as stress and poor husbandry, are believed to cause an increase in parasite numbers, resulting in diarrhea and potentially death. Signs of giardiasis in pet chinchillas can include a cyclic sequence of appetite loss and diarrhea, associated with a declining body and fur condition. The organism is usually not enteroinvasive, and so blood in the feces is uncommon. Most infected chinchillas have complete blood count values within reference limits. Recently weaned juvenile chinchillas, immunosuppressed animals, and those living in crowded environments appear to be at highest risk of showing clinical disease.[74,75] *Giardia*-infected chinchillas are a potential reservoir for zoonotic transmission.[74,76,77]

Diagnosis

Giardia cysts are shed intermittently, and repeated fecal analysis may be needed to detect cysts. In addition, cysts can deteriorate in fecal flotation solutions, leading to false-negative results. A variety of different *Giardia*-detection tests have been evaluated for use in animals. Despite the improved specificity, there is no one test that can be performed on a single fecal sample that has 100% sensitivity. Even more problematic is the lack of an assay with high positive predictive value for clinical giardiasis. This problem arises from the high background prevalence of infection in clinically healthy animals.

Fecal Microscopy: Direct Smear and Concentration Techniques

Giardia trophozoites can be observed in direct smears of unstained fecal specimens, using light microscopy. A small amount of fresh diarrheic feces is mixed with a drop of normal saline solution on a microscope slide and covered with a coverslip. A refrigerated sample or one examined several hours after collection probably will contain no living organisms At ×100, their rapid motion identifies trophozoites, but their structural characteristics should be observed at ×400. Trophozoites are rarely found in formed feces. Further testing with *Giardia* antigen tests or polymerase chain reaction (PCR) can be used to differentiate the organisms if cytology is inconclusive. Although they also inactivate the parasites, the application of Lugol solution, methylene blue, or acid-methyl green to the wet mount helps in the visualization of the internal structures of the trophozoites. If trophozoites are not seen on the direct smear, examination for cysts should be performed by zinc-sulfate flotation.

Fecal Enzyme-Linked Immunosorbent Assay

The use of an antigen–enzyme-linked immunosorbent assay (ELISA) (Remel ProSpecT microplate assay [Thermo Fisher Scientific, Lenexa, KS, USA]) for detection of Giardia in chinchilla feces has been reported.[78] However, the sensitivity and specificity for this test in chinchillas has not been determined and the significance of a positive ELISA is of questionable clinical significance, as clinically normal chinchillas can also shed Giardia in the feces.[70,71] Quantification of fecal cyst or trophozoite numbers in animals with diarrhea appears to be more clinically relevant in determining if an infection with Giardia is related to the clinical signs.

Fecal PCR

Assemblage-specific PCR is clinically and epidemiologically beneficial, as mixed genetic group infections are likely to be missed using conventional PCR approaches.[74] However, the assignment of isolates to specific Giardia assemblages is not always consistent because alternate genes can give different results.[79] Thus, some chinchilla isolates can be genotyped as "potentially zoonotic" by one gene but as "host specific" with another. Another problem is that the available primers do not consistently amplify Giardia DNA. Sometimes individual isolates can be amplified at one locus but not at another, whereas other isolates may have the opposite PCR pattern.[79] Giardia PCR assay results can also be falsely negative because of the presence of PCR inhibitors in feces and so should not be used as the sole means of confirming Giardia infection. Because of the inconsistent findings in single genes, use of multilocus genotyping is recommended.[80,81]

Treatment

In most healthy chinchillas, infection appears to be self-limiting; however, treatment will lessen the duration of clinical signs and prevent transmission.

Chinchillas with giardiasis can be treated with metronidazole, tinidazole, or fenbendazole. Nitroimidazole drugs (eg, metronidazole, tinidazole) are highly effective in humans. A 5-day to 7-day course of metronidazole can be expected to cure more than 90% of individuals (data from humans, dogs, and cats), and a single dose of tinidazole, ronidazole, or ornidazole will cure a similar number.[82–85] Efficacy and safety studies have not been performed with these drugs on chinchillas, so all doses are extrapolations from humans, or occasionally dogs and cats. Furthermore, it is unknown if these compounds eradicate Giardia completely or only inhibit cyst production for a time; hence, treated animals may remain a source of chronic cyst shedding.

Treat all animals in contact and thoroughly disinfect the environment to prevent reinfection. Replace wooden cage interior parts, such as resting boards. Giardia cysts remain infectious for up to several weeks in a cool and humid environment.

Because Giardia infection may be difficult to eliminate, the primary goal is to resolve diarrhea. The treatment protocol used may need to be varied according to each individual patient. Additionally, control measures should be instituted to attempt to avoid reinfection. In chinchillas with persistent diarrhea and detection of Giardia in feces, an extensive workup should be undertaken to evaluate for other underlying disorders that may aid in the perpetuation of clinical disease.

ACKNOWLEDGMENTS

The authors thank Arno Wuenschmann, Dr med. vet., Dipl. ACVP (University of Minnesota) for providing photographs for this article, as well as Drury Reavill, DVM, Dipl. ABVP (avian), Dipl. ACVP (Zoo/Exotic Pathology Service) for providing information on neoplastic and cardiac diseases of chinchillas.

REFERENCES

1. Bekyurek T, Liman N, Bayram G. Diagnosis of sexual cycle by means of vaginal smear method in the chinchilla (*Chinchilla lanigera*). Lab Anim 2002;36(1): 51–60.
2. Weir BJ. The management and breeding of some more hystricomorph rodents. Lab Anim 1970;4(1):83–97.
3. Jordan WJ. Sterility in *Chinchilla lanigera*. Kleintierpraxis 1965;10:243–4 [in German].
4. Kraft H. Diseases of chinchillas. Neptun City (NJ): T.F.H. Publications Inc; 1987.
5. Ward ML, Morrison LR, Else RW, et al. Endometritis in the chinchilla: 3 Cases (2003-2006). Belfast (United Kingdom): British Small Animal Veterinary Congress; 2007.
6. Kottwitz J. Stump pyometra in a chinchilla. Exotic Dvm 2006;8(5):24–8.
7. Granson H, Carr AP, Parker D, et al. Cystic endometrial hyperplasia and chronic endometritis in a chinchilla. J Am Vet Med Assoc 2011;239(2):233–6.
8. Lucena RB, Giaretta PR, Tessele B, et al. Diseases of chinchilla (*Chinchilla lanigera*). Pesqui Vet Bras 2012;32(6):529–35.
9. Cote E. Clinical veterinary advisor. 2nd edition. St Louis (MO): Elsevier; 2010.
10. Aiello SE, Moooo MA. The Merck veterinary manual. 10th edition. Whitehouse Station (NJ): Merck Sharp & Dohme Corp; 2012.
11. Hansen D. Chinchilla. In: Goebel T, Ewringmann A, editors. Heimtierkrankheiten. Stuttgart (Germany): Verlag Eugen Ulmer; 2005. p. 100–18.
12. Kirinus JK, Krewer C, Zeni D, et al. Outbreak of systemic listeriosis in chinchillas. Cienc Rural 2010;40(3):686–9.
13. Wideman WL. *Pseudomonas aeruginosa* otitis media and interna in a chinchilla ranch. Can Vet J 2006;47(8):799–800.
14. Mans C, Donnelly TM. Disease problems of chinchillas. In: Quesenberry KE, Carpenter JW, editors. Ferrets, rabbits, and rodents: clinical medicine and surgery. St Louis (MO): Saunders-Elsevier; 2012. p. 311–25.
15. Roos TB, Shackelford RM. Some observations on the gross anatomy of the genital system and two endocrine organs and body weights in the chinchilla. Anat Rec 1955;123(3):301–11.
16. Layne JN. The glans penis and baculum of the rodent *Dactylomys dactylinus desmarest*. Mammalia 1960;24(1):87–92.
17. Dellmann HD. On the anatomy of the male sex organs in the chinchilla. Z Anat Entwicklungsgesch 1962;123:137–54 [in German].
18. Doerning BJ, Brammer DW, Rush HG. *Pseudomonas aeruginosa* infection in a *Chinchilla lanigera*. Lab Anim 1993;27(2):131–3.
19. Fehr M. Chinchilla. In: Fehr M, Sassenburg L, Zwart P, editors. Krankheiten der Heimtiere. 6th edition. Hannover (Germany): Schluetersche; 2005. p. 183–212 [in German].
20. Johnson CA. Disorders of the penis, prepuce and testes. In: Nelson RW, Couto CG, editors. Manual of small animal internal medicine. 2nd edition. St Louis (MO): Elsevier; 2005.

21. MacPhail CM. Surgery of the reproductive and genital systems. In: Fossum TW, editor. Small animal surgery. 4th edition. St Louis (MO): Elsevier; 2012. p. 780–855.
22. Jones RJ, Stephenson R, Fountain D, et al. Urolithiasis in a chinchilla. Vet Rec 1995;136(15):400.
23. Newberne PM. Urinary calculus in a chinchilla. North Am Vet 1952;33:334.
24. Spence S, Skae K. Urolithiasis in a chinchilla [letter]. Vet Rec 1995;136(20):524.
25. Osborne CA, Albasan H, Lulich JP, et al. Quantitative analysis of 4468 uroliths retrieved from farm animals, exotic species, and wildlife submitted to the Minnesota Urolith Center: 1981 to 2007. Vet Clin North Am Small Anim Pract 2009;39(1):65–78.
26. Hansen S. Investigations on calcium metabolism, growth, attrition and composition of the incisors with varying dietary calcium content and gnawing material in chinchillas (C. lanigera). Hannover (Germany): Institut fuer Tierernaehrung, Tierärztliche Hochschule Hannover; 2012.
27. Daniel HJ 3rd, Fulghum RS, Brinn JE, et al. Comparative anatomy of Eustachian tube and middle ear cavity in animal models for otitis media. Ann Otol Rhinol Laryngol 1982;91(1 Pt 1):82–9.
28. Bakaletz LO. Chinchilla as a robust, reproducible and polymicrobial model of otitis media and its prevention. Expert Rev Vaccines 2009;8(8):1063–82.
29. Browning GC, Granich MS. Surgical anatomy of the temporal bone in the chinchilla. Ann Otol Rhinol Laryngol 1978;87(6 Pt 1):875–82.
30. Hanamure Y, Lim DJ. Anatomy of the chinchilla bulla and Eustachian tube: I. Gross and microscopic study. Am J Otol 1987;8(3):127–43.
31. Brown C. Middle ear sample collection in the chinchilla. Lab Anim (NY) 2007; 36(9):22–3.
32. Corbeel L. What is new in otitis media? Eur J Pediatr 2007;166(6):511–9.
33. Giebink GS. Otitis media: the chinchilla model. Microb Drug Resist 1999;5(1): 57–72.
34. Lovdahl M, Steury J, Russlie H, et al. Determination of ciprofloxacin levels in chinchilla middle ear effusion and plasma by high-performance liquid chromatography with fluorescence detection. J Chromatogr B Biomed Sci Appl 1993;617(2): 329–33.
35. Chan KH, Swarts JD, Doyle WJ, et al. Efficacy of a new macrolide (azithromycin) for acute otitis media in the chinchilla model. Arch Otolaryngol Head Neck Surg 1988;114(11):1266–9.
36. Babl FE, Pelton SI, Li Z. Experimental acute otitis media due to nontypeable Haemophilus influenzae: comparison of high and low azithromycin doses with placebo. Antimicrobial Agents Chemother 2002;46(7):2194–9.
37. Alper CM, Doyle WJ, Seroky JT, et al. Efficacy of clarithromycin treatment of acute otitis media caused by infection with penicillin-susceptible, -intermediate, and -resistant Streptococcus pneumoniae in the chinchilla. Antimicrobial Agents Chemother 1996;40(8):1889–92.
38. Kawana M, Kawana C, Giebink GS. Penicillin treatment accelerates middle ear inflammation in experimental pneumococcal otitis media. Infect Immun 1992; 60(5):1908–12.
39. Jekl V, Knotek Z. Evaluation of a laryngoscope and a rigid endoscope for the examination of the oral cavity of small mammals. Vet Rec 2007;160(1):9–13.
40. Jekl V, Hauptman K, Knotek Z. Quantitative and qualitative assessments of intraoral lesions in 180 small herbivorous mammals. Vet Rec 2008;162(14):442–9.
41. Crossley AD. Dental disease in chinchillas (PhD thesis). Manchester (United Kingdom): Department of Dental Medicine and Surgery, University of Manchester; 2003.

42. Crossley DA, Dubielzig RR, Benson KG. Caries and odontoclastic resorptive lesions in a chinchilla (*Chinchilla lanigera*). Vet Rec 1997;141(13):337–9.
43. Crossley DA. Dental disease in chinchillas in the UK. J Small Anim Pract 2001; 42(1):12–9.
44. Wiggs RB, Lobprise HB. Periodontology. In: Wiggs RB, Lobprise HB, editors. Veterinary dentistry: principles and application. Philadelphia: Lippincott-Raven; 1997. p. 186–231.
45. Dumitrescu AL. Antibiotics and antiseptics in periodontal therapy. Berlin: Springer; 2011.
46. Zetner K, Rothmueller G. Treatment of periodontal pockets with doxycycline in beagles. Vet Ther 2002;3(4):441–52.
47. Tyrrell KL, Citron DM, Jenkins JR, et al. Periodontal bacteria in rabbit mandibular and maxillary abscesses. J Clin Microbiol 2002;40(3):1044–7.
48. Pignon C, Sanchez-Migallon Guzman D, Sinclair K, et al. Evaluation of heart murmurs in chinchillas (*Chinchilla lanigera*): 59 cases (1996-2009). J Am Vet Med Assoc 2012;241(10):1344–7.
49. Linde A, Summerfield NJ, Johnston M, et al. Echocardiography in the chinchilla. J Vet Intern Med 2004;18(5):772–4.
50. Hoefer HL, Crossley DA. Chinchillas. In: Meredith A, Redrobe S, editors. BSAVA manual of exotic pets. 4th edition. Quedgeley (Gloucester): British Small Animal Veterinary Association; 2002. p. 65–75.
51. Keagy HF, Keagy EH. Epizootic gastroenteritis in chinchillas. J Am Vet Med Assoc 1951;117(886):35–7.
52. Löliger HC. Pathology of necrotic enterocolitis in chinchillas following infection with *Pseudomonas pyocyanea*. Kleintierpraxis 1961;6:41–8 [in German].
53. Devos A, Viaene N, Spanoghe L, et al. Pathogenesis and treatment of *Pseudomonas aeruginosa* infection in chinchillas and guinea-pigs. Vlaams Diergeneeskundig Tijdschrift 1966;35:369–79 [in Dutch].
54. Halen P, Pohl P, Thomas J. [Septicemia caused by *Pseudomonas* in mink and chinchillas]. Ann Med Vet 1966;110(6):397–406 [in French].
55. Favati V, Marranghini M. *Pseudomonas aeruginosa* infection in chinchillas. Treatment with a new antibiotic, gentamicin sulphate. Zooprofilassi 1968;23(6–7): 277–86 [in Italian].
56. Soldati G. Outbreak of *Pseudomonas aeruginosa* infection in chinchillas. Nuova Vet 1972;48(4):240–2 [in Italian].
57. Menchaca ES, Moras EV, Martin AM, et al. Infectious diseases of the chinchilla. IV. *Pseudomonas aeruginosa*. Gaceta Veterinaria 1980;42(348):96–102 [in Spanish].
58. Brem M. Investigations about the diseases of the gastrointestinal tract in the chinchilla (Dr. med. vet. thesis). Munich (Germany): Medizinische Tierklinik, Ludwig-Maximilians Universität; 1982.
59. Mathieu X, Duran JC, Rivas M. Normal bacterial flora of the wild *Chinchilla lanigera silvestre*. Rev Latinoam Microbiol 1982;24(2):77–82 [in Spanish].
60. Miller LG, Finegold SM. Normal bacterial flora of the chinchilla [abstract]. Abstr Gen Meet Am Soc Microbiol 1967;67:66.
61. Spanoghe L. The significance of *Pseudomonas aeruginosa* infections in animals [abstract]. Antonie Van Leeuwenhoek 1984;50(3):290.
62. Soncini R, Epstein B. Diseases of the chinchilla in Argentina. Universidad Nacional de La Plata. Revista de la Facultad de Ciencias Veterinarias 1968;10(22): 19–21 [in Spanish].
63. Lazzari AM, Vargas AC, Dutra V, et al. Infectious agents isolated from *Chinchilla laniger*. Cienc Rural 2001;31(2):337–40 [in Portuguese].

64. Hirakawa Y, Sasaki H, Kawamoto E, et al. Prevalence and analysis of *Pseudomonas aeruginosa* in chinchillas. BMC Vet Res 2010;6:52.
65. Mena KD, Gerba CP. Risk assessment of *Pseudomonas aeruginosa* in water. Rev Environ Contam Toxicol 2009;201:71–115.
66. George SE, Kohan MJ, Walsh DB, et al. Acute colonization study of polychlorinated biphenyl-degrading pseudomonads in the mouse intestinal-tract—comparison of single and multiple exposures. Environ Toxicol Chem 1989;8(2):123–31.
67. Stewart PS, Costerton JW. Antibiotic resistance of bacteria in biofilms. Lancet 2001;358(9276):135–8.
68. Newberne PM. An outbreak of bacterial gastroenteritis in the South American chinchilla. North Am Vet 1953;34:187–8, 191.
69. Shelton GC. Giardiasis in the chinchilla. II. Incidence of the disease and results of experimental infections. Am J Vet Res 1954;15(54):75–8.
70. Eidmann S. Studies on the etiology and pathogenesis of fur damage in the chinchilla [Dr. med. vet.]. Hannover (Germany): Institut fur Pathologie, Tierarztliche Hochschule; 1992 [in German].
71. Fialho CG, Oliveira RG, Teixeira MC, et al. Comparison of protozoan infection between chinchillas (*Chinchilla lanigera*) from a commercial breeding facility in southern Brazil and chinchillas from a natural reserve in Chile. Parasitología Latinoamericana 2008;63(1–4):85–7 [in Portuguese].
72. Veronesi F, Piergili Fioretti D, Morganti G, et al. Occurrence of *Giardia duodenalis* infection in chinchillas (*Chincilla lanigera*) from Italian breeding facilities. Res Vet Sci 2012;93(2):807–10.
73. Gurgel AC, Sartori AD, de Araujo FA. Protozoan parasites in captive chinchillas (*Chinchilla lanigera*) raised in the State of Rio Grande do Sul, Brazil. Parasitología Latinoamericana 2005;60(3–4):186–8.
74. Levecke B, Meulemans L, Dalemans T, et al. Mixed *Giardia duodenalis* assemblage A, B, C and E infections in pet chinchillas (*Chinchilla lanigera*) in Flanders (Belgium). Vet Parasitol 2011;177(1–2):166–70.
75. Fehr M. Diarrheal diseases in the chinchilla associated with *Giardia* infection?. Rodentia 2002;2:50–1 [in German].
76. Karanis P, Ey PL. Characterization of axenic isolates of *Giardia intestinalis* established from humans and animals in Germany. Parasitol Res 1998;84(6): 442–9.
77. Schönball U. Case report: Giardiasis in a chinchilla—possible source of infection for human being?. Kleintierpraxis 1992;37(11):785–8 [in German].
78. Pantchev N, Globokar-Vrhovec M, Beck W. Endoparasites from indoor kept small mammals and hedgehogs. Laboratory evaluation of fecal, serological, and urinary samples (2002-2004). Tierarztl Prax Ausg K Kleintiere Heimtiere 2005; 33(4):296–306 [in German].
79. Caccio SM, Ryan U. Molecular epidemiology of giardiasis. Mol Biochem Parasitol 2008;160(2):75–80.
80. Lebbad M, Mattsson JG, Christensson B, et al. From mouse to moose: multilocus genotyping of *Giardia* isolates from various animal species. Vet Parasitol 2010; 168(3–4):231–9.
81. Scorza AV, Ballweber LR, Tangtrongsup S, et al. Comparisons of mammalian *Giardia duodenalis* assemblages based on the beta-giardin, glutamate dehydrogenase and triose phosphate isomerase genes. Vet Parasitol 2012;189(2–4): 182–8.
82. Gardner TB, Hill DR. Treatment of giardiasis. Clin Microbiol Rev 2001;14(1): 114–28.

83. Scorza AV, Lappin MR. Metronidazole for the treatment of feline giardiasis. J Feline Med Surg 2004;6(3):157–60.

84. Abbitt B, Huey RL, Eugster AK, et al. Treatment of giardiasis in adult Greyhounds, using ipronidazole-medicated water. J Am Vet Med Assoc 1986;188(1):67–9.

85. Fiechter R, Deplazes P, Schnyder M. Control of *Giardia* infections with ronidazole and intensive hygiene management in a dog kennel. Vet Parasitol 2012;187(1–2): 93–8.

Hyperthyroidism and Hyperparathyroidism in Guinea Pigs (*Cavia porcellus*)

João Brandão, LMV[a], Claire Vergneau-Grosset, DVM[b],
Jörg Mayer, DVM, MSc, Dipl. ABVP (ECM), Dipl. ECZM (small mammal)[c],*

KEYWORDS

- Guinea pig • Cavia porcellus • Thyroid • Parathyroid • Pathology
- Diagnostic testing • Treatment

KEY POINTS

- Diseases of the cavian thyroid and parathyroid have been documented in the scientific literature.
- Clinical signs of a thyroid or parathyroid disorder can be subtle and varied.
- The diagnosis of a true or primary thyroid or parathyroid malfunction can be challenging but should be done in a systematic fashion, as is done with other mammals.
- Treatment of the diagnosed condition can vary and ranges from medical management instead of surgery or radioactive therapy.
- Currently, thyroid and/or parathyroid disease might be a clinically underdiagnosed condition due to inadequate representation in the literature.

HYPERTHYROIDISM

Hyperthyroidism or thyrotoxicosis is a disease process with multiple causes and manifestations characterized by elevated thyroxine (T4) and/or triiodothyronine (T3) serum levels with reduced thyrotropin (TSH) concentrations.[1–4] In humans, the most common cause of thyrotoxicosis is Graves disease, an autoimmune condition in which autoantibodies stimulate the thyrotropin receptors leading to overproduction of T4 and T3.[1]

The thyroid gland activity is controlled by the hypothalamus-pituitary-thyroid axis. The hypothalamus produces thyroid-releasing hormone that stimulates the pituitary to produce TSH that, in turn, stimulates the thyroid gland to produce thyroid hormones, mainly T3 and T4. The stimulation or suppression of this pathway is

[a] Veterinary Clinical Sciences, School of Veterinary Medicine, Louisiana State University, Skip Bertman Drive, Baton Rouge, LA 70803, USA; [b] Companion Avian and Exotic Animal Medicine, University of California, 1 Shields Avenue, Davis, CA 95616, USA; [c] College of Veterinary Medicine, University of Georgia, 501 DW Brooks Drive, Athens, GA 30602, USA
* Corresponding author.
E-mail address: mayerj@uga.edu

Vet Clin Exot Anim 16 (2013) 407–420
http://dx.doi.org/10.1016/j.cvex.2013.01.001
1094-9194/13/$ – see front matter © 2013 Elsevier Inc. All rights reserved.
vetexotic.theclinics.com

controlled by a negative feedback mechanism. Secondary hyperthyroidism, also called thyrotropin-induced hyperthyroidism or central hyperthyroidism, has been described in great detail in human medical literature.[5–8] This condition is caused by a primary TSH-secreting pituitary tumor, which leads to an elevation of thyroid hormone secretion; although in some cases it may cause hypothyroidism.[7–9] Although TSH-secreting pituitary tumors are rare, adenomas are the most commonly reported pituitary neoplasias, whereas carcinomas are unusual.[6,10–12] If the abnormal production of T3 and T4 occurs due an abnormal behavior of the thyroid alone, this is diagnosed as primary hyperthyroidism or simply hyperthyroidism.

Hyperthyroidism has been described in several animal species; it is the most common endocrine disease in cats.[13] Feline hyperthyroidism was first reported in the 1970s and the condition seems to mainly affect middle-aged to older cats without breed and sex predisposition.[13–15] Only one case of juvenile hyperthyroidism in an 8-month old domestic shorthaired cat can be found in the scientific literature to date.[10] In this case, a diffuse thyroid hyperplasia was detected on histopathology.[10] In general, hyperthyroidism in cats is usually caused by a benign thyroid adenoma or a diffuse adenomatous hyperplasia.[16] In most cases of hyperthyroidism in cats, a goiter or a thyroid gland hyperplasia can be detected.[13] Hyperthyroidism has been described in dogs but it is rare.[17]

Among exotic species, hyperthyroidism has been rarely described. In avian species, only one case of naturally occurring hyperthyroidism has been reported in a wild barred owl (*Strix varia*) due to a productive thyroid follicular carcinoma.[18] In reptiles, hyperthyroidism has been described in a green iguana (*Iguana iguana*) and in a leopard gecko (*Eublepharis macularius*).[19,20]

Primary hyperthyroidism has been described in guinea pigs for several decades but this disease is not commonly reported in most textbooks; therefore, clinicians may not be aware of this condition leading to a potential underdiagnosis of this condition in the English-speaking community.[21] Furthermore, if incomplete necropsies are performed in which the thyroid gland is not collected, the diagnosis of primary thyroid disease will not occur. Recently, thyroid neoplasias have been reported to be one of the most common neoplasias (3.6%) detected in guinea pigs by one laboratory service.[22] Of the 19 cases reported, 8 were macrofollicular thyroid adenoma, 5 follicular thyroid carcinoma, 3 papillary thyroid adenoma, 1 thyroid cystadenoma, 1 follicular-compact thyroid carcinoma, and 1 small cell thyroid carcinoma.[22] No scientific data exists to assess age predisposition of the condition; however, it seems that mainly animals more than 3 years of age are affected with a possible predisposition toward female guinea pigs.[23]

The clinical signs in the guinea pigs affected by thyroid disease causing hyperthyroidism seem to be similar to other species. The most common clinical signs are hyperesthesia, hyperactivity, and polyphagia with paradoxic poor body condition or progressive weight loss.[23] In the case of a goiter formation, a palpable mass at the ventral cervical area may be noticed on palpation. Diarrhea or soft feces, polyuria and/or polydipsia, progressive alopecia, and tachycardia are inconsistently reported.[23]

Reference intervals of thyroid hormones have been reported in guinea pigs in the scientific literature.[24,25] In one study, significant differences were detected between females and castrated males, but no significant differences were detected between intact and castrated males or females and intact males.[24] In another study in which total T4 reference intervals were determined using a point-of-care T4 enzyme immunoassay (T4 and Cholesterol Reagent Disk; Abaxis Inc, Union City, CA, USA), no significant differences were detected between age (2 vs 8 months), sex, housing type, and sampling protocol.[25] Although this study demonstrated repeatability, results were not compared with the gold standard via radioimmunoassay methodology.[25] Future studies may be necessary to compare and correlate the values obtained by different methodologies. However, in the authors' opinion, the use of this point-of-care methodology may be a useful tool for screening and initial assessment of the thyroid function of pet guinea pigs using a commonly available and cost-effective analyzer.

Not all cases of hyperthyroidism will cause an increase of the total hormone levels and occasional elevations of thyroid values may be caused by other conditions. It has been shown that stress can cause a significant decrease of thyroid hormones in guinea pigs.[26] In other species, unrelated sickness may induce a euthyroid sick syndrome in which the total hormones will be lower and, therefore, hiding a possible hyperthyroid status.[16] In early or mild hyperthyroidism, the total thyroid values may be within normal limits.[16]

In other animal species and humans, free thyroid hormone measurement is commonly used to assess thyroid function. Free hormones (ie, free T4 and/or free T3 or fT4 and/or fT3) are the active form of the thyroid hormones and have been shown to be more reliable than total values for conditions such as hypothyroidism.[27] In cases of euthyroid sick syndrome or nonthyroidal illness syndrome, the total hormones may be below normal levels, whereas the free thyroid values are less likely to be affected.[28] In cases of hyperthyroidism, an elevated value of total hormones seems to be a reliable method of diagnosis, although measurement of free thyroid values may confirm the suspected condition. To date, only one reference interval study for free thyroid hormones in guinea pigs can be found in the scientific literature.[29] In this study, no significant difference of free T4 or free T3 was detected between adult males and adult pregnant and nonpregnant females.[29]

Another important tool to assess thyroid function is endogenous TSH. In the situation of a primary TSH-producing pituitary tumor, the blood TSH level is elevated, which leads to an overstimulation of the thyroid. In cases of primary hyperthyroidism, the endogenous TSH blood level should be normal to low. The high level of thyroid hormones in the blood stream should provide a negative feedback to the hypothalamus-pituitary-thyroid axis, which, in turn, should downregulate the production of thyroid hormones. In the case of a true thyroid overproduction, the thyroid gland should continue to produce high levels of hormones independently of low or normal levels of TSH. In humans, TSH and fT4 measurement provide the most complete laboratory diagnostic information.[1] To the authors' knowledge, reference intervals for TSH in guinea pigs have not been established.

A definitive diagnosis of hyperthyroidism should not be based on a single thyroid hormone level measurement. Although laboratory tests may be highly suggestive of thyrotoxicosis, some common conditions may cause elevated thyroid values. For example, scurvy in guinea pigs has been shown to increase radioiodine-131 (^{131}I) uptake by the thyroid, which suggests that thyroid activity is higher in guinea pigs with low levels of vitamin C.[30] Therefore, in suspected cases of hyperthyroidism, other diagnostic tools should be used to confirm the suspicion, along with confirmatory laboratory results.

DIAGNOSIS
Physical Examination

If a mass is detected on the ventral aspect of the neck on physical examination, goiter should be considered even though this finding is not pathognomonic of hyperthyroidism. Other common clinical signs include weight loss regardless of normal appetite or hyperphagia, hyperactivity, hyperesthesia, and tachypnea. Diarrhea or soft feces, polyuria and/or polydipsia, progressive alopecia, and tachycardia are inconsistently reported.

Laboratory Test

In the case of a suspected case of hyperthyroidism, several hormones can be quantified to identify hyperactivity of the thyroid gland. A full thyroid panel can be submitted to an endocrinology laboratory. In the authors' opinion, a full thyroid panel should include total T3 (TT3) and total T4 (TT4) by radioimmunoassay, free T3 (fT3) and free T4 (fT4) by equilibrium dialysis. Several reference interval studies have been published recently. **Table 1** compiles reference intervals for several thyroid hormones for pet and research guinea pigs. To the authors' knowledge, no commercially available endocrinology laboratory has validated thyroid panels for guinea pigs.

Imaging

Imaging techniques may provide a better assessment of the thyroid gland. Ultrasonographic examination of the thyroid is commonly used in dogs and has been assessed in terms of its use for diagnosis of thyroid neoplasia.[31] Other imaging techniques used to diagnose thyroid neoplasias include CT and MRI. A recent study compared the sensitivity and specificity of ultrasound, CT, and MRI in dogs to diagnose thyroid carcinomas.[32] In this study, CT had higher specificity (100%), whereas MRI had higher sensitivity (93%) in diagnosing thyroid carcinoma.[32]

In cases in which goiter is noted, cytologic analysis of a fine-needle aspirate (FNA) of the swollen thyroid may provide the diagnosis of thyroid neoplasia. If a goiter is not present or palpable, an ultrasound-guided FNA may be needed to collect samples. If the clinical signs and blood work diagnostic tests are suggestive of hyperthyroidism but the cytologic sample is nondiagnostic, surgical biopsies may be needed. In the

Table 1
Reference intervals of total thyroxine (TT4), total triiodothyronine (TT3), free thyroxine (fT4) and free triiodothyronine (fT3) of guinea pigs (*Cavia porcellus*)

Target Population	TT4 (µg/dL)	TT3 (ng/dl)	fT4 (ng/dl)	fT3 (ng/dl)	Methodology
Laboratory	4.04 (2.26–5.82)[a]	—	—	—	Enzyme immunoassay[25]
Pet	4.17 (3.01–5.33)[a]	—	—	—	Enzyme immunoassay[25]
Laboratory	—	—	1.17 ± 0.09[b]	—	Unknown[82]
Pet	2.1 (1.1–5.2)[a]	—	—	—	Chemiluminescence[24]
Laboratory	2.5–3.2[c]	39–44[c]	1.26–2.03[c]	0.221–0.260[c]	Radioimmunoassay[29]
Unknown	4.54 ± 0.443[b]	31.7 ± 1.4[b]	0.67 ± 0.57[b]	0.224 ± 0.108[b]	Radioimmunoassay[83]
Unknown	Males 2.9 ± 0.6[b] Females 3.2 ± 0.7[b]	Males 39 ± 17[b] Females 44 ± 10[b]	—	—	Unknown[84]

Collected from the available literature. Information on the different target populations (laboratory vs pet guinea pigs) and methodology used to determine values are provided when information was available in the cited study.
[a] Values are provided as mean values and reference interval.
[b] Values are provided as mean and standard error of the mean.
[c] Values are provided as reference interval.

authors' opinion, complete removal of the thyroid tissue for biopsies is not advisable. Because of the significance of the thyroid hormones for homeostasis and normal metabolism, future hormone-replacement therapy is needed with complete removal of the thyroid. Total thyroidectomy most likely will induce a hypothyroid status, which can be controlled by immediate T4 replacement and monitoring.[33,34] Partial thyroidectomy may provide adequate samples for the histologic diagnosis of thyroid neoplasias. Immunohistochemistry as a diagnostic tool has been used in human and veterinary medicine, including guinea pigs.[22,35–38]

The use of scintigraphy for assessment of the thyroid gland has been described in animals and humans.[39,40] It can be used to detect both local and metastatic and/or ectopic thyroid tissue.[39] Scintigraphy allows a visual identification of functional tissue because of the selective uptake of different radionuclides and may provide the diagnosis of hyperthyroidism before laboratory tests are consistently abnormal.[16,39,40] The use of different isotopes has been described: [131]I, radioiodine-123, or 99 mTc-pertechnetate.[23,39]

In the absence of advanced diagnostic tests, diagnosis based on clinical history, clinical findings, response to a trial therapy and thyroid levels may be sufficient to identify a suspected case of hyperthyroidism.

Differential Diagnosis

The detection of a ventral neck mass on physical examination in a guinea pig should be suggestive of a thyroid neoplasia or hyperplasia, although other neoplasias, as well as granulomas, abscesses, and lymph node hyperplasia, need to be considered. Subcutaneous neck abscess formation can be caused by several causes, such as bite wounds, penetration of hay through the oral mucosa and subsequent migration, and cervical lymphadenitis.[41] Cervical lymphadenitis is said to be the most common cause of asymmetrical submandibular swelling, which is most commonly caused by *Streptococcus zooepidemicus*.[42] In cases of hyperthyroidism, the owners commonly report that the animal appears to lose weight although the food intake is unchanged or even increased. Weight loss is commonly caused by dietary causes (eg, food competition, poor nutrition, food deprivation), nondietary causes (eg, dental disease; bulla osteitis, otitis, or facial nerve paralysis; caseous lymphadenitis; gastrointestinal ileus or obstruction; cystic calculi), increased metabolic demand (eg, infectious process, cavian leukemia, metabolic disease, pregnancy) or nutrient malabsorption (gastrointestinal ileus, metabolic disease, dysbiosis).[43] In the authors' opinion, weight loss detected in most of the differentials previously mentioned are usually seen as a consequence of hypophagia, whereas, in hyperthyroidism, the weight loss is a consequence of increased metabolic rate.

TREATMENT

As in any endocrinopathy, the main objective of treatment is to normalize the levels of the circulating hormones. In the case of hyperthyroidism, the main objective of the treatment should be reducing the thyroid hormone levels. Several treatment options are currently available for the practitioner.

Medical Treatment

Antithyroid drugs are fairly simple molecules called thionamides. The primary effect is to inhibit thyroid hormone synthesis by interfering with the thyroid peroxidase-mediated iodination of tyrosine residues in the thyroglobulin.[44] These drugs can be used to control hyperthyroidism caused either by a neoplasm or by hormonal overproduction. A pharmacokinetic study of propylthiouracil (PTU) in guinea pigs has shown that plasma levels are reached after 2 hours and have similar pharmacologic characteristics to humans.[23,45]

The most common drugs to be used in cats are methimazole and carbimazole. In humans, both methimazole and PTU are rapidly absorbed in the gastrointestinal tract with a peak at 1 to 2 hours.[44] Although methimazole is similar to PTU, the former tends to be free in the serum, whereas the latter is 80% to 90% bound to albumin.[23,44] In humans, methimazole is considered to be 10-fold more potent and longer acting than PTU but seems to be equally effective.[40,46] Although no studies on guinea pigs are available, the use of the feline dose for various drugs seems to be effective in controlling clinical signs of hyperthyroidism. In guinea pigs, anecdotal use of methimazole (0.5–2 mg/kg orally once to twice a day) or carbimazole (1–2 mg/kg orally once a day) seem to be effective. The dose selection should be based on routine thyroid level measurement.[23] As with other trial therapies, the dose of the different medications should be adapted to each case. Regular thyroid level rechecks are needed and dose correction should be performed accordingly.

The use of some of these drugs in pregnant female guinea pigs has caused goitrous changes in the off-spring due to placental permeability.[17] In experimental settings, technetium-99 m d, 1-hexamethyl propylene amine oxime has been shown to cross the placenta and radioactivity was detected mostly in the liver and brain of the fetus.[47]

Radiation Therapy

Although not reported as a treatment for pet guinea pigs, this therapeutic option has been described both in humans and dogs. In older publications, anecdotal observations suggested that thyroid tumors were resistant to radiation; however, more recent studies seem to indicate that external beam radiation is a good alternative.[48,49] Radiation is advisable in the case of incomplete surgical excision. Both palliative and curative protocols have been reported. In dogs, a dose of 46.8 to 48 Gy over 12 fractions (3 times a week) has been reported.[50] Palliative treatment with four once-weekly fractions of 9 Gy of 4 MeV x-rays provided a median survival time of 96 weeks (mean 85 weeks, range 6–247 weeks) in 13 dogs.[51] This study suggests that palliative radiation should be considered for the control of invasive thyroid carcinomas in dogs.[51] The objective of palliative radiation is to increase the quality of life of the patient and it should be considered in cases in which surgical removal is not recommended or evidence of metastasis have been detected.[49] There is no report of the use of radiation therapy in guinea pigs. It is unclear if the responsiveness of thyroid tumors in this species is similar to that of dogs or what is the median survival time after curative or palliative treatments. To apply adequate radiation levels to the neoplastic tissue, the surrounding normal tissue may be inadvertently affected and cause acute and late side effects.[52,53] In humans, the reported side effects during the treatment period were erythema, dry or moist desquamation, and mucositis of the esophagus, trachea, and larynx. Late toxicity side effects, although infrequent, include skin telangiectasia and skin pigmentation.[54] Dogs develop similar signs (eg, dry to moist skin desquamation, hair loss, mucositis) but may also have permanent alopecia and hair color change.[49]

Surgical Thyroidectomy

If complete bilateral excision of the thyroid glands is performed, hormonal replacement therapy will be necessary for the remainder of the guinea pig's life. Although side effects and consequences of the thyroidectomy should be considered, surgical thyroidectomy is still one of the treatment options with best prognosis for a nonmetastatic productive or benign thyroid neoplasm. One specific surgical approach using electric cautery has been described for guinea pigs.[55] The investigators report recurrent laryngeal nerve damage and incomplete gland removal as possible complications, which are similar to side effects in humans.[55] Among 124 thyroidectomies, 52 animals had accidental incomplete thyroidectomies, which allowed thyroid regrowth within 2 to 3 months postsurgery.[55] Thyroid regrowth is a concern both for research purposes when hypothyroidism needs to be maintained and for clinical cases in which surgical thyroidectomy is used for the treatment of hyperthyroidism. The accidental removal of the parathyroid glands is a common complication of thyroidectomy; however, in guinea pigs, these glands may not be attached to the thyroid so it may be less of a concern.[55–57] However, care should still be taken to avoid removal of the parathyroid glands. The location of the parathyroid tissue in relationship to the thyroid tissue in the guinea pig has been described.[57] The investigators recommend reviewing these important anatomic details before performing surgery. For more information on the anatomic location of the parathyroid glands, see discussion on hyperparathyroidism above.

Radioiodine Treatment

Radioactive isotopes have been used to treat hyperthyroidism in guinea pigs. In humans, concerns with possible oncogenic effects and ophthalmopathies have been associated with the use of radioactive isotopes.[46] Several isotopes have been described in humans but ^{131}I is the only one reported for clinical control of hyperthyroidism.[23] This chemical emits β and γ radiation, but only the β particles cause destruction of the follicular cells resulting in histopathological changes, including epithelial swelling and necrosis, edema, and leukocyte infiltration, followed by gland fibrosis leading to destruction of most of the thyroid gland.[46] ^{131}I can be administered either subcutaneously or intravenously.[23] In humans with Graves disease, after oral administration of ^{131}I most radionuclide is localized in the thyroid gland.[46] In cats, the radioiodine will be primarily concentrated in the hyperplastic and neoplastic tissue, whereas the normal tissue only receives a small dose of radiation because the tissue is suppressed.[58] In one study, approximately one out of five hyperthyroid cats had multiple areas of hyperfunctional thyroid tissue and/or intrathoracic hyperfunctional thyroid tissue for which surgical thyroidectomy would not be curative.[59]

This treatment may be the best therapeutic option because it can result in long-term control of the disease. It is potentially curative, affecting productive tissue (thyroid and ectopic tissue) and, to a lesser extent, the nonfunctional tissue. It does not affect the parathyroids (common complication of surgery), is less invasive than surgery, and has a higher success rate.[23,58] In humans, the dose of ^{131}I is based on the size of the gland and is calculated using the following formula: dose (MCi) = (μCi of ^{131}I/g of thyroid × estimated thyroid weight)/24-h radioiodine uptake.[46] In guinea pigs, the dose of 1 MCi given subcutaneously has been reported to have achieved good clinical results, although further studies are needed to assess the effectiveness of the dose and possible side effects.[23]

OTHER CONSIDERATIONS
Anesthesia

For most of the treatments and diagnostic tests, the patients will need to be anesthetized. Therefore, it is important to consider the implications of anesthesia in hyperthyroid patients. The preoperative, intraoperative, and postoperative complications, as well as preventive therapies for humans with hyperthyroidism undergoing anesthesia, have been published. It is advisable to attempt to control the thyroid function and establish an euthyroid status before any procedure requiring anesthesia. In humans and animals, correlation between thyroid diseases and cardiac conditions has been reported.[60–62] Dogs with induced hyperthyroidism had increased heart rates and increased T-wave amplitudes but did not have fractional shortening or ventricular hypertrophy, which has been reported in cats, rats, and humans.[62] In another study, 13 out of 30 dogs developed cardiac failure as a sequela of exogenous hyperthyroidism.[63] It is suggested that, in humans with hyperthyroidism, the use of ketamine may cause severe hypertension and tachycardia.[23] Therefore, in humans, beta-blockers are often administered before surgery to reduce the heart rate, thus providing symptomatic relief and cardiac protection.[64] One of the main concerns with thyroidectomy in humans is the difficult intubation due to tracheal displacement caused by a mass effect. Fiberoptic intubation is recommended in challenging cases.[64] Postoperatively, the main concerns involve hematoma, laryngeal and pharyngeal edema with subsequent respiratory obstruction, tracheal collapse, hypocalcaemia, pain, and nausea.[64]

Thyroid Storm

A thyrotoxic or thyroid storm is a life-threatening condition characterized by an exacerbation of clinical thyrotoxicosis; it has been described in humans and cats.[65–67] It is suggested that in humans a thyroid storm may occur due to thyroid surgery, administration of iodine, discontinuation of antithyroid medication, decreased production of T4-binding proteins, or iatrogenic cause (ie, palpation of the thyroid gland and administration of T4).[65,68] A conclusive diagnosis of thyroid storm is difficult because there may not be a significant difference between an uncomplicated thyrotoxicosis and a thyroid storm.[65] Although not described in guinea pigs, clinicians should consider this condition in the event of a rapid and unexpected deterioration of a patient previously diagnosed or suspected of hyperthyroidism.

HYPERPARATHYROIDISM

Hyperparathyroidism has been suspected anecdotally in guinea pigs; however, there are only two reports of fibrous osteodystrophy suspected to be associated with secondary nutritional hyperparathyroidism in the peer-reviewed literature.[69–71] Fibrous osteodystrophy has been reported in a 10-month old female guinea pig, 2-year-old male guinea pig, and a male 1-year-old Satin guinea pig.[70,71] Fibrous osteodystrophy is a condition caused by primary or secondary hyperparathyroidism and results in increased osteoclastic resorption of bone and replacement by fibrous tissue.[69]

Embryologically, the parathyroid glands develop from the endodermal lining of the third and fourth pharyngeal pouch and move toward the thyroid gland lateromedially.[72,73] In the guinea pig, small groups of the parathyroid cells are enclosed in the thyroid lobes and in surrounding areas.[74]

Ionized calcium, phosphate, and magnesium concentrations are maintained by vitamin D3 and by two polypeptide hormones, parathyroid hormone (PTH) and calcitonin.[72] The main actions of PTH are to promote bone resorption, increase renal calcium reabsorption, decrease renal phosphate reabsorption, and stimulate 1,25-dihydroxyvitamin D synthesis from 25-hydroxyvitamin D by the kidneys.[75] In return, a high ionized calcium concentration exerts a negative feedback on the parathyroid gland. This negative feedback is lost in primary hyperparathyroidism. Guinea pig PTH is an 84–amino acid single-chain polypeptide, which is synthesized, stored, and secreted by the parathyroid glands.[76] In addition to its role in calcium metabolism, PTH causes relaxation of smooth muscle in the cardiovascular system, gastrointestinal tract, gallbladder, trachea, uterus, and vas deferens.[76,77]

Radioimmunoassay is the primary method for measurement of serum or plasma PTH concentration in laboratory animals.[75] ELISA-kits are also available for research purposes and measure guinea pig serum PTH (Kamiya Biomedical Company, Seattle, WA, USA). However, both these methods measure biologically inactive fragments of PTH found in circulation in addition to the active hormone.[75] Half-life of middle and C-terminal PTH fractions, which are inactive portions, are 10-fold to 20-fold longer than the active N-terminal fraction. The two-site PTH assay used in human medicine detects only complete PTH peptides in circulation by using two different polyclonal antibodies. N-terminal PTH being assayed are incubated simultaneously with the antibodies, thus creating a sandwich with the intact hormone.[78] However, to date, these kits are not commercially available.

Normal PTH concentrations have been described in rats but not in other rodents to the authors' knowledge.[72,75] Normal PTH concentrations observed in rats varied with strain and gender; therefore, it is likely that reference intervals should be established for each gender and strain of guinea pigs.

Vitamin D deficiency, calcium malabsorption, or other calcium metabolism disturbances may play a role in the onset of disease.[69,71] Diets with a low calcium to phosphorus ratio (Ca:P) have been reported to reduced growth rates, stiffness of joints, and calcification of soft tissues. They may also affect the uptake of magnesium and potassium.[79] Other investigators have seen guinea pigs presented with this disease that were purposely placed on low-calcium diets to prevent urolithiasis.[69] Breeders in Europe and the United States also report this disease in the Satin type receiving an appropriate diet, suggesting an inherited factor in this line of guinea pigs.[69,70]

Clinical signs in the affected guinea pigs consisted of difficulty walking and lethargy.[70,71] Generalized osteopenia of the axial and appendicular skeleton as demonstrated by a double cortical line sign was noted on radiographs.[71] However, in these case reports, PTH concentrations were not determined antemortem and parathyroid glands were not sampled postmortem.[70,71] In the case reported in a Satin guinea pig, all tested biochemical parameters were within reference intervals, including calcium, phosphorous, renal parameters, alanine transaminase, glutamate dehydrogenase, and T4 concentrations.[70] A mild leucocytosis was noted on complete blood cell count (17,800/uL, reference interval 7–14,000/uL).[70] Unfortunately, a necropsy was declined by the owner so the precise pathogenesis of the fibrous osteodystrophy in this case was not established.[69,70] In another case report, fibrous osteodystrophy associated with pathologic femoral fractures were diagnosed postmortem based on histologic lesions and osteodensitometric measurement compared with a control guinea pig.[71] Otitis media, dental malocclusion, and degenerative joint disease of coxofemoral and stifle joints were also noted radiographically and confirmed postmortem, which could either be incidental findings or could be associated with the hyperparathyroidism.[71] Because no renal lesions were detected, and based on the imbalanced low Ca:P ratio of the diet, the investigators suspected a nutritional cause.[71] However, primary hyperparathyroidism was not ruled out because the parathyroid glands were not obtained at necropsy in these three cases.[70,71] Paraneoplastic hyperparathyroidism, associated with parathyroid related hormone was not ruled out either, although no neoplastic lesion was detected postmortem.[71]

Diagnosis should be based on dietary history, physical examination findings, radiographic findings, plasma total and ionized calcium concentrations, serum 25-hydroxyvitamin D, and PTH concentrations, although no reference intervals are established in guinea pigs to date.[69] Necropsy findings include severely thinned trabecular bone, marked osteoclastic activity, resorption of cortical bone, and extensive replacement with fibrous connective tissue and hyperplastic parathyroid glands.[69] This disease must be differentiated from hypovitaminosis C because the clinical signs can appear similar.[69]

Treatment is aimed at normalizing Ca:P ratios.[69] The diet should contain 0.3% to 0.4% magnesium, 0.4% to 1.4% potassium, 0.9% to 1.1% calcium, and 0.6% to 0.7% phosphorus.[80] The correct Ca:P ratio is 1.5 to 1. Oral calcium glubionate therapy has been recommended, as well as supplementation of vitamin D and increased exposure to sunlight empirically.[69] Osteoporosis associated with oversupplementation with cod liver oil has also been reported in guinea pigs. Therefore, vitamin D supplementation should be used with caution at 1,600 IU/kg of food as a maximum dose.[69,80] Pain management should be provided and can include opioid medications for skeletal pain as well as antiinflammatory medications.[69] Supportive care, including assisted feeding and fluids should also be provided as needed. In the initial case report, supportive care including antiinflammatory drugs, antibiotics, and dietary support was attempted for 2 weeks in both guinea pigs before euthanasia was elected.[71] In the published case in a Satin guinea pig, risedronate sodium (Actonel, Sanofi-Aventis, Germany) was prescribed empirically at 0.25 mg per guinea pig every 24 hours orally.[70] Risedronate is a bisphosphonate component prescribed in osteoporotic human patients. Risedronate can suppress bone turnover, increase bone mass, and reduce fracture risk, and acts by reducing osteoclast activity leading to apoptosis of osteoclasts.[81] However the therapeutic dose is unknown in guinea pig. The Satin guinea pig survived 2.5 years after diagnosis of osteofibrosis.[70] Prognosis of secondary nutritional hyperparathyroidism has been reported as guarded without aggressive supportive care.[69]

ACKNOWLEDGMENTS

The authors thank Dr Michelle Hawkins for her insightful comments about hyperparathyroidism in guinea pigs.

REFERENCES

1. Franklyn JA, Boelaert K. Thyrotoxicosis. Lancet 2012;379:1155–66.
2. Seigel SC, Hodak SP. Thyrotoxicosis. Med Clin North Am 2012;96:175–201.
3. McDermott MT. Hyperthyroidism. Ann Intern Med 2012;157:ITC1–16.
4. Bahn RS, Burch HB, Cooper DS, et al. Hyperthyroidism and other causes of thyrotoxicosis: management guidelines of the American Thyroid Association and American Association of Clinical Endocrinologists. Endocr Pract 2011;17:456–520.
5. Clore JN, Sharpe AR, Sahni KS, et al. Thyrotropin-induced hyperthyroidism: evidence for a common progenitor stem cell. Am J Med Sci 1988;295:3–5.
6. Gesundheit N, Petrick PA, Nissim M, et al. Thyrotropin-secreting pituitary adenomas: clinical and biochemical heterogeneity. Case reports and follow-up of nine patients. Ann Intern Med 1989;111:827–35.
7. Beck-Peccoz P, Brucker-Davis F, Persani L, et al. Thyrotropin-secreting pituitary tumors. Endocr Rev 1996;17:610–38.
8. Beck-Peccoz P, Persani L, Asteria C, et al. Thyrotropin-secreting pituitary tumors in hyper- and hypothyroidism. Acta Med Austriaca 1996;23:41–6.
9. Gershengorn MC, Weintraub BD. Thyrotropin-induced hyperthyroidism caused by selective pituitary resistance to thyroid hormone. A new syndrome of "inappropriate secretion of TSH". J Clin Invest 1975;56:633–42.
10. Gordon JM, Ehrhart EJ, Sisson DD, et al. Juvenile hyperthyroidism in a cat. J Am Anim Hosp Assoc 2003;39:67–71.
11. Mixson AJ, Friedman TC, Katz DA, et al. Thyrotropin-secreting pituitary carcinoma. J Clin Endocrinol Metab 1993;76:529–33.

12. Brucker-Davis F, Oldfield EH, Skarulis MC, et al. Thyrotropin-secreting pituitary tumors: diagnostic criteria, thyroid hormone sensitivity, and treatment outcome in 25 patients followed at the National Institutes of Health. J Clin Endocrinol Metab 1999;84:476–86.
13. Peterson ME, Randolph JF, Mooney CT. Endocrine diseases. In: Sherding RG, editor. The cat: diseases and clinical management. 2nd edition. New York: Churchill Livingston Inc; 1994. p. 1403–506.
14. Thoday KL, Mooney CT. Historical, clinical and laboratory features of 126 hyperthyroid cats. Vet Rec 1992;131:257–64.
15. Mooney CT. Feline hyperthyroidism. In: Ettinger SJ, Feldman EC, editors. Textbook of veterinary internal medicine: diseases of the dog and the cat. 7th edition. St Louis (MO): Elsevier Saunders; 2010. p. 1761–79.
16. Broome MR. Thyroid scintigraphy in hyperthyroidism. Clin Tech Small Anim Pract 2006;21:10–6.
17. Peterson RR, Young WC. The problem of placental permeability for thyrotrophin, propylthiouracil and thyroxine in the guinea pig. Endocrinology 1952;50:218–25.
18. Brandao J, Manickam B, Blas-Machado U, et al. Productive thyroid follicular carcinoma in a wild barred owl (*Strix varia*). J Vet Diagn Invest 2012;24:1145–50.
19. Hernandez-Divers SJ, Knott CD, MacDonald J. Diagnosis and surgical treatment of thyroid adenoma-induced hyperthyroidism in a green iguana (*Iguana iguana*). J Zoo Wildl Med 2001;32:465–75.
20. Boyer T, Wallack S, Bettencourt A, et al. Hyperthyroidism in a leopard gecko, *Eublepharis macularius*, and radioiodine (I-131) treatment. Proc Assoc Reptilian Amphibian Vets, South Padre Island, TX 2010;53.
21. Ewringmann A, Glöckner B. Leitsymptome bei Meerschweinchen, Chinchilla und Degu. Diagnostischer Leitfaden und Therapie. 1st edition. Stuttgart (Germay): Enke publishing; 2005.
22. Gibbons PM, Garner MM, Kiupel M. Morphological and immunohistochemical characterization of spontaneous thyroid gland neoplasms in guinea pigs (*Cavia porcellus*). Vet Pathol 2012. [Epub ahead of print].
23. Mayer J, Wagner R, Taeymans O. Advanced diagnostic approaches and current management of thyroid pathologies in Guinea pigs. Vet Clin North Am Exot Anim Pract 2010;13:509–23.
24. Muller K, Muller E, Klein R, et al. Serum thyroxine concentrations in clinically healthy pet guinea pigs (Cavia porcellus). Vet Clin Pathol 2009;38:507–10.
25. Fredholm DV, Cagle LA, Johnston MS. Evaluation of precision and establishment of reference ranges for plasma thyroxine using a point-of-care analyzer in healthy guinea pigs (*Cavia porcellus*). J Exot Pet Med 2012;21:87–93.
26. Brown-Grant K, Pethes G. The response of the thyroid gland of the guinea-pig to stress. J Physiol 1960;151:40–50.
27. Scott-Moncrieff JC. Hypothyroidism. In: Ettinger SJ, Feldman EC, editors. Textbook of veterinary internal medicine: diseases of the dog and the cat. 7th edition. St Louis (MO): Elsevier Saunders; 2010. p. 1751–61.
28. Chopra IJ. Clinical review 86: euthyroid sick syndrome: is it a misnomer? J Clin Endocrinol Metab 1997;82:329–34.
29. Castro MI, Alex S, Young RA, et al. Total and free serum thyroid hormone concentrations in fetal and adult pregnant and nonpregnant guinea pigs. Endocrinology 1986;118:533–7.
30. Beaton GH, Hellebust DM, Paul W, et al. The effect of scurvy on thyroid activity in the guinea pig. J Nutr 1960;70:321–8.
31. Taeymans O. Thyroid ultrasound in dogs: a review. Ultrasound 2009;17:137–43.

32. Taeymans O, Penninck DG, Peters RM. Comparison between clinical, ultrasound, CT, MRI, and pathology findings in dogs presented for suspected thyroid carcinoma. Vet Radiol Ultrasound 2013;54(1):61–70.

33. Gough IR, Wilkinson D. Total thyroidectomy for management of thyroid disease. World J Surg 2000;24:962–5.

34. Efremidou EI, Papageorgiou MS, Liratzopoulos N, et al. The efficacy and safety of total thyroidectomy in the management of benign thyroid disease: a review of 932 cases. Can J Surg 2009;52:39–44.

35. Cheung CC, Ezzat S, Freeman JL, et al. Immunohistochemical diagnosis of papillary thyroid carcinoma. Mod Pathol 2001;14:338–42.

36. Patnaik AK, Lieberman PH. Gross, histologic, cytochemical, and immunocytochemical study of medullary thyroid carcinoma in sixteen dogs. Vet Pathol 1991;28:223–33.

37. Prasad ML, Pellegata NS, Huang Y, et al. Galectin-3, fibronectin-1, CITED-1, HBME1 and cytokeratin-19 immunohistochemistry is useful for the differential diagnosis of thyroid tumors. Mod Pathol 2005;18:48–57.

38. Ramos-Vara JA, Miller MA, Johnson GC, et al. Immunohistochemical detection of thyroid transcription factor-1, thyroglobulin, and calcitonin in canine normal, hyperplastic, and neoplastic thyroid gland. Vet Pathol 2002;39:480–7.

39. Lass P, Kaniuka S. Feline hyperthyroidism. The contribution of nuclear medicine. Hell J Nucl Med 2005;8:145–8.

40. Muller AF, Berghout A, Wiersinga WM, et al. Thyroid function disorders—guidelines of the Netherlands Association of Internal Medicine. Neth J Med 2008;66:134–42.

41. Beaufrere H, Sickafoose L. Abscesses. In: Oglesbee B, editor. Blackwell's five-minute veterinary consult: small mammals. Chichester (West Sussex): Wiley-Blackwell; 2011. p. 26–228.

42. Tully TN. Cervical lymphadenitis. In: Oglesbee B, editor. Blackwoll'o fivo minute veterinary consult: small mammals. Chichester (West Sussex): Wiley-Blackwell; 2011. p. 240–2.

43. Antinoff N. Weight Loss and cachexia. In: Oglesbee B, editor. Blackwell's five-minute veterinary consult: small mammals. Chichester (West Sussex): Wiley-Blackwell; 2011. p. 342–3.

44. Cooper DS. Antithyroid drugs. N Engl J Med 2005;352:905–17.

45. Benker G, Reinwein D. Pharmacokinetics of antithyroid drugs. Klin Wochenschr 1982;60:531–9.

46. Rivkees SA, Sklar C, Freemark M. Clinical review 99: the management of Graves' disease in children, with special emphasis on radioiodine treatment. J Clin Endocrinol Metab 1998;83:3767–76.

47. Owunwanne A, Omu A, Patel M, et al. Placental binding and transfer of radiopharmaceuticals: technetium-99 m d, 1-HMPAO. J Nucl Med 1998;39:1810–3.

48. Barber LG. Thyroid tumors in dogs and cats. Vet Clin North Am Small Anim Pract 2007;37:755–73, vii.

49. Mayer MN, MacDonald VS. External beam radiation therapy for thyroid cancer in the dog. Can Vet J 2007;48:761–3.

50. Pack L, Roberts RE, Dawson SD, et al. Definitive radiation therapy for infiltrative thyroid carcinoma in dogs. Vet Radiol Ultrasound 2001;42:471–4.

51. Brearley MJ, Hayes AM, Murphy S. Hypofractionated radiation therapy for invasive thyroid carcinoma in dogs: a retrospective analysis of survival. J Small Anim Pract 1999;40:206–10.

52. Mazzarotto R, Cesaro MG, Lora O, et al. The role of external beam radiotherapy in the management of differentiated thyroid cancer. Biomed Pharmacother 2000;54: 345–9.

53. Thrall DE. Biological principles of radiation therapy. In: Morrison WB, editor. Cancer in dogs and cats: medical and surgical management. 2nd edition. Baltimore (MD): Williams & Wilkins; 1998. p. 375–88.
54. Brierley JD, Tsang RW. External-beam radiation therapy in the treatment of differentiated thyroid cancer. Semin Surg Oncol 1999;16:42–9.
55. Kromka MC, Hoar RM. An improved technic for thyroidectomy in guinea pigs. Lab Anim Sci 1975;25:82–4.
56. Birchard SJ. Thyroidectomy and parathyroidectomy in the dog and cat. Probl Vet Med 1991;3:277–89.
57. Walter WG, Baldwin DE. Observations on the parathyroid glands of guinea pigs affected with metastatic calcification. Can J Comp Med Vet Sci 1963;27: 140–6.
58. Peterson ME. Radioiodine treatment of hyperthyroidism. Clin Tech Small Anim Pract 2006;21:34–9.
59. Harvey AM, Hibbert A, Barrett EL, et al. Scintigraphic findings in 120 hyperthyroid cats. J Feline Med Surg 2009;11:96–106.
60. Fadel BM, Ellahham S, Ringel MD, et al. Hyperthyroid heart disease. Clin Cardiol 2000;23:402–8.
61. Klein I, Danzi S. Thyroid disease and the heart. Circulation 2007;116:1725–35.
62. Hoey A, Page A, Brown L, et al. Cardiac changes in experimental hyperthyroidism in dogs. Aust Vet J 1991;68:352–5.
63. Piatnek-Leunissen D, Olson RE. Cardiac failure in the dog as a consequence of exogenous hyperthyroidism. Circ Res 1967;20:242–52.
64. Bacuzzi A, Dionigi G, Del Bosco A, et al. Anaesthesia for thyroid surgery: perioperative management. Int J Surg 2008;6(Suppl 1):S82–5.
65. Sarlis NJ, Gourgiotis L. Thyroid emergencies. Rev Endocr Metab Disord 2003;4: 129–36.
66. Tolbert MK, Ward CR. Feline focus-feline thyroid storm: rapid recognition to improve patient survival. Compend Contin Educ Vet 2010;32:E1–6.
67. Ward CR. Feline thyroid storm. Vet Clin North Am Small Anim Pract 2007;37: 745–54, vii.
68. Yoon SJ, Kim DM, Kim JU, et al. A case of thyroid storm due to thyrotoxicosis factitia. Yonsei Med J 2003;44:351–4.
69. Hawkins MG, Bishop CR. Disease problems of guinea pigs. In: Quesenberry KE, Carpenter JW, editors. Ferrets, rabbits, and rodents: clinical medicine and surgery. 3rd edition. St Louis (MO): Elsevier/Saunders; 2012. p. 295–310.
70. Rapsch Dahinden C, Klawitter A, Sagawe J, et al. [Course of Osteodystrophia fibrosa generalisata in a Satin guinea pig]. Schweiz Arch Tierheilkd 2009;151: 233–7 [in German].
71. Schwarz T, Stork CK, Megahy IW, et al. Osteodystrophia fibrosa in two guinea pigs. J Am Vet Med Assoc 2001;219:63–6, 49.
72. Reimers TJ. Hormones. In: Loeb WF, Quimby FW, editors. The clinical chemistry of laboratory animals. 2nd edition. Philadelphia: Taylor & Francis; 1999. p. 455–99.
73. Yamasaki M. Comparative anatomical studies on the thyroid and thymic arteries. III. Guinea pig (*Cavia cobaya*). J Anat 1995;186(Pt 2):383–93.
74. Zabel M, Surdyk J, Biela-Jacek I. Immunocytochemical study of the distribution of S-100 protein in the parathyroid gland of rats and guinea pigs. Histochemistry 1986;86:97–9.
75. DePaolo LV, Masoro EJ. Endocrine hormones in laboratory animals. In: Loeb WF, Quimby FW, editors. The clinical chemistry of laboratory animals. 1st edition. New York: Pergamon Press; 1989. p. 279–308.

76. Motomura Y, Chijiiwa Y, Iwakiri Y, et al. Interactive mechanisms among pituitary adenylate cyclase-activating peptide, vasoactive intestinal peptide, and parathyroid hormone receptors in guinea pig cecal circular smooth muscle cells. Endocrinology 1998;139:2869–78.

77. Kline LW, Benishin CG, Pang PK. Parathyroid hormone (PTH) and parathyroid hormone-related protein (PTHrP) relax cholecystokinin-induced tension in guinea pig gallbladder strips. Regul Pept 2000;91:83–8.

78. Feldman EC, Nelson RW. Hypercalcemia and primary hyperthyroidism. In: Feldman EC, Nelson RW, editors. Canine and feline endocrinology and reproduction. 3rd edition. St Louis (MO): Saunders; 2004. p. 659–715.

79. O'Dell BL, Morris ER, Pickett EE, et al. Diet composition and mineral balance in guinea pigs. J Nutr 1957;63:65–77.

80. Hollamby S. Rodents: neurological and musculoskeletal disorders. In: Keeble E, Meredith A, editors. BSAVA manual of rodents and ferrets. Gloucester (United Kingdom): British Small Animal Veterinary Association; 2009. p. 161–8.

81. Khedr NF, El-Ashmawy NE, El-Bahrawy HA, et al. Modulation of bone turnover in orchidectomized rats treated with raloxifene and risedronate. Fundam Clin Pharmacol 2012. [Epub ahead of print].

82. Binah O, Rubinstein I, Gilat E. Effects of thyroid hormone on the action potential and membrane currents of guinea pig ventricular myocytes. Pflugers Arch 1987; 409:214–6.

83. Anderson RR, Nixon DA, Akasha MA. Total and free thyroxine and triiodothyronine in blood serum of mammals. Comp Biochem Physiol A Comp Physiol 1988;89: 401–4.

84. Quimby FW. The clinical chemistry of laboratory animals. 2nd edition. Philadelphia: Taylor & Francis; 1999.

Gastrointestinal Disease in Guinea Pigs and Rabbits

Julie DeCubellis, DVM, MS[a],

Jennifer Graham, DVM, DABVP (Avian/Exotic Companion Mammal), DACZM[a,b],*

KEYWORDS

- Gastrointestinal disease • Rabbit • Guinea pig • Stasis • Enteritis • GDV
- Liver torsion

KEY POINTS

- Dental disease is a commonly encountered problem in guinea pigs and rabbits.
- Even minor changes in the diet or digestive process can lead to significant gastrointestinal (GI) disease in guinea pigs and rabbits.
- Diarrheal disease is common and frequently results from alterations in intestinal microflora balance.
- Several cases of dilatation have been documented in guinea pigs.
- Rabbits secrete higher levels of gastric acid and pepsin than do rats and guinea pigs, likely contributing to their higher incidence of gastric ulceration.
- Signs of lead toxicity in rabbits include neurologic presentations, such as seizures, torticollis, and blindness, but more common signs may be nonspecific and include anemia, anorexia, loss of body condition, and GI stasis.
- One of the authors has documented 16 cases of liver torsion in rabbits at a single referral institution in 5 years.

DENTAL DISEASE, GASTROINTESTINAL STASIS, AND DYSBIOSIS IN GUINEA PIGS AND RABBITS

Dental disease is a commonly encountered problem in guinea pigs and rabbits. Guinea pig and rabbit teeth are elodont (continuously growing/erupting), aradicular (open rooted), and hypsodont (long-crowned) and contain incisors and cheek teeth (premolars and molars). With insufficient wear, particularly from low-fiber, low-abrasion diets,

The authors have nothing to disclose.

[a] Department of Zoological Companion Animal Medicine, Cummings School of Veterinary Medicine, Tufts University, 200 Westboro Road, North Grafton, MA 01536, USA; [b] Department of Comparative Medicine, University of Washington School of Medicine, 1959 Northeast Pacific Street, Seattle, WA 98195, USA

* Corresponding author. Department of Zoological Companion Animal Medicine, Cummings School of Veterinary Medicine, Tufts University, 200 Westboro Road, North Grafton, MA 01536, USA.

E-mail address: Jennifer.Graham@Tufts.edu

molar crowns elongate and alter the slope of the occlusal plane, eventually creating sharp points that inhibit closure, often resulting in secondary incisor elongation.[1] Malocclusion also results from diets deficient in vitamin C in guinea pigs because it is critical for gingival health and anchoring of teeth. Trauma, infection, and genetics are also implicated. Dental disease can lead to oral ulcerations, infection, abscess formation, and tongue entrapment in guinea pigs. Guinea pigs are more sensitive to subtle occlusal changes than rabbits, and even mild disease can lead to anorexia and malnutrition.[2] Buccal ulcerations generally form along the upper arcades and lingual ulcerations along the lower arcades in rabbits. Congenital deformities can also result in malocclusion and produce dental disease at several months of age. In rabbits with mandibular prognathism, most commonly seen in dwarf rabbits, misalignment causes overgrowth of unopposed incisors, with upper incisors curving inward and upward toward the roof of the mouth and lower incisors curving outward and upward, sometimes into the upper lip or nose.[1,3,4]

Clinical signs of primary dental disease include anorexia, dysphagia, excessive salivation and drooling, weight loss, emaciation, and changes in fecal appearance and quantity. The presence of facial masses, excessive swelling, exophthalmos, and purulent nasal discharge suggests secondary infection/abscess formation. Animals with anorexia or dysphagia from a systemic disease, or with ocular disease restricting feeding, can develop secondary dental disease.[4] Diagnosis requires a routine physical examination, including thorough oral examination of the incisors, cheek teeth, periapical structures, bone, tongue, and oral mucosa. Complete dental examinations require extraoral radiographic studies from multiple projections (lateral, obliques, ventrodorsal, and rostrocaudal) using high-definition (mammography) film[5] as well as a thorough examination with patients under anesthesia, assisted by oral endoscopy, when available.[6] Diagnosis of periapical disease and abscess can be aided by CT, when available.[7]

Dental correction involves shortening of overgrown teeth, restoring the occlusal plane, extracting any diseased teeth, and treating abscessation. Dental procedures[8] and anesthetic and analgesic considerations[4,8,9] have recently been reviewed. Surgical treatment must be combined with medical therapy to manage pain, restore health (hydration, diet correction, and vitamin C supplementation for guinea pigs), and minimize infection as well as the risk of postoperative GI stasis.[2] Long-term management of dental disease includes providing a high-fiber diet with Timothy grass hay (ad lib),[10] adequate vitamin C for guinea pigs (10–30 mg/d), and regular rechecks with tooth trimming as needed.

Guinea pigs are less prone than rabbits to develop periapical infections and osteomyelitis, although they frequently present with more advanced disease and poor prognosis.[11] Periapical infection, abscessation and/or osteomyelitis of the surrounding bones are common sequelae in rabbits with dental disease. Treatment typically requires extraction, opening and excising an entire abscess capsule, careful débridement of bone, marsupialization with secondary closure, and packing the surgical site. Antibiotic therapy should be based on culture and sensitivity results and can include combinations of oral and/or injectable agents as well as impregnated beads.[11]

GASTROINTESTINAL HYPOMOTILITY AND STASIS

GI stasis is a common problem in guinea pigs and rabbits. The GI tract is specialized for its high-fiber herbivorous diet; even minor changes in the diet or digestive process can lead to significant GI disease. GI stasis has a multifactorial etiology. In animals receiving an adequate diet, GI stasis can result from reduced intake secondary to one of several or a combination of factors causing anorexia, including dental disease, dysphagia, pain, anxiety, environmental changes, infection, dysbiosis, neoplasia, chronic disease, drug effects (anesthetics, anticholinergics, opioids, and antibiotics), obstruction/foreign bodies, and accidental or forced restriction (preoperative fasting). Restricted water intake and activity also impair adequate processing of dietary fiber and promote stasis. In addition to reducing intake, chronic stress causes increased catecholamine signaling, acting on the enteric nervous system to impair intestinal motility. Once initiated, dysmotility leads to reduced colonic transit, with decreased fecal output, increased dehydration of intestinal contents, dehydration of gastric contents with trichobezoar formation, impaired cecal fermentation, and disruption of the enteric microflora, creating a cycle of further anorexia and worsening stasis.[12,13] In severe cases, stasis leads to partial or complete obstruction or accumulation of gas within the GI tract (bloat) that can be a life-threatening emergency (discussed later). Clinical signs of GI stasis can include decreased or absent fecal material, anorexia, bruxism, pain with abdominal palpation, decreased GI sounds, dehydration, abdominal distension, gastric tympany, and respiratory or cardiovascular compromise.[14] Severely ill rabbits progress to hypovolemic shock with reduced blood pressure and altered mentation.

Diagnosis requires a thorough history, physical examination, and abdominal imaging (radiographs and/or ultrasound). Radiographic studies of the abdomen in 2 views are essential for examining gastric contents, colonic fecal contents, and, most importantly, severe gas/fluid accumulation suggestive of obstruction, which constitutes a surgical emergency.[15] Trichobezoars are an uncommon cause of stasis in guinea pigs but also require surgical intervention.[16] Laboratory studies (complete blood cell count, biochemistry, and urinalysis) can be helpful for determination of an underlying cause of anorexia, but most have only nonspecific findings of dehydration or possibly elevated hepatic enzymes from developing hepatic lipidosis.[17]

Routine GI stasis is treated with comprehensive supportive care (aggressive fluid hydration, pain management, and assisted nutrition) best performed in a hospital setting for close monitoring. Animals should be kept warm in a dark, quiet place to minimize stress. Fluid replacement is achieved with warmed fluids (25–35 mL/kg every 8 hours) and can be given orally or subcutaneously [SC]), although animals with severe dehydration require more aggressive intravenous (IV) fluids. Anxiety can be minimized with injectable midazolam (0.25–0.5 mg/kg IV/intramuscular [IM]) and pain controlled with analgesics, such as buprenorphine (0.01–0.05 mg/kg, IM or SC every 4–6 hours), which can later be transitioned to meloxicam after adequate hydration (0.2 mg/kg IM/SC/by mouth every 24 hours in guinea pigs and 0.2–1 mg/kg IM/SC/by mouth every 24 hours in rabbits). Once obstruction has been ruled out, prokinetic agents, including metoclopramide (0.5 mg/kg SC/by mouth every 8–12 hours) and/or cisapride (0.5 mg/kg by mouth every 8–12 hours) can be used. Simethicone (20 mg/kg by mouth every 8–12 hours) can be used to reduce gas distension and ranitidine (2 mg/kg IV every 24 hours, 2–5 mg/kg by mouth every 12 hours) used in cases with prolonged anorexia where gastric ulceration is likely. Nutritional support is essential and can be performed by syringe feeding (15 mL/kg every 8 hours) of an herbivore critical care formulation. Prolonged nutritional support can be provided by nasogastric tube. Antibiotics should only be used in cases complicated by enterotoxemia and bacterial enteritis.[17–19]

Dysbiosis and Antibiotic-associated Enterotoxemia

Diarrheal disease is common and frequently results from alterations in the intestinal microflora balance,[20] or dysbiosis, ranging from mild changes causing soft stools, to pathogenic bacterial overgrowth with more significant enteritis, to life-threatening enterotoxemia. The gut flora is sensitive to any type of environmental change. Frequent causes of dysbiosis include poor diet, hypomotility, stress, toxins, and antibiotic use. Low-fiber, high-carbohydrate diets are the primary risk factor for several reasons: (1) formation of dense masses that prohibit adequate digestion and sterilization by the low pH gastric juice and enzymes; (2) reduced hindgut motility (discussed previously), delaying clearance of luminal bacteria and fermentation byproducts, causing an altered cecal pH and fermentation environment that favors the growth of pathogenic species; and (3) carbohydrate-rich diets that provide a readily available source of luminal glucose for opportunistic organisms, such as *Escherichia coli* and *Clostridium* spp.[12,21] Systemic illness and stress, also acting to reduce motility, can precipitate dysbiosis. Indiscriminate antibiotic use, particularly with narrow-spectrum agents that selectively target beneficial gram-positive bacteria (penicillins, amoxicillin ± clavulanic acid, cephalosporins, ampicillin, clindamycin, and lincomycin), creates optimal conditions for overgrowth of pathogenic species. Chloramphenicol, trimethoprim/sulfas, and fluoroquinolones are least likely to damage the microflora, and there is a decreased risk with parenteral versus oral administration.[14,22]

Overgrowth of *C spiroforme* in rabbits causes an often-fatal enterotoxemia due to elaboration of bacterial toxin. Although adults with dysbiosis can develop enterotoxemia, weanlings are most susceptible due to their poorly established flora and high gastric pH. Newborns can also develop toxemia from toxin secreted into the milk of infected mothers.[12] Recently, it has been demonstrated that *C spiroforme* toxin (binary actin-ADP-ribosylating, iota-like toxin) gains access to enterocytes via the lipolysis-stimulated lipoprotein receptor, which is also used by the *C difficile* transferase and *C perfringes* iota toxins, causing a secretory diarrhea.[23,24] In acute infections, rabbits develop watery diarrhea, possibly with blood, that soils the perineum and legs. They become anorexic and decline over 2 to 4 days into a moribund state with hypovolemic shock, leading to death. On necropsy, the cecum, the primary reservoir for bacterial growth, is often covered with petechial and ecchymotic hemorrhage that can spread into the appendix and proximal colon. The mucosa can also contain hemorrhage, thick mucus, gas, or pseudomembranes.[25]

In young rabbits (7–14 weeks of age), bacterial dysbiosis and resultant cecal hyperacidity can lead to the proliferation of enteric goblet cells with voluminous mucus production, causing a mucoid enteritis.[26] Although the exact cause is unclear, the disease is predominantly found in intense breeding colonies and is uncommon in pet rabbits. Affected animals have anorexia and develop lethargy, weight loss, and cecal impaction.[25]

Clinical symptoms of antibiotic associated enterotoxemia begin 1 to 5 days after antibiotic administration, and include anorexia, dehydration, and hypothermia; diarrhea may or may not be present. Diagnosis is based on clinical history and clinical signs and can be confirmed with polymerase chain reaction or ELISA-based commercial tests for *C difficile* toxin. Treatment of dysbiosis/enteritis/enterotoxemia involves aggressive supportive care and correction of hypomotility. Correction of dehydration and nutritional deficiencies are critical, as is providing a warm, safe environment with adequate analgesia. For cases of enteritis caused by bacterial overgrowth, fecal bacterial culture and sensitivity can be helpful to guide antiobiotic therapy with broad-spectrum agents, including trimethoprim-sulfamethoxazole (30 mg/kg by mouth every 12 hours) or enrofloxacin (15 mg/kg by mouth every 24 hours). For enterotoxemia, a dual approach of metronidazole (20 mg/kg every 12 hours) and cholestyramine (2 g/20 mL water every 24 hours by gavage) can be used to treat *Clostridium* infection and bind its toxin, although *C spiroforme* has widespread intrinsic and acquired antimicrobial resistance.[27,28] Chloramphenicol (50 mg/kg by mouth every

8 hours) can be used to attempt to suppress *Clostridial* overgrowth.[14,22] Preventing dysbiosis with a high-fiber diet and reducing stress is key to prevention. Attempts to correct the dysbiosis have anecdotal success, including transfaunation and commercial probiotics containing *Lactobacillus* spp, although controlled studies to document their utility are lacking.[29] Exterotoxemia is best avoided by judicious antibiotic use in guinea pigs and rabbits.

Gastrointestinal Disease in the Guinea Pig

Gastric dilation and volvulus

GI stasis can result in the accumulation of gas within the GI tract (bloat), particularly in the stomach and cecum, prompting a surgical emergency. Gastric dilation-volvulus (GDV) is a rare, life-threatening complication of this gas accumulation, with such a high mortality that is frequently diagnosed at necropsy. Although far less common than in other species (human, canine, and swine), several cases have been documented in guinea pigs,[30–33] many involving breeding females in laboratory colonies. The authors have had 3 recent cases of GDV in guinea pigs at their institution (**Fig. 1**).

Clinical signs of gastric dilation are similar to those found with GI stasis, although more severe symptoms, such as dyspnea, cyanosis, tachycardia, and cardiovascular shock, may also be present.[30] When gastric tympany is present and/or there is evidence of gastric dilation on imaging, decompression is achieved by passing a large red rubber tube into the stomach through the oral cavity. A needle used as a trocar can be passed percutaneously, although this carries a risk of gastric or cecal rupture or peritonitis. If GDV is suspected, emergent surgical intervention is required to reduce the volvulus. After surgical intervention, medical management per GI stasis is used. Simethicone can be used to enhance gas absorption but only after aggressive hydration to avoid a potential foreign body from dehydrated simethicone.[18]

Bacterial enteritis

Although dietary factors (low fiber and excess carbohydrates) can cause soft stools in all guinea pigs, diarrhea from bacterial enteritis is usually seen in weanlings, pregnant sows, and immunocompromised/chronically stressed adults. The most common cause is *C piliforme* (Tyzzer disease), transmitted by fecal-oral route. Infected animals progress rapidly from onset of lethargy, anorexia, and diarrhea to acute death. Antemortem diagnosis is generally not possible because *C piliforme* is an intracellular bacterium that does not grow in culture. At necropsy, infections are marked by intestinal inflammation

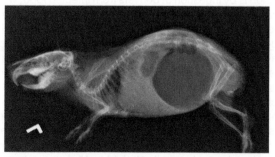

Fig. 1. Lateral radiographic projection of a guinea with a caudally displaced gastric dilatation volvulus. There is also mineralized material in the caudal region suggestive of urolithiasis. The owners declined emergency surgery and this guinea pig died within 3 hours of instituting supportive care measures.

and patchy hepatic necrosis. Treatment has not proved beneficial, and prevention is best achieved by good husbandry and stress reduction, especially during weaning.[14,34]

Salmonellosis from *S typhimurium* and *S enteritidis* are less-frequent causes of bacterial enteritis but are highly lethal with greater than 50% mortality. Transmission is generally from contaminated food or water, although fecal transmission also occurs. Infected animals exhibit anorexia, weight loss, light-colored feces with or without diarrhea, weakness, depression, and poor grooming. Infected pregnant sows have a high incidence of abortion. Physical examination frequently reveals hepatosplenomegaly (with punctate necrotic foci in the viscera at necropsy) and conjunctivitis. Salmonella can be cultured from the feces. Because infected animals can become asymptomatic carriers of this zoonotic disease, treatment is not recommended. Preventive measures include thorough disinfection of the environment and proper storage and washing of all fresh fruits and vegetables offered.[14,35]

Other causes of bacterial enteritis include *Yersinia pseudotuberculosis*, *E coli*, *C perfringes*, *Pseudomonas aeruginosa*, *Citrobacter freundii*, *Listeria monocytogenes*, and *Lawsonia intracellularis*. *Y pseudotuberculosis* can cause distinct clinical presentations: an acute, rapidly fatal (28–48 h) septicemic form; a chronic diarrheal disease with wasting and death within weeks; and a nonfatal infection marked by abscesses of the head and neck lymph nodes. *Y pseudotuberculosis* can also cause abscess formation in the ileum, cecum, mesenteric lymph nodes, liver, and omentum. Treatment is not advised, because it can induce an asymptomatic carrier state and promote zoonotic transmission.[22,35] *E coli* infection/overgrowth is particularly virulent in weanlings and is marked by anorexia, diarrhea, depression, wasting, and death. At necropsy, yellow fluid and gas are found in the intestines, and there is often focal hepatic necrosis.[35] *L intracellularis* is most often found in swine but can also infect rodents, including guinea pigs. The intracellular organism infects enteric epithelial cells, causing a proliferative enteropathy marked by diarrhea, wasting, and eventual death.[36]

Parasitic disease

GI helminth infections are predominately due to the guinea pig roundworm, *Paraspidodera uncinata*. The nematode develops and resides in the cecum and colon but does not invade the mucosa. Typical oxyurid eggs are shed in the feces, and ingestion leads to infection within 3 to 5 days. Infections are often mild and subclinical, although heavy infections lead to anorexia, diarrhea, weight loss, and poor coat. Treatment is with ivermectin (0.2 mg/kg SC) and prevention by effective sanitation.[22,34]

Cryptosporidium wrairi is a protozoan that targets the small intestine epithelial brush border. Transmission is by ingestion of oocysts from infected food, water, and fomites. Infections are marked by diarrhea, weight loss, rectal prolapse, potbellied appearance, and a greasy coat. Although immunocompetent animals generally recover within 4 weeks and develop resistance, weanlings, juveniles, and immunosuppressed animals often have a more severe course with mortality approaching 50%. Oocysts can be diagnosed on fecal examination, and organisms may be seen on histopathology. Oocysts can be destroyed with 5% ammonia or extremes of temperature. Cryptosporiodosis is potentially zoonotic.

Eimeria caviae is an intestinal coccidian of guinea pigs that is generally nonpathogenic but can cause significant disease in weanlings. Infections are more common in breeding colonies due to overcrowding, poor husbandry, and concurrent disease. Watery diarrhea and pasty stools usually start 10 to 13 days postexposure to oocysts and can last 4 to 5 days. This is accompanied by anorexia and lethargy and is frequently fatal. Fecal analysis can provide a diagnosis, and treatment with sulphonamides is effective when combined with sanitation (10% ammonia kills oocysts) and housing improvements.[37] *Balantidium caviae*, *Trichomonas caviae*, and *Giardia duo-denalis* are other generally nonpathogenic protozoans found in guinea pigs.

Fecal impaction

Fecal impaction is predominately identified in older guinea pigs, especially boars. The exact cause is unknown, but inguinal gland infections, loss of muscle tone, and reduced coprophagy have all been implicated. Animals present with straining and have a large, foul-smelling impacted mass of feces and sebaceous secretions within a large, flaccid vent opening. Therapeutic interventions include dietary changes to increase fiber, mineral oil, and repeated manual evacuations using a cotton-tipped applicator. Long-term therapy is generally required.[14,22]

Hepatic lipidosis

Hepatic lipidosis is a rapidly developing, fatal complication of anorexia, especially in obese guinea pigs. A pathogenic mobilization and uptake of fatty acids for glucose generation is a likely cause, although the mechanisms are unclear. Significant hepatic damage can occur within 48 hours; thus, anorexia for 12 hours or more is an emergency requiring nutritional support.[14]

Neoplasia

Neoplasms of the GI tract are rare in guinea pigs but can mimic clinical findings of more common GI disorders. Lymphosarcomas, adenocarcinomas of the stomach and cecum, and GI stromal tumors have been reported.[38]

Gastrointestinal Disease in the Rabbit

Gastric ulceration

Rabbits secrete higher levels of gastric acid and pepsin than do rats and guinea pigs, likely contributing to their higher incidence of gastric ulceration.[39] In a review of 1000 rabbit postmortem examinations, Hinton[40] reported 7.3% with gastric ulcers. The majority occurred in the fundus and without significant surrounding reaction, suggesting a stress response to other illness. The link between stress and ulcers can be experimentally demonstrated in rabbits by intraperitoneal injections of epinephrine, because rabbits serve as a model organism for ulcers.[41] Similarly, hypovolemic shock can induce gastric ulcers in rabbits in a matter of hours.[42] In Hinton's review, 2% of the rabbits had solitary peptic ulcers, the majority of which were perforated and found in females dying in the peripartum period.[40]

Rabbits with gastric ulcers frequently present with anorexia and evidence of pain, such as bruxism. In more severe or perforated disease there may be clinical signs of anemia and shock. Physical examination may reveal acute abdomen with peritoneal signs. Radiographic imaging or ultrasonography is helpful to eliminate other causes, such as obstruction, neoplasia, or foreign body. Although endoscopy can provide direct visualization of ulcers, many animals are not sufficiently stable for an anesthetized procedure.[13] Treatment should be aimed at controlling any underlying diseases, providing hydration and analgesia (discussed previously), mucosal protection with sucralfate, and acid blockade with ranitidine (2 mg/kg IV every 24 hours or 2–5 mg/kg by mouth every 12 hours).

Cecal impaction

Altered cecocolonic motility, as well as diets high in fine-particle indigestible fiber (such as psyllium), can cause dehydration and compaction of cecal and colonic contents into hard lumps, or cecoliths. Cecoliths are the most common cause of lower intestinal obstruction, most frequently in the sacculated colon. Frequently, this is a chronic problem and rabbits have a history of anorexia, abdominal pain, and failure to thrive. Many are also positive for *Encephalitozoon cuniculi*, suggesting a possible link.[12]

Clinical presentation correlates with severity of the obstruction and ranges from anorexia and abdominal pain to moribund animals requiring emergent attention. Cecoliths are readily palpable on physical examination, and abdominal imaging is helpful to gauge intestinal obstruction. Treatment involves SC or IV fluid therapy, analgesia (buprenorphine, 0.03–0.05 mg/kg SC/IV every 6–12 hours), and careful enemas to advance fecal contents without destroying the damaged colonic mucosa. Animals should initially be fed foods with a high water content supplemented with grass hay for fiber and can later be supplemented with canned pumpkin (1 tbsp every 12 hours) to boost water content.[12]

Dysautonomia

Dysautonomia is a rare idiopathic, progressive loss of autonomic system function. It was successfully documented in the rabbit after studies of animals with presumed mucoid enteropathy.[43,44] Clinical features are consistent with autonomic dysfunctions, including dry mucous membranes, mydriasis, urinary incontinence, bradycardia, proprioceptive deficits, cecal impaction, and loss of anal sphincter tone. Anorexia and depression are common. A presumptive diagnosis is made by the clinical findings, and radiography is helpful to document megaesophagus, aspiration pneumonia, and a dilated, impacted colon. Definitive diagnosis requires histologic documentation of chromolytic degeneration of autonomic neurons. Supportive care is provided, although the prognosis is poor in rabbits.

Bacterial enteritis

Bacterial enteritis from enteropathogenic *E coli* can cause large outbreaks in weaning commercial rabbits but is not reported in pet rabbits. The bacteria attach to cecal and colonic epithelial cells and cause effacement of the surface microvilli, inhibiting colonic absorption and causing watery diarrhea. Severity depends on the age of the rabbit and serotype, although mortality can be more than 50%. On necropsy, the cecal wall may have characteristic longitudinal, paintbrush hemorrhages. A presumptive diagnosis is made by isolation of *E coli* on fecal cultures, although serotyping is not commercially available. Supportive care as well as antimicrobial therapy with trimethoprim-sulfamethoxazole (30 mg/kg by mouth every 12 hours) or enrofloxacin (10 mg/kg by mouth every 12 hours) pending culture sensitivity results.[45,46]

Enteritis caused by *C piliforme* (Tyzzer disease), a motile gram-variable spore-forming obligate intracellular bacterium, is found in many species of small mammals, including rabbits and guinea pigs. Infected animals, in particular weanlings, progress rapidly from onset of lethargy, anorexia, and watery diarrhea to acute death. Adults may have a more chronic course. Antemortem diagnosis is generally not possible because *C piliforme* is an intracellular bacterium that does not grow in culture. At necropsy, infections are marked by patchy necrosis in the liver and proximal colon and degenerative lesions of the myocardium. Treatment has not proved beneficial, and prevention is best achieved by disinfection (spores are killed with 0.3% sodium hypochlorite solution or 80°C heat for 30 min), good husbandry, and stress reduction, especially during weaning.[12]

Proliferative enteritis caused by *L intracellularis*, an intracellular, gram-negative, curved-to-spiraled bacterium, is most often found in swine but can also be found in rabbits and rodents. The intracellular organism infects enteric epithelial cells, causing a proliferative enteropathy marked by diarrhea and wasting.[36] It is most common in weanlings (2–4 months) and can be treated with chloramphenicol (30–50 mg/kg by mouth/SC every 12 hours for 7–14 days) because macrolide antibiotics, used to treat *L intracellularis* in other species, are not recommended for use in rabbits.[12]

Viral diseases

Oral papillomatosis Rabbit oral papillomatosis virus infection seems restricted to laboratory rabbits, especially New Zealand white rabbits, causing benign oral papillomas on the ventral surface of the tongue. Rarely, papillomas occur elsewhere in the mouth, and there is 1 report of a concomitant conjunctival papilloma.[47] Papillomas start as small millimeter-sized sessile lesions and can grow into larger (3–5 mm) clusters of pedunculated papules. The lesions are benign and can persist for as long as 145 days.[48]

Rabbit enteric coronavirus The virus was discovered as a cause of rapidly fatal enteritis in young (3–10 weeks) laboratory rabbits.[49] Infected rabbits develop lethargy, diarrhea, abdominal swelling, pleural effusion, and cardiomyopathy and invariably die within 24 hours. At necropsy, the intestine is fluid-filled and the villi are effaced. The virus has hemagglutination activity and can be detected in the feces. A divergent coronavirus strain has recently been identified in game rabbits in Asia.[50]

Rotavirus Rotavirus is highly infectious with a high morbidity and variable (generally low) mortality. Weanling rabbits (2–4 months) are most susceptible, and disease severity is increased with coinfection with another enteric pathogen.[51] Antibodies to rotavirus are found in laboratory, commercial, and pet rabbits, indicating it can infect most strains.[52] Infection impairs the sodium solute pumps on the enterocyte surface, impairing reabsorption.[53] Rotavirus infections are marked by anorexia, dehydration, and green-yellow watery diarrhea. The intestines become distended and congested, with petechial hemorrhages, chronic inflammation, and villous atrophy. Diagnosis requires virus identification, and treatment is with supportive care.

Rabbit hemorrhagic disease virus This calicivirus of the genus *Lagovirus* affects only European rabbits. It was first described in China in 1984 and rapidly spread throughout Asia, Australia, and New Zealand and into Europe, with rare outbreaks in the United States and elsewhere.[54] Transmission is via direct contact (shed into urine, feces, and respiratory secretions), fomite contamination, and even by intermediate insect vectors. The disease occurs in rabbits over 2 months of age, in part due to its binding to the histo-blood group antigens H, A, and B type 2 oligosaccharides, which are present on the surface of mature respiratory and intestinal epithelial cells.[55] The virus replicates in the liver, causing severe hepatic necrosis and eventual death from disseminated intravascular coagulation. The clinical presentation and course varies from a peracute disease lasting only 12 to 36 hours, followed by sudden death, to an acute or subacute febrile illness with anorexia, diarrhea (or constipation), neurologic, and other systemic symptoms, lasting a few days to weeks, to a persistent/latent disease with continued virus shedding.

Laboratory studies demonstrate a worsening lymphopenia and thrombocytopenia, with eventual prolonged prothrombin and thrombin times. At necropsy, there is extensive hepatic necrosis, splenomegaly, pulmonary hemorrhage, and evidence of disseminated intravascular coagulation. The virus cannot be cultured; thus, diagnosis requires molecular testing.[54] Rabbit hemorrhagic disease virus is a reportable disease. Vaccination programs using attenuated vaccines have had mixed results. A recombinant vaccine has recently been developed and should assist prevention in endemic areas.[56] The virus can be inactivated with 0.5% sodium hypochlorite or 1% formalin.

Parasitic diseases

Coccidiosis Coccidia are the most common parasites of the rabbit GI tract and, although they cause significant disease in young (<6 months old) rabbits, they can be incidentally found in fecal studies in adult rabbits. Of the 12 species of the genus *Eimeria*, *E stiedae* is exclusive to the liver, with the rest causing intestinal disease. Hepatic coccidiosis is ubiquitous in commercial rabbitries and can be fatal in young rabbits by obstructing liver function. Severe disease is marked by anorexia, diarrhea, abdominal bloating, and icterus. Biochemical tests confirm hepatic disease, with aspartate aminotransferase, alanine aminotransferase, bile acids, and total bilirubin elevations. On necropsy, the liver is studded with nodular, encapsulated abscesses. Oocysts can be identified in bile or feces.

Intestinal coccidiosis is common in rabbits of all ages and most often associated with *E perforans* infection. Subclinical infection is common, and disease severity varies with age (worse under 6 months), species of *Eimeria*, parasite burden, and condition of the rabbit (stress, poor husbandry, and poor diet). Significant disease is marked by diarrhea with possible mucus or blood, dehydration, and weight loss. Intussusception is a complication of severe disease. Diagnosis depends on histopathology and/or fecal identification. Molecular assays have been developed to identify intestinal *Eimeria* spp.[57] In addition to supportive care, sulfa drugs are most effective at limiting multiplication. Sulfadimethoxine (15 mg/kg by mouth every 12 hours) or trimethoprim-sulfamethoxazole (30 mg/kg by mouth every 12 hours) can be used for 10 days of therapy. Recovering rabbits develop lifelong immunity.[12]

Cryptosporidiosis *Cryptosporidium parvum* infects the small intestine and causes a self-limited diarrheal illness (4–5 days duration) in young rabbits (peak, 30–40 days old). Illness is accompanied by anorexia, depression, and dehydration. The organism can be identified on histopathology. Other than supportive care, there is no effective treatment. Recently, reports of rabbit *Cryptosporidium* spp causing zoonotic disease in humans have been reported in several countries.[58]

Nematodes *Passalurus ambiguous*, the rabbit pinworm, is found in most rabbits, and even large parasite burdens are not pathogenic. Adult worms reside in the cecum and colon, and transmission is direct by ingestion of eggs during cecotrophy. Diagnosis is often routine by identification of worms or eggs in the feces, although identification should not prompt treatment in most cases. When treatment is necessary, benzimidazoles, such as fenbendazole (10–20 mg/kg by mouth, repeated in 10–14 days), are effective.[12]

Aflatoxicosis

Aflatoxins produced by the fungi, *Aspergillus flavus* and *Aspergillus parasiticus*, cause liver and biliary damage in rabbits. Rabbits are the most sensitive species to these toxins and serve as an animal model for aflatoxicosis.[59] Outbreaks occur from contaminated feed and are accompanied by anorexia, depression, and weight loss, progressing to icterus and death within 3 to 4 days.[60] On necropsy, livers are congested with periportal and ductal fibrosis, sinusoidal dilation, and hepatocyte degenerative changes. Treatment involves removal of contaminated feed and supportive care.

Neoplasia

GI neoplasms in rabbits include epithelial and smooth muscle tumors. Epithelial tumors include gastric adenocarcinoma, papilloma of the sacculus rotundus, papillomas of the rectal squamocolumnar junctional mucosa, and metastatic tumors, especially uterine adenocarcinoma. Smooth muscle tumors include leiomyoma and leiomyosarcoma of the stomach and intestines. Clinically, these tumors can present as intestinal obstruction.[61] Biliary tumors, such as bile duct adenoma and carcinoma, are reported in the rabbit.[62]

Lead Toxicity

Signs of lead toxicity in rabbits include neurologic presentations, such as seizures, torticollis, and blindness, but more common signs may be nonspecific and include anemia, anorexia, loss of body condition, and GI stasis.[63] Lead toxicity should be a differential in rabbits that chew baseboards or paint in older houses and have nucleated red cells or basophilic stippling on blood smears. Lead levels greater than 10 µg/dL are diagnostic for lead poisoning.[63] The authors diagnose at least 1 to 2 cases of lead toxicity in rabbits annually and signs usually involve GI stasis or loose stools (**Fig. 2**).[64] Affected rabbits can be treated with calcium ethylenediaminetetraacetic acid (30 mg/kg SC every 12 hours for 5–7 days) in addition to supportive care for GI stasis. Debilitated animals should be hospitalized for more intensive supportive care but stable animals can be treated at home with SC injections given by the owner. The source of lead should be determined and eliminated from the rabbit's environment to prevent further intoxication.

Colonic Entrapment

Partial colonic entrapment and chronic recurring GI stasis may result from adhesions after ovariohysterectomy.[64] Practitioners should keep this differential in mind if seeing a recently spayed female rabbit with recurring ileus. A mass effect may be palpated in the region of adhesions and colonic segments cranial to the area of entrapment may be dilated. Radiographs and ultrasound can be helpful to assess these patients and surgical exploratory is indicated in patients with significant disease. Due to the delicate nature of the rabbit intestinal tract, prognosis may be poor if there is significant accompanying colonic pathology.

Liver Lobe Torsion

One of the authors (JG) has documented 16 cases of liver torsion in rabbits at a single referral institution in 5 years.[64–66] Rabbits with this condition present with nonspecific signs of GI stasis and some have cranial abdominal pain or an abnormally placed liver lobe on abdominal palpation. Because signs can be nonspecific, it is advisable to perform blood work on all rabbits presenting with nonspecific signs of GI stasis. If liver enzymes are elevated, abdominal ultrasound is recommended. Ultrasound reveals lack of blood flow in the affected liver lobe on color flow Doppler (**Fig. 3**) and is diagnostic for liver lobe torsion. Prompt surgical removal of the affected lobe is advisable if

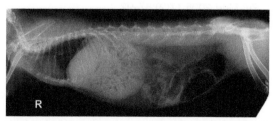

Fig. 2. Lateral radiographic projection of a rabbit with lead toxicosis (lead >65 µg/dL; normal <10 µg/dL). This rabbit presented with a 2-week history of diarrhea that had been refractory to antibiotic therapy by the referring veterinarian. Note that this radiograph is consistent with nonspecific GI stasis and no metallic densities are seen on the films.

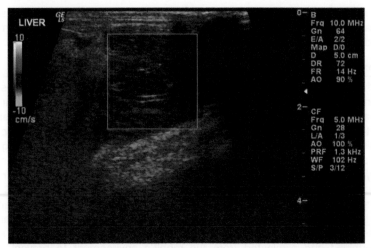

Fig. 3. Ultrasound image of a rabbit with a caudate liver lobe torsion. The box surrounds the torsed lobe and demonstrates a lack of blood flow in the affected liver lobe on color flow Doppler. Note the surrounding hyperechoic fat, a common finding seen on ultrasound of liver lobe torsions in rabbits.

the patient is stable for surgery.[65] If an owner declines surgery, supportive care measures alone (fluids, syringe feeding, prokinetic agents, analgesics, and antibiotics, if indicated) are still indicated. The author (JG) has documented survival in 3 of 6 rabbits with liver lobe torsion treated with supportive care measures alone.

REFERENCES

1. Reiter AM. Pathophysiology of dental disease in the rabbit, guinea pig, and chinchilla. J Exo Pet Med 2008;17(2):70–7.
2. Capello V. Diagnosis and treatment of dental disease in pet rodents. J Exo Pet Med 2008;17(2):114–23.
3. Harcourt-Brown FM. The progressive syndrome of acquired dental disease in rabbits. J Exo Pet Med 2007;16(3):146–57.
4. Lennox AM. Diagnosis and treatment of dental disease in pet rabbits. J Exo Pet Med 2008;17(2):107–13.
5. Gracis M. Clinical technique: normal dental radiography of rabbits, guinea pigs, and chinchillas. J Exo Pet Med 2008;17(2):78–86.
6. Hernandez-Divers SJ. Clinical technique: dental endoscopy of rabbits and rodents. J Exo Pet Med 2008;17(2):87–92.
7. Capello V, Cauduro A. Clinical technique: application of computed tomography for diagnosis of dental disease in the rabbit, guinea pig, and chinchilla. J Exo Pet Med 2008;17(2):93–101.
8. Lennox AM. Clinical technique: small exotic companion mammal dentistry–anesthetic considerations. J Exo Pet Med 2008;17(2):102–6.
9. Wenger S. Anesthesia and analgesia in rabbits and rodents. J Exo Pet Med 2012; 21(1):7–16.
10. Clauss M. Clinical technique: feeding hay to rabbits and rodents. J Exo Pet Med 2012;21(1):80–6.
11. Capello V. Clinical technique: treatment of periapical infections in pet rabbits and rodents. J Exo Pet Med 2008;17(2):124–31.

12. Olglesbee BL, Jenkins JR. Rabbits: gastrointestinal diseases. In: Quesenberry KE, Carpenter JW, editors. Ferrets, rabbits, and rodents: clinical medicine and surgery. 3rd edition. St Louis (MO): Saunders Elsevier; 2012. p. 193–204.
13. Reusch B. Rabbit gastroenterology. Veterinary Clin North Am Exot Anim Pract 2005;8(2):351–75.
14. Hawkins MG, Bishop CR. Disease problems of guinea pigs. In: Quesenberry KE, Carpenter JW, editors. Ferrets, rabbits, and rodents: clinical medicine and surgery. 3rd edition. St Louis (MO): Saunders Elsevier; 2012. p. 295–310.
15. Harcourt-Brown TR. Management of acute gastric dilation in rabbits. J Exo Pet Med 2007;16(3):168–74.
16. Theus M, Bitterli F, Foldenauer U. Successful treatment of a gastric trichobezoar in a Peruvian guinea pig (cavia aperea porcellus). J Exo Pet Med 2008;17(2):148–51.
17. Lichtenberger M, Lennox A. Updates and advanced therapies for gastrointestinal stasis in rabbits. Veterinary Clin North Am Exot Anim Pract 2010;3(3):525–41.
18. Hawkins MG, Graham JE. Emergency and critical care of rodents. Vet Clin North Am Exot Anim Pract 2007;10(2):501–31.
19. Tamura Y. Current approach to rodents and patients. J Exo Pet Med 2010;19(1):36–55.
20. Rosenthal KL, Harris J, Rankin S. Molecular analysis of the gastrointestinal microbiota of Oryctolagus cuniculus. Proceedings. In Proceedings of the Association of Avian Veterinarians (AAV)/Association of Exotic Mammal Veterinarians (AEMV) Annual Conference. Seattle (WA): AAV/AEMV; 2011. p. 153.
21. Johnson DH. The gastrointestinal tract of the rabbit: health and disease (part II). Proceedings. In: Proceeding of the American Board of Veterinary Practitioners (ABVP) Symposium. San Antonio (TX): ABVP; 2012.
22. Johnson DH. The gastrointestinal tract of the guinea pig: health and disease. Proceedings. In: Proceedings of the American Board of Veterinary Practitioners (ABVP) Symposium. San Antonio (TX): ABVP; 2012.
23. Xia Y, Hu HZ, Pothoulakis C, et al. Clostridium difficile toxin A excites enteric neurones and suppresses sympathetic neurotransmission in the guinea pig. Gut 2000;46(4):481–6.
24. Papatheodorou P, Wilczek C, Nölke T, et al. Identification of the cellular receptor of Clostridium spiroforme toxin. Infect Immun 2012;80(4):1418–23.
25. Harcourt-Brown F. Textbook of rabbit medicine. 1st edition. Oxford (UK): Alden Press; 2002. p. 284, 285.
26. Haligur M, Ozmen O, Demir N. Pathological and ultrastructural studies on mucoid enteropathy in new zealand rabbits. J Exo Pet Med 2009;18(3):224–8.
27. Lipman NS, Weischedel AK, Connars MJ, et al. Utilization of cholestyramine resin as a preventative treatment for antibiotic (clindamycin)-induced enterotoxaemia in the rabbit. Lab Anim 1992;26:1–8.
28. Agnoletti F, Ferro T, Guolo A, et al. A survey of Clostridium spiroforme antimicrobial susceptibility in rabbit breeding. Vet Microbiol 2009;136(1–2):188–91.
29. Wasson K, Criley JM, Clabaugh MB, et al. Therapeutic efficacy of oral lactobacillus preparation for antibiotic-associated enteritis in guinea pigs. Contemp Top Lab Anim Sci 2000;39(1):32–8.
30. Dudley ES, Boivin GP. Gastric volvulus in guinea pigs: comparison with other species. J Am Assoc Lab Anim Sci 2011;50(4):526–30.
31. Keith JC Jr, Rowles TK, Warwick KE, et al. Acute gastric distention in guinea pigs. Lab Anim Sci 1992;42(4):331–2.
32. Lee KJ, Johnson WD, Lang CM. Acute gastric dilation associated with gastric volvulus in the guinea pig. Lab Anim Sci 1977;27(5 Pt 1):685–6.

33. Mitchell EB, Hawkins MG, Gaffney PM, et al. Gastric dilation-volvulus in a guinea pig (Cavia porecllus). J Am Anim Hosp Assoc 2010;46(3):174–80.

34. Ward ML. Rodents: digestive system disorders. In: Keeble E, Meredith A, editors. BSAV manual of rodents and ferrets. Gloucester (United Kingdom): British Small Animal Veterinary Association; 2009. p. 123–41.

35. Percy DH, Barthold SW. Guinea pig. In: Percy DH, Barthold SW, editors. Pathology of laboratory rodents and rabbits. 2nd edition. Ames (IA): Blackwell Publishing; 2001. p. 209–47.

36. Lawson GH, Gebhardt CJ. Proliferative enteropathy. J Comp Pathol 2000;122: 77–100.

37. Elsheikha H, Brown P, Skuse A. Death and diarrhea in guinea pigs (Cavia porcellus). Lab Anim 2009;38(6):189–91.

38. Jelinek F, Hron P, Hozmanova F. Gastrointestinal stromal tumor in a guinea pig: a case report. Acta Vet Brno 2009;78:287–91.

39. Redfern JS, Lin HJ, McArthur KE, et al. Gastric acid and pepsin secretion in conscious rabbits. Am J Physiol 1991;261:G295–304.

40. Hinton M. Gastric ulceration in the rabbit. J Comp Pathol 1980;90:475–81.

41. Man WK, Silcocks PB, Wales R, et al. Histology of experimental stress ulcer: the effects of cimetidine on adrenaline gastric lesions in the rabbit. Br J Exp Pathol 1981;62(4):411–8.

42. Collin BJ. Stress ulcer induced by hypovolemic shock in female rabbit. Anat Histol Embryol Zentral Vet 1977;6(1):94.

43. Van der Hage M, Dorrestein GM. Cecal impaction in the rabbit: relationship with dysautonomia. Paper presented at the 6th World Rabbit Conference Lempdes. France, July 9–12, 1996. p. 77–80.

44. Whitwell K, Needham J. Mudoid enteropathy in UK rabbits: dysautonomia confirmed. Vet Rec 1996;139:323–4.

45. Blanco JE, Blanco M, Blanco J, et al. Prevalence and characteristics of enteropathogenic Escheria coli with the eae gene in diarrhoeic rabbits. Microbiol Immunol 1997;41(2):77–82.

46. Swennes AG, Buckley EM, Parry NM, et al. Enzootic enteropathogenic Escheria coli infection in laboratory rabbits. J Clin Microbiol 2012;50(7):2353–8.

47. Munday JS, Aberdein D, Squires RA, et al. Persistent conjunctival papilloma due to oral papillomavirus infection in a rabbit in New Zealand. J Am Assoc Lab Anim Sci 2007;46(5):69–71.

48. Sundberg JP, Junge RE, El Shazly MO. Oral papillomatosis in New Zealand white rabbits. Am J Vet Res 1985;46:664–8.

49. LaPierre J, Marsolais G, Pilon P, et al. Preliminary report on the isolation of a - coronavirus in the intestine of the laboratory rabbit. Can J Microbiol 1980;26: 1204–8.

50. Lau SK, Woo PC, Yip CC, et al. Isolation and characterization of a novel Betacoronavirus subgroup A coronavirus, rabbit coronavirus HKU14, from domestic rabbits. J Virol 2012;86(10):5481–96.

51. Ciarlet M, Gilger MA, Barone C, et al. Rotavirus disease, but not infection and development of intestinal histopathological lesions, is age restricted in rabbits. Virology 1998;251(2):343–60.

52. DiGiacomo RF, Thouless ME. Epidemiology of naturally occurring rotavirus infection in rabbits. Lab Anim Sci 1986;36(2):153–6.

53. Halaihel N, Lievin V, Alvarado F, et al. Rotavirus infection impairs intestinal brush-border membrane Na+ - solute cotransport activities in young rabbits. Am J Physiol Gastrointest Liver Physiol 2000;279(3):G587–96.

54. Abrantes J, Van Der Loo W, Le Pendu J, et al. Rabbit hemorrhagic disease (RHD) and rabbit haemorrhagic disease virus (RHDV): a review. Vet Res 2012;43(12): 1–19.

55. Nystrom K, Le Gall-Reculé G, Grassi P, et al. Histo-blood group antigens act as attachment factors of rabbit hemorrhagic disease virus infection in a virus strain-dependent manner. PLoS Pathog 2011;7:e1002188.

56. Wang X, Qiu L, Hao H, et al. Adenovirus-based oral vaccine for rabbit hemorrhagic disease. Vet Immunol Immunopathol 2012;145(1–2):277–82.

57. Oliveira UC, Fraga JS, Licois D, et al. Development of molecular assays for the identification of the 11 Eimeria species of the domestic rabbit (Oryctolagus cuniculus). Vet Parasitol 2011;176(2–3):275–80.

58. Chalmers RM, Robinson G, Elwin K, et al. Cryptosporidium sp. rabbit genotype, a newly identified human pathogen. Emerg Infect Dis 2009;15(5):829–30.

59. Clark JD, Jain AV, Hatch RC, et al. Experimentally induced chronic aflatoxicosis in rabbits. Am J Vet Res 1980;41(11):1841–5.

60. Krishna L, Dawra RK, Vaid J, et al. An outbreak of aflatoxicosis in Angora rabbits. Vet Hum Toxicol 1991;33(2):159–61.

61. Harcourt-Brown FM. Gastric dilation and intestinal obstruction in 76 rabbits. Vet Rec 2007;161(12):409–14.

62. DeCubellis J, Kruse AM, McCarthy RJ, et al. Billiary cystadenoma in a rabbit (Oryctolagus cuniculus). J Exo Pet Med 2010;19(2):177–82.

63. Fisher PG, Carpenter JW. Neurologic and musculoskeletal diseases. In: Quesenberry KE, Carpenter JW, editors. Ferrets, rabbits, and rodents: clinical medicine and surgery. 3rd edition. St Louis (MO): Saunders Elsevier; 2012. p. 245–56.

64. Graham JE. GI stasis in rabbits: when it's not just "ileus". Proceedings. In: Proceedings of the Association of Avian Veterinarians (AAV) Symposium. Louisville (KY): AAV; 2012. p. 71–4.

65. Stanke NJ, Graham JE, Orcutt CJ, et al. Successful outcome of hepatectomy as treatment for liver lobe torsion in four domestic rabbits. J Am Vet Med Assoc 2011;238(9):1176–83.

66. Graham JE. Liver lobe torsion in rabbits. Proceedings. In: Proceedings of the Association of Avian Veterinarians (AAV) Symposium. Louisville (KY): AAV; 2012. p. 83.

Viral Infections of Rabbits

Peter J. Kerr, BVSc, PhD[a],

Thomas M. Donnelly, BVSc, DipVP, DipACLAM, DipABVP(ECM)[b],*

KEYWORDS

- Borna disease virus • Caliciviridae infections • Coronavirus infections
- Herpesviridae infections • Papillomavirus infections • Poxviridae infections
- Rabbits • Rabies virus • Rotavirus infections

KEY POINTS

- Rabbit hemorrhagic disease is caused by a calicivirus and is characterized by fulminant hepatitis with a fatality rate of more than 90% in adult rabbits. It is not present in the United States. It is spread by direct contact between rabbits, by flies feeding on carcasses, and experimentally by fleas and mosquitoes. A single-dose vaccination of inactivated virus at 8 to 12 weeks followed by an annual booster is generally protective.

- Myxomatosis is a lethal, generalized viral disease of rabbits. It is endemic in wild rabbit populations and in *Sylvilagus* spp. It commonly occurs in the Pacific states of the United States in warmer months. The virus is spread passively on the mouthparts of mosquitoes and fleas. Outbreaks in farmed, laboratory, and pet rabbits result from spillover in wild rabbit populations. A single-dose vaccination of inactivated virus at 8 to 12 weeks followed by an annual booster is generally protective.

- Rabbit fibroma virus is endemic in *Sylvilagus* spp in North America. It is spread by mosquitoes and causes a cutaneous fibroma at the inoculation site with no systemic signs of disease. The fibroma generally regresses within 3 to 4 weeks of infection. It is one of the most common causes of cutaneous neoplasms in pet rabbits.

- Cottontail rabbit papillomavirus, also known as Shope papillomavirus, is a cause of papillomas (warts) on nonhaired or thinly haired skin of rabbits. In 66% to 80% of infected rabbits, papillomas develop into carcinomas 8 to 14 months later. The virus is spread from *Sylvilagus* spp to rabbits by mosquitoes. Infection is uncommon.

- Rabbit oral papillomavirus occurs naturally in rabbits and is widespread among domestic rabbits in Europe and the Americas, particularly young animals. The papillomas are localized mostly on the underside of the tongue and usually regress spontaneously within a few weeks to a few months.

- The multifactorial enteritis complex of juvenile rabbits can be caused by bacteria, viruses, and parasites. Several different viruses have been isolated from rabbits with diarrhea, such as rotavirus, coronavirus, and astrovirus. Whether natural outbreaks of enteritis can be caused by these viral agents alone or in conjunction with other pathogens (eg, *Clostridia* spp, *Escherichia coli*, and coccidia) is not clear.

---

[a] CSIRO Entomology, GPO Box 1700, Canberra, ACT 2601, Australia; [b] The Kenneth S. Warren Institute, 712 Kitchawan Road, Ossining, NY 10562, USA
* Corresponding author.
E-mail address: smallpets@tomvet.com

Vet Clin Exot Anim 16 (2013) 437–468
http://dx.doi.org/10.1016/j.cvex.2013.02.002
1094-9194/13/$ – see front matter © 2013 Elsevier Inc. All rights reserved.

INTRODUCTION

Viral diseases in rabbits are infrequently encountered by clinicians seeing pet rabbits in North America. Occasionally myxomatosis may be seen. The situation is different in Europe and Australia where myxomatosis and rabbit hemorrhagic disease, the major viral diseases affecting European rabbit (Oryctolagus cuniculus) populations are endemic. This review considers viruses affecting rabbits by their clinical significance. Viruses of major and minor clinical significance are described, and viruses of laboratory significance are mentioned.

VIRAL INFECTIONS OF MAJOR CLINICAL SIGNIFICANCE
Rabbit Hemorrhagic Disease Virus: Rabbit Hemorrhagic Disease

Introduction

Rabbit hemorrhagic disease (RHD) was first described in China in 1984 in a shipment of Angora rabbits (Oryctolagus cuniculus) from East Germany. The disease is characterized by fulminant hepatitis with a case fatality rate of more than 90% in adult rabbits. RHD is caused by a calicivirus termed Rabbit Hemorrhagic Disease Virus (RHDV) (Family: Caliciviridae; Genus: lagovirus), which since 1985 has spread to or emerged in Europe in wild and domestic rabbits, and in domestic rabbits in Asia, the Middle East, North Africa, and the Americas. RHDV was deliberately released in Australia and New Zealand as a biologic control for European rabbits and is now established in the wild in these countries (Table 1).[1]

The United States has experienced 4 sporadic incursions of RHDV, the first of which occurred in Iowa in 2000.[2] In 2001, an outbreak of RHD was reported in Utah and was traced to a shipment and subsequent outbreak in Illinois.[3] A second isolated outbreak occurred in 2001 in New York and is suspected to have resulted from the importation

Table 1
Viral infections of rabbits

	Disease Caused
• Viruses of Major Clinical Significance	
Rabbit hemorrhagic disease virus	Rabbit hemorrhagic disease
Myxoma virus	Myxomatosis
• Viruses of Minor Clinical Significance	
Rabbit fibroma virus (Shope fibroma virus)	Rabbit fibromatosis
Lapine rotavirus	Rotaviral infection (Rotaviral diarrhea)
Cottontail rabbit papillomavirus (Shope papillomavirus)	Rabbit papillomatosis
Rabbit oral papillomavirus	Oral papillomatosis
Herpesvirus: Herpes simplex	Herpes encephalitis
Herpesvirus: Leporid-4	Systemic herpesvirus infection
• Viruses of Laboratory Significance	
Astrovirus	Enteric disease (?)
Bornavirus	Borna disease
Rabies virus	Rabies
Vaccinia virus	Rabbitpox (Rabbit plague)
Pleural effusion disease virus (infectious cardiomyopathy virus)	Pleural effusion disease and cardiomyopathy
Rabbit enteric coronavirus	Coronaviral enteritis

of rabbit meat from China.[4] The most recent outbreak of RHD was in 2005 and occurred in Indiana.[5] Each outbreak was contained, and was the result of a separate but indeterminable introduction of RHDV rather than from a single virus lineage.[4]

Caliciviruses closely related to RHDV, but generally avirulent or of low virulence, have been identified in domestic and wild rabbits in Europe[6,7] and Australia[8–10] and domestic rabbits in the United States (Michigan rabbit calicivirus)[11] and their presence inferred by serology in rabbit populations on various islands[12,13] and New Zealand.[14] These viruses have been termed rabbit caliciviruses (RCVs) to distinguish them from the lethal RHDV. Viral monitoring indicates that more virulent variants of RCVs, which are genetically distinct from RHDV, are emerging in Europe.[15,16] A related lagovirus, European Brown Hare Syndrome virus (EBHSV), emerged in Europe around the same time as RHDV but does not cause disease in European rabbits. EBHSV may not be as species-specific as RHDV.[1]

Epidemiology
RHDV is specific for European rabbits (*Oryctolagus cuniculus*). Probably all ages are susceptible to infection but young rabbits less than 4 weeks of age rarely develop lethal disease. This age-based protection is lost between 4 and 12 weeks of age.[17] There is no gender predisposition. Young rabbits may be more susceptible to an emergent virulent variant of RCV.[15]

RHDV is infectious by virtually all routes of administration but oronasal infection is probably the most common natural route of infection; conjunctival inoculation by flies may also be important.

Infected rabbits shed RHDV in all secretions. The virus is robust and persists for prolonged periods particularly in rabbit carcasses or on fomites.[18,19] RHDV is spread by direct contact between rabbits or indirectly between susceptible rabbits and carcasses or contaminated environments. It is spread by flies feeding on carcasses, which contain very high concentrations of virus particularly in the liver, and experimentally can be spread mechanically by fleas and mosquitoes.[20,21] Because of the extreme concentrations of virus in carcasses, predator or scavenger species of birds and mammals may also aid spread in the wild, as virus can pass both unchanged and infectious through the gut, and be shed in the feces.

Strong seasonality may be present in wild populations, where most adults have survived infection and are subsequently immune. During the breeding season, as young rabbits gradually lose protection provided by maternal antibody, they provide a susceptible population for RHDV to spread. Epidemics in wild rabbits provide the potential for virus to spread into farmed or domestic rabbits via insects, fomites, or direct contact.

Epidemiology of RHDV, both in wild and farmed rabbits, may be strongly influenced by the circulation of RCV strains, which in some circumstances can provide cross-protection to RHDV.[6,8,22–26]

Clinical presentation
Peracute disease There is sudden death with no premonitory signs; rabbits may be observed grazing normally immediately before death (**Fig. 1**A). Death can occur within 30 to 36 hours of oral infection and as early as 24 hours after injection of virus.

Acute disease Rabbits appear quiet and reluctant to move; they may have an elevated temperature and raised heart and respiratory rates for 24 hours before death. Death usually occurs within 48 to 72 hours after infection.

Subacute disease In subacute disease, there are signs of liver failure, including icterus (see **Fig. 1**C); death occurs over days to several weeks.

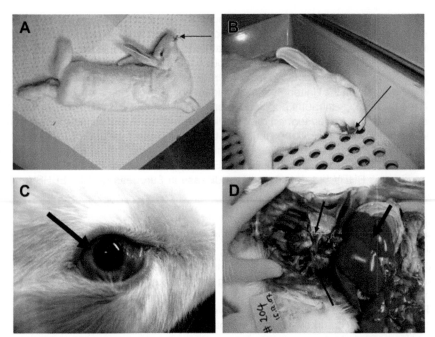

Fig. 1. Rabbits with rabbit hemorrhagic disease. (*A*) Rabbit that died of RHD during a convulsion. Notice how food is still in the mouth (*arrow*). (*B*) Blood from nose and mouth (*arrow*) of a rabbit that died of acute RHD. (*C*) Icteric iris (*arrow*) in albino rabbit with chronic RHD. (*D*) Necropsy of a rabbit that died of RHD. Notice the pale liver (*thick arrow*) and hemorrhages in the lungs (*thin arrows*). (*Courtesy of* Tanja Strive, PhD, CSIRO Entomology, Black Mountain, Australia.)

Subclinical disease A small proportion of infected adult rabbits clears the virus and seroconverts with few or no clinical signs of disease. Young rabbits less than 4 to 5 weeks of age rarely develop disease following infection, although they shed virus, may have a raised temperature, and deaths do occur.

History There is sudden death in adult or subadult rabbits, possibly preceded by 24 hours of quietness/depression with elevated respiratory rate and temperature. Lateral recumbency, coma, and convulsions may be observed before death. Blood from the nose or hematuria may be present (see **Fig. 1**B). In rabbitries, an epidemic with extreme mortality rates in adult and subadult rabbits but not in very young rabbits is typical.

Clinical examination Depression, elevated temperature (up to 42°C), raised respiratory rate, convulsions, ataxia, posterior paresis, and central nervous system depression may occur. Hematuria, bloody diarrhea, and blood from the nares or mouth may be present (see **Fig. 1**B). Pronounced jaundice may be seen in rabbits that have survived more than a few days after infection.

Pathophysiology
RHDV replicates to high titers in the liver, inducing acute hepatic necrosis and fulminant liver failure (see **Fig. 1**D); disseminated intravascular coagulation, hepatic encephalopathy and nephrosis may occur because of the acute hepatic necrosis.[27,28]

Diagnosis

Initial database Leukopenia (lymphopenia and neutropenia) with moderate reduction in thrombocytes but normal erythrocyte numbers[29]; elevated liver enzymes: serum alanine amino transferase (ALT), aspartate amino transferase (AST), lactate dehydrogenase (LDH); alkaline phosphatase (AP) and γ-glutamyltransferase (GGT) are dramatically elevated by 36 to 48 hours after infection; increased serum bilirubin; hypoglycemia; hyperlipidemia; significantly elevated blood urea nitrogen (BUN) and creatinine; increased prothrombin time and decreased factor V and factor VII are all present by 36 to 48 hours after infection.[28–32]

Advanced/confirmatory testing

Necropsy Pale, swollen liver with pronounced lobular pattern and possible focal hemorrhages may be the only major necropsy finding (see **Fig. 1**D). Additional findings include very enlarged, dark spleen; dark-colored kidneys; congested or hemorrhagic lungs with fluid/froth in the trachea (see **Fig. 1**D); hyperemic tracheal mucosa; and ecchymotic and petechial hemorrhages in intestinal and bladder walls and in subcutaneous tissues.

Histopathology Histopathology includes coagulative necrosis of hepatocytes at the periphery of the lobule; thrombi in renal and pulmonary blood vessels (disseminated intravascular coagulation); nephrosis; and lymphocyte depletion from spleen. Subacute cases may show signs of liver regeneration with connective tissue and bile duct proliferation and large, pale-staining binucleate hepatocytes.[27,33]

Virology RHDV cannot be grown in tissue culture. Reverse transcriptase polymerase chain reaction (RT-PCR) is the most common diagnostic tool. Viral RNA can be detected in most tissues, including blood, but the highest concentration is in the liver. Low levels of RHDV RNA can persist for prolonged periods in rabbits that survive infection[34–36] and, depending on the specificity of the assay, nonpathogenic RCV strains may cross-react, so care is needed in interpretation of RT-PCR results in the absence of liver pathology. Hemagglutination of human red blood cells is used as a diagnostic test for RHDV, but not all strains hemagglutinate, and the assay is much less sensitive than RT-PCR; capture enzyme-linked immunosorbent assay (ELISA) using clarified liver homogenates can also be used to demonstrate virus but again is much less sensitive than RT-PCR. Immunostaining of liver sections or impression smears using specific monoclonal antibodies can be used to detect RHDV antigen.[37] Electron microscopy on liver homogenates can demonstrate calicivirus particles in negative stained preparations.[37]

Serology Infected juvenile rabbits or surviving adults develop very high titers of antibody to RHDV capsid protein. Indirect and competition ELISAs are used to demonstrate specific serum antibody to RHDV and isotype ELISAs can be used to demonstrate IgG, IgM and IgA.[37] Hemagglutination inhibition tests can also be used but have largely been replaced by ELISA because of the increased sensitivity and convenience. Serologic cross-reaction with avirulent RCVs occurs, so care is needed when interpreting serologic results.[38] Competition ELISA is more specific than indirect or isotype ELISAs.

Treatment

There is no specific treatment; supportive care only. Experimentally, treatment with melatonin (starting at the time of infection) or cardiotrophin (starting at 12 hours post infection) reduced liver damage, and cardiotrophin also increased survival rates.[39–42] Vaccination in the face of an outbreak is used in rabbitries to bring the disease under control, as vaccinated animals quickly develop protective immunity. Infected rabbits should be isolated to prevent transmission.

Prognosis and outcome
Prognosis is extremely guarded. Most clinically affected rabbits will die; subacutely infected animals may survive depending on the degree of liver damage and damage to other tissues; chronic liver disease including cirrhosis may result.

Prevention
Vaccination using an adjuvanted, inactivated whole virus vaccine is generally protective. A single dose at 8 to 12 weeks is followed by an annual booster. The vaccine manufacturer's recommendations should be followed. It is not clear if maternal antibody interferes with earlier vaccination but if this is necessary, it may be advisable to give a booster at 10 to 12 weeks of age. Antigenic variants of RHDV/RCV that overcome vaccination have been reported.[15,16,43]

A combined inactivated RHDV vaccine plus a live myxoma virus vaccine in a single-dose formulation is available (Dercunimix, Merial, Lyons, France). A recombinant Myxoma virus vaccine expressing the RHDV capsid protein has recently been released (Nobivac Myxo-RHD, MSD-Animal Health, Hoddesdon, Hertfordshire, UK) as a combined live vaccine to provide protection against myxomatosis and RHDV.[44] A single dose is recommended in rabbits older than 5 weeks of age.

Incoming rabbits should always be quarantined to prevent introduction of disease.

Myxoma Virus: Myxomatosis

Introduction
Myxoma virus (MYXV) (Subfamily: Chordopoxvirinae; Genus: *leporipoxvirus*) causes the lethal, generalized disease myxomatosis in domestic and wild European rabbits (*Oryctolagus cuniculus*). The virus naturally circulated in tapeti *(Sylvilagus brasiliensis)* in South America; however, following deliberate introductions into Australia and Europe as a biologic control for wild European rabbits, MYXV now is endemic in wild European rabbit populations and can spill over into farmed, laboratory, and pet rabbits. MYXV has also been successfully introduced into Chile and Argentina to control feral European rabbits. A closely related virus, often called Californian myxoma virus, is found in *Sylvilagus bachmani* (brush rabbit) in the Pacific states of the United States and the Baja peninsula of Mexico (**Table 2**). This virus is also highly lethal in European rabbits.[45]

Table 2
Lagomorph viruses: transmission between *Oryctolagus* and *Sylvilagus* and severity of induced disease

Virus	*Oryctolagus* European Rabbit		*Sylvilagus* American Cottontail
• Poxviridae			
Myxoma virus	Myxoma	⬅	Fibroma[a]
Rabbit (Shope) fibroma virus	Fibroma, mild	⬅	Fibroma, severe[a]
• Papillomaviridae			
Cottontail rabbit (Shope) papilloma virus	Papilloma, SQC 75%	⬅	Papilloma, SQC 25%[a]
Oral papilloma virus	Oral papilloma[a]	➡	Oral papilloma

Abbreviation: SQC, squamous cell carcinoma.
[a] Natural host.

Epidemiology

Myxomatosis is essentially a disease of European rabbits, although European hares may rarely develop generalized disease.[46] There is no age or sex predilection but very young rabbits may die without obvious myxomatosis. Passively transmitted maternal antibody may modify the disease outcome in young rabbits born to immune does.[47]

The virus is spread passively on the mouthparts of biting arthropods, predominantly mosquitoes and fleas (but also Culicoides midges and lice), that probe through the virus-rich cutaneous lesions when seeking a blood meal. The virus does not replicate in the vector.[48]

Contact spread from rabbit to rabbit may also occur from virus shed in ocular and nasal secretions or from the surface of eroded skin lesions[46]; virus is also potentially present in semen and genital secretions. Oral infection is very inefficient so conjunctival or nasal inoculation is probably necessary for transmission. Aerosol transmission is inefficient but virus is readily transmitted on fomites, such as water bottles or feeders, or by handlers.

In Europe and Australia, wild European rabbits act as reservoirs for MYXV and mosquitoes can transmit the virus to domestic rabbits. Where there is close proximity between wild and domestic rabbits, fleas and direct contact may also transmit virus.

In South America, vector transmission from *S brasiliensis* to farmed, laboratory, or pet rabbits occurs.[46] Similar spillover occurs from *S bachmani* in the Pacific states of the United States and Mexico.[49–53]

Seasonality is driven by the availability of vectors and the epidemiology of the disease in wild rabbits. In rabbitries, introduction of rabbits carrying the disease (including vaccinated rabbits) has led to epidemics.[54] Introduced semen may also pose a risk.[55]

Clinical presentation
Disease forms

Peracute myxomatosis Peracute myxomatosis may present as sudden deaths with only mild or no clinical signs of myxomatosis, particularly with Californian MYXV infections. Neurologic signs, such as convulsions, have been described.[46] In Australia, some field strains cause acute pulmonary edema in domestic rabbits. Death typically occurs 7 to 15 days after infection.

Acute myxomatosis Acute myxomatosis is the classic mucocutaneous form of myxomatosis with multiple skin lesions (**Fig. 2**A); a second amyxomatous form with fewer skin lesions has been described in Europe.[55–58] Australian field isolates may also present as essentially amyxomatous in domestic rabbits. Case fatality rates are nearly 100%, but in some individuals, the disease course may be prolonged. Death typically occurs 10 to 15 days after infection.

Subacute myxomatosis Natural selection in European rabbits in Australia and Europe has seen the emergence of attenuated field strains of MYXV.[59,60] These viruses cause typical myxomatosis but with a protracted course (see **Fig. 2**B); case fatality rates may be less than 50% to more than 95%, with deaths occurring from 10 to 30 plus days after infection. Survivors may be left with chronic respiratory disease.

History and physical examination Very early cases present with slight eyelid swelling, conjunctivitis, and thickened ears (see **Fig. 2**A); temperatures may be elevated above 40°C but this is variable. Depending on the virulence of the virus, this may be 5 to

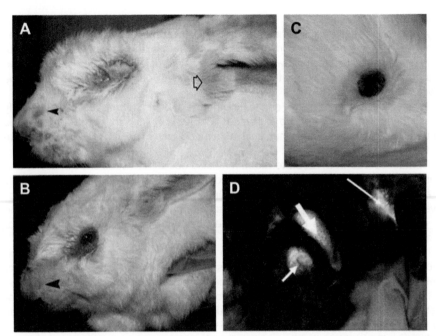

Fig. 2. Clinical appearance of rabbits with myxomatosis. (*A*) Acute myxomatosis caused by virulent myxoma virus. Skin lesions are present on the nose (*solid arrowhead*). The base of the ear is swollen (*open arrowhead*) and the eyes are closed with mucopurulent conjunctivitis. (*B*) Rabbit infected with attenuated strain of myxoma virus. The eyelid margins are red and swollen and serous discharge is present. Swelling is noted around the face and nose (*arrowhead*). (*C*) Scabbed skin lesion (approximately 2.5-cm diameter) at primary infection site. (*D*) Swollen testis (*broad arrow*); swollen genital opening (*short arrow*); secondary skin lesions (*narrow arrow*). ([*A, B*] *From* Best SM, Kerr PJ. Coevolution of host and virus: the pathogenesis of virulent and attenuated strains of myxoma virus in resistant and susceptible European rabbits. Virology 2000;267(1):36–48; with permission.)

10 days after infection. Careful examination may reveal a 1-cm to 2-cm diameter, raised, reddened primary cutaneous lesion, but the size and thickness of this varies enormously with the strain of virus (see **Fig. 2**C).

Later in the disease course, rabbits present with swollen eyelids and mucopurulent blepharoconjunctivitis in which the eyes may be partially or completely closed by the eyelid swelling (there is no involvement of the eye itself). The face is swollen and the ears swollen and drooping or just thickened, particularly around the base (see **Fig. 2**A).

Mucopurulent nasal discharge is common and the nasal passages may be occluded causing a gasping, stertorous respiration with extension of the head and neck.

Severe swelling of the anogenital region is typical and in males, orchitis and epididymitis together with gross swelling of the scrotum occur (see **Fig. 2**D).[61]

In the classic mucocutaneous form of myxomatosis, cutaneous lesions ranging from a few millimeters to 5 to 6 cm in diameter and from 1 to 20 mm high occur over the eyelids, face, ears, and scrotum and late in the disease can be palpated over the body, legs, and feet. In late infections, or in recovering rabbits, the surface of the cutaneous lesions may be hemorrhagic, black, or scabbing (see **Fig. 2**C).

Popliteal and prescapular lymph nodes are grossly enlarged and readily palpable. Temperatures may be as high as 41°C but often drop below normal before death.

Rabbits may continue to eat and drink until quite late in the disease course but severe weight loss is common and dehydration may occur.

Pathophysiology

Virus inoculated into the dermis/epidermis by biting arthropods replicates locally in macrophages/dendritic cells and then in epidermal cells.[62] Proliferation of the epidermal cells and mucoid swelling of the underlying dermis forms the raised primary lesion that is sometimes referred to as a myxoma or tumor. From the primary site, MYXV is transported to the draining lymph node where it replicates in T cells, macrophages, and other cells, causing almost complete loss of T cells. From the draining lymph node, it disseminates in lymphocytes and possibly macrophage/monocytes to distal tissues, such as lungs, spleen, testes, skin, and mucocutaneous sites, such as eyelids. Virus replication at distal skin sites causes the secondary cutaneous lesions found over the body.[62–64]

The cause of death in acute classic myxomatosis is obscure; major organs are typically not severely damaged.[65] MYXV profoundly suppresses innate and adaptive immune responses, although low titers of IgM and IgG and even neutralizing antibody can be detected before death.[45,64,66–70] Secondary bacterial infections of the conjunctivae, upper respiratory tract, and lungs are typical in rabbits that survive longer than 10 to 14 days after infection and may be the major cause of death in rabbits infected with subacute strains of MYXV. Rabbits free of *Pasteurella multocida* and *Bordetella bronchiseptica* appear to have fewer complications before death, but even these may have lobar pneumonia at necropsy.

Diagnosis

Clinical signs of classic myxomatosis are fairly clear-cut, although bacterial upper respiratory tract infections can cause confusion and misdiagnosis.[55] Hematology is generally unremarkable: neutrophilia, lymphopenia, and lymphocytosis can all be seen at different stages depending on the virulence of the virus.

Necropsy findings are largely limited to the external lesions and features already described, and depend on the time of death and the underlying virulence of the virus. The cutaneous lesions are clearly separated from the underlying tissue and have a glistening, mucoid appearance on the cut surface. Lymph nodes are grossly enlarged, sometimes hemorrhagic, and may have a watery consistency on section. The spleen is generally 2 to 3 times normal size and often dark-colored. In males, scrotal edema of 0.5 to 1.0 cm may be obvious on incising the skin. In peracute cases, pulmonary edema may be the cause of death with the trachea and bronchi full of froth and fluid, and the lungs dripping fluid. Hemorrhages on serosal membranes and intestinal and stomach walls may be present in some cases.

Confirmatory testing Histopathology of cutaneous lesions is characterized by cellular proliferation and cell death.[71] In the epidermis, the epidermal cells proliferate, enlarge, and undergo ballooning degeneration; the underlying dermis is edematous with complete disruption of the connective tissue architecture; the endothelium of the small blood vessels is disrupted by large stellate or polygonal "myxoma cells." These cells appear to migrate from the blood vessels into the dermis where they are often surrounded by polymorphs. In infections with virulent virus, there may be an influx of polymorphs into the dermis, particularly at the base but lymphocytes are rarely present.[62] In lymphoid tissues, complete loss of lymphocytes from both B-cell and T-cell zones can occur together with proliferation of reticular cells that obliterate the sinuses; disruption of the small blood vessels by myxoma cells is similar to that in the epidermis and polymorphs may be prominent. The presence of virus can be confirmed by immunostaining of epidermal sections from the nodular lesions or eyelids. Negative-stained electron microscopy can be used to identify virus eluted from skin sections.[72]

PCR, using specific oligonucleotide primers for MYXV, can be done on DNA extracted from biopsies, conjunctival swabs, or tissues collected at necropsy. Virus titers in blood are generally low but the white cell fraction could be used for PCR in early/acute cases. A 1-mm dermal punch biopsy from a lesion yields sufficient DNA for diagnostic PCR.

MYXV can be readily cultured from cutaneous lesions or eyelids (biopsied or collected at necropsy) or from conjunctival swabs. The virus grows in various rabbit cell lines, including RK-13 and SIRC, and other mammalian cell lines, such as Vero and BGMK, and on the chorioallantoic membrane of embryonated chicken eggs. Tissues and swabs in 1:1 glycerol/saline or glycerol/phosphate-buffered saline can be stored at −20°C for some weeks before processing but for prolonged storage should be kept at −80°C.

Specific antibody can be detected as early as 6 to 10 days after infection using ELISA and persists for at least 12 months. Other serologic assays include complement fixation, virus neutralization, and gel immunodiffusion; these are less sensitive than ELISA.[72] Gel immunodiffusion can also be used to detect viral antigen.

Differential diagnosis
- Bacterial respiratory tract infections (eg, pasteurellosis)
- Bacterial conjunctivitis/keratoconjunctivitis
- Rabbit systemic herpesvirus infection, a recently described virus (leporid 4 herpesvirus) in North America causing swollen head, mucopurulent conjunctivitis, nodular hemorrhagic skin lesions, and respiratory distress.[73]

Treatment
At present, no specific treatment exists for myxomatosis. If the decision is made to attempt treatment, careful monitoring is necessary to avoid prolonging suffering. The aims of treatment should be to provide nursing support, control secondary infections, and minimize distress. Cessation of food and water intake, ongoing severe weight loss, or rectal temperature below 38°C is grounds for euthanasia.

Infected rabbits should be kept warm. There is evidence that high temperatures ameliorate the effects of attenuated viruses[74]; food intake and hydration should be carefully monitored. Broad-spectrum antibiotics, such as fluoroquinolones, potentiated sulfonamides, or tetracyclines, could be used but there is no clear evidence supporting their use and antibiotic treatment had no impact on the disease caused by virulent virus.[75] For analgesia, buprenorphine 0.03 mg/kg twice daily has been used in acute myxomatosis but appeared to have little impact on rabbit behavior compared with untreated rabbits.[76]

An orally active derivative of cidofovir, CMX001, has activity against MYXV in vitro (G. McFadden, personal communication, 2009) and against the orthopoxvirus rabbitpox in rabbits in vivo but is available only experimentally.[45,77,78]

Prognosis and outcome
Highly virulent strains of MYXV have essentially 100% case fatality rates in domestic rabbits. Attenuated strains of MYXV may have case fatality rates of less than 50% to more than 95%, but the clinical course of the disease is prolonged. Rabbits infected with attenuated strains may recover over 2 to 3 weeks; in these rabbits, the cutaneous lesions become circumscribed and clearly demarcated from the surrounding skin, scab, and dry out, often leaving a scarred "moth-eaten" appearance of the face and ears. Chronic respiratory disease, such as snuffles, is common in surviving rabbits;

some surviving rabbits do not gain weight and may have more serious underlying secondary infections, such as bacterial pneumonia. Even in apparently recovered rabbits, it is not unusual to find complete consolidation of cranial lung lobes at necropsy.

Prevention

Vaccination Immunization with live attenuated strains of MYXV (e.g. Dervaximyo SG33, Merial, Lyons, France) or the heterologous rabbit fibroma virus (RFV) (Nobivac Myxo, MSD-Animal Health, Hoddesdon, Hertfordshire, UK) is used to protect rabbits against myxomatosis in Europe.[79] The homologous live vaccines appear to provide longer lasting protection than vaccination with RFV but some have been associated with immunosuppression in young rabbits. This has led to recommendations to vaccinate initially with RFV followed by a boost with attenuated MYXV.[80,81] The Australian federal government does not permit commercial use of myxomatosis vaccines in domestic rabbits in Australia.

Neither type of vaccine provides 100% protection against high-dose challenge and protection can be quite short-lived (3–12 months). Vaccinated rabbits can become infected on challenge and shed virus.

Other preventive measures
- Prevention of contact with wild rabbits and screening of cages/buildings to prevent mosquito transmission. Elimination of other vectors, such as rabbit fleas, lice, and mites.
- Quarantine of incoming rabbits to prevent introduction of rabbits incubating the disease. Even vaccinated rabbits should be quarantined.
- Isolation of suspected clinical cases and in-contact rabbits until diagnosis is confirmed.

VIRAL INFECTIONS OF MINOR CLINICAL SIGNIFICANCE
Rabbit Fibroma Virus (Shope Fibroma Virus): Rabbit Fibromatosis

Introduction
Rabbit fibroma virus (RFV) (Subfamily: Chordopoxvirinae; Genus: *leporipoxvirus*) circulates in Eastern cottontail rabbits (*Sylvilagus floridanus*) in North America (see **Table 2**). It is genetically and antigenically closely related to myxoma virus, but in European rabbits (*Oryctolagus cuniculus*) RFV normally causes only a cutaneous fibroma at the inoculation site with no systemic signs of disease. In suckling rabbits, more generalized disease and death usually occur.[82,83] RFV is used as a live virus heterologous vaccine against myxomatosis.[79,84]

Epidemiology
RFV causes cutaneous fibromas in *S floridanus* usually on the feet (**Fig. 3A**), legs, or muzzle[85]; virus is spread passively on the mouthparts of biting arthropods (predominantly mosquitoes) that probe through the fibroma seeking a blood meal; fleas can transmit the virus but experimentally seemed relatively inefficient.[86,87] European rabbits may be infected by mosquitoes (or possibly by fleas if in close contact with Eastern cottontail rabbits) from this natural reservoir of the virus. The highest risk is during the autumn when large populations of infected cottontail rabbits and mosquitoes may coexist. The virus is reported in the Eastern and Midwest states of the United States, including Texas, and in Ontario, Canada.[46,88] Experimentally, mosquito transmission from immunocompetent European rabbits is inefficient, despite high titers of virus in the fibroma, so the European rabbit is essentially a dead-end host and virus

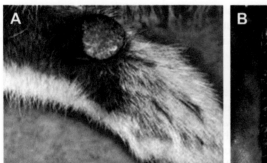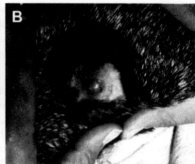

Fig. 3. (*A*) Nodular fibromatous growth on forepaw of Eastern cottontail rabbit naturally infected with rabbit (Shope) fibroma virus. (*B*) Experimentally induced Shope fibroma on the dorsum of a pigmented rabbit 21 days post inoculation. The fibroma is freely movable in the subcutaneous tissue. ([A] *Image from* Department of Veterinary Pathology, Armed Forces Institute of Pathology, Washington, DC.)

spread from either naturally infected or vaccinated rabbits would be unlikely.[48,89,90] However, suckling rabbits or immunosuppressed adult rabbits in which the immune response fails to clear the fibroma can act as sources for mosquito transmission.[90,91] Direct rabbit-to-rabbit spread does not occur,[82] but mechanical spread between rabbits is theoretically possible. Virus dropped into the conjunctivae or nose will infect rabbits. Natural outbreaks in commercial rabbitries have been reported in the United States.[88,92] In a 16-year retrospective study of cutaneous neoplasms in pet rabbits from the University of Pennsylvania veterinary school, 10.5% of skin tumors were RFV-induced fibromas.[93]

Clinical presentation
Skin nodules 0.5 to 6.0 cm in diameter are typically found on the forepaws, ears, and head. There may be multiple discrete nodules, freely moveable with no underlying tissue connections (see **Fig. 3**B). Usually no systemic signs of illness occur except in suckling rabbits where more generalized disease and death may ensue.[82,83,88] The fibromas generally resolve within 3 to 4 weeks of infection.[84]

Pathophysiology
There is a solid tumorlike nodule, glistening and mucoid on cut surface; it may be necrotic in the center with scabbing of overlying epidermis. Histologically, it is described as a fibroxanthosarcomalike tumor.[94,95]

Diagnosis
Diagnosis is made from clinical appearance and history; histopathology; virus isolation (RFV is readily cultured in rabbit cell lines, such as RK-13 or SIRC, and on the chorioallantoic membrane of embryonated chicken eggs); demonstration of poxvirus particles using thin-section electron microscopy on fibroma sections; or amplification of RFV DNA using PCR on DNA extracted from fibroma tissue collected at necropsy or biopsy.

Treatment
No treatment is normally necessary.

Prognosis and outcome
In all but suckling rabbits or experimentally immunosuppressed rabbits, the disease is not normally significant.

Prevention
Shield lactating does and their litters from mosquitoes.

Lapine Rotavirus: Rotaviral Enteritis

Introduction
Rotaviruses (Family: Reoviridae) are a major cause of diarrhea in intensively reared animals throughout the world. Essentially, every species of domestic animal and bird harbors at least one indigenous rotavirus that typically is responsible for causing diarrhea in newborn animals. The clinical signs, diagnosis, and epidemiology of disease are similar in all species; the severity of disease ranges from subclinical, through enteritis of varying severity, to death.

The classification of rotaviruses is based on genotypic and serologic analyses. Variation in the group-specific capsid antigen on VP6 defines the 6 major groups A to F. Rabbit rotaviruses are typically group A rotaviruses.[96–98] Differentiation into serotypes is based on neutralization tests. Because both outer capsid proteins (VP4 and VP7) carry type-specific epitopes recognized by neutralizing antibodies, a binary system of classification of serotypes has developed, similar to that used for influenza viruses. For example, in group A rotaviruses, 14 G serotypes have been defined on the basis of differences in VP7, and 14 P serotypes based on differences in VP4.[99]

Epidemiology
Rotavirus is an important and common disease agent in commercial rabbitries. It is rarely diagnosed in pet rabbits. Serologic surveys of commercial rabbitries in Europe[100–104] and North America,[105,106] laboratory research rabbits,[107] Eastern cottontail rabbits (*S floridanus*),[108] and hares (*Lepus* spp)[108,109] indicate lapine rotaviruses are widespread. In many commercial rabbitries, rotavirus infection is likely enzootic, as rotaviruses can survive in feces for several months.

Rotaviruses are excreted in the feces of infected animals in high titer (up to 10^{11} viral particles per gram); shedding of virus can occur for 6 to 8 days from the second to fifth day postinfection.[110] Some rotaviruses are highly resistant to chlorination, and can survive for long periods in water, so that water-borne transmission is also a risk.[111]

Most viruses with multisegmented double-stranded RNA genomes, such as rotavirus, are included in the family Reoviridae. Because of their segmented RNA genomes, reassortment of genome segments among different strains of rotavirus is common, as is a high rate of RNA mutations in individual genes.[112] The resulting genetic shift and drift leads to a remarkable diversity of rotaviruses, reflected by the numerous serotypes and strains of virus. Consequently, infection with new strains of rotavirus is common in breeding facilities.

Clinical presentation
Rotavirus infection in rabbits younger than 2 weeks old is characterized by voluminous, soft to liquid feces.[113] Some affected animals are only moderately depressed, and often continue to suckle or drink milk.[106,110] Rabbits older than 2 weeks of age typically do not show diarrhea because of the fluid absorptive capability of the cecum.[113] Other factors, particularly reduced colostrum intake, but also infections with other enteric pathogens, such as *Escherichia coli*, poor hygiene, chilling, and overcrowding, contribute to the severity of disease.[104,105] Young animals may die because of dehydration or secondary bacterial infection.

During epizootic infections, suckling rabbits may experience high mortality. During enzootic infections, suckling rabbits receive maternal antibody transplacentally, and experience low mortality but high morbidity.[114]

Pathophysiology

Rotavirus infections cause intestinal malabsorption and maldigestion by destruction of the terminally differentiated enterocytes lining the tips of the intestinal villi. Rotaviruses replicate in mature enterocytes lining intestinal villi, especially in the jejunum and ileum. Damaged villi become shortened and covered with undifferentiated epithelial cells that migrate from the crypts. These cells secrete reduced levels of disacchari- dases (eg, lactase); lactose and other disaccharides accumulate in the lumen causing an osmotic drain and attracting fluid into the lumen.[113,115,116] The neonatal bowel is especially susceptible to infection, because of the slow epithelial turnover rate and the high proportion of terminally differentiated epithelium, and is less able to carry out glucose-coupled sodium transport[116] and chloride secretion.[115]

Undigested lactose in the milk promotes bacterial growth and exerts a further osmotic effect; both mechanisms contribute to the diarrhea. In young rabbits, bacte- rial superinfection with E coli and other bacteria (eg, Clostridia spp) and coccidia have an additive effect and contribute to the multifactorial enteritis complex of juvenile rabbits.[103,105,117] Mortality can often be high in commercial rabbitries.

Diagnosis

Diagnosis is based on history, age, and characteristic gross and microscopic features. Electron microscopy still allows rapid diagnosis, as virus particles are plentiful in the feces of affected animals, and have a highly distinctive wheel-like appearance (from the Latin rota = wheel). ELISA is a more practicable and more sensitive method for detection of rotaviruses in feces in most laboratories. A commercial human rotavirus antigen detection kit has been shown to be effective in laboratory rabbits because of its ability to detect rotavirus antigen in feces.[118] The specificity of enzyme immunoas- says can be manipulated by selecting either group-specific or serotype-specific or broadly cross-reactive antibodies as capture and/or indicator antibodies in an antigen-capture assay. Rotaviruses are difficult to isolate in cell culture.[119]

Diagnostic tests that identify the viral genome in RNA extracted directly from feces include polyacrylamide gel electrophoresis, which can distinguish rotavirus groups A, B, and C by RNA electropherotype pattern alone.[112] RT-PCR assay allows the use of primer pairs appropriate for the degree of specificity desired (rotavirus groups based on VP6, or G and P genotypes based on VP7 and VP4).[112] These tests are generally used to make necessary distinctions in molecular epidemiologic studies to identify reassortant viruses and potential interspecies transmission. The rate of success of any diagnostic test for rotavirus is significantly affected by the time of sample collec- tion; samples collected beyond 48 hours after onset of diarrhea are of limited value.[101]

Treatment

Supportive care, including warmth, is critical. Recovery in severely dehydrated rabbits can be aided by administering oral electrolyte solutions containing glucose shortly after the onset of diarrhea.[104] In severe cases that are likely to be "enteritis complex," the value of antibiotics is questionable.

Prognosis and outcome

Prognosis is affected by superinfection with other intestinal pathogens.[103,113,117] Rotavirus antigen has been detected from healthy rabbits (specimens taken one day after weaning and 1 week later) in about 15% of commercial Italian rabbitries.[103]

Prevention

Although the management of intensive rearing units for farmed rabbits can be improved to reduce the incidence of disease, there is little likelihood that improved hygiene alone can completely control rotavirus infections. Local immunity in the small intestine is more important than systemic immunity in providing resistance to infection; rotavirus antibodies present in immune colostrum and milk are critical in protecting neonates.[114,120] Although much of the colostral antibody enters the circulation, serum antibody levels are not as critical for protection. Inoculation of the dam with inactivated or attenuated rotavirus vaccines promotes higher levels of antibody in the colostrum and milk, and a longer period of antibody secretion in milk, with a corresponding decrease in the incidence of disease in neonates.[121]

Cottontail Rabbit Papillomavirus (Shope Papillomavirus): Rabbit Papillomatosis

Introduction
Cottontail rabbit papillomavirus (CRPV), also commonly known as Shope papillomavirus (Family: Papillomaviridae) is a cause of papillomas (warts) in rabbits. Classic studies on viral oncogenesis were performed in the 1930s[122–124] with CRPV.

Epidemiology
The natural host is the cottontail rabbit (*Sylvilagus* spp) (see **Table 2**).[125] CRPV causes natural disease uncommonly in domestic rabbits.[126,127] Insect vectors (eg, mosquitoes) are probably the cause of mechanical spread of virus from cottontail rabbits to domestic rabbits.

Clinical presentation
CRPV papillomas occur most frequently on nonhaired or thinly haired skin, such as eyelids and ears. In CRPV papillomas, the normal process of keratinization is altered, as evidenced by the hyperkeratosis, parakeratosis, and fragmentation of the horny layer. Consequently, lesions range from a pedunculated, cornified surface overlying a fleshy central area (early papilloma) to multiple conical/cylindrical hornlike masses of firm keratin 3 to 5 mm in diameter and 0.5 to 2.0 cm in length (cutaneous horns) **(Fig. 4)**.

Pathophysiology
Warts induced by CRPV in both cottontail rabbits[125] and European rabbits often progress to carcinomas. Virus replication occurs only in the cottontail rabbit,[128] and not the European rabbit, although one strain of CRPV has been shown to replicate at low levels in European rabbits.[129] In domestic rabbits, the tissue surrounding an inoculation site (either experimentally or naturally by mosquitoes) is clinically and histologically normal, but contains viral DNA at low levels detectable by PCR. The latent virus is able to form warts from mild skin irritation.[130] Ultraviolet irradiation will also induce warts, which is why the lesions are typically found on the ears, lips and eyelids: areas without much fur that are exposed to sunlight.[131] Different mRNA transcripts are present (E1 protein, E2 protein, E6 protein, E7 protein, L1 protein, and L2 protein transcripts) in latent viruses. Only E6 and E7 oncoprotein transcripts can be induced to form papillomas.[132] The papillomas develop into carcinomas 8 to 14 months later in 25% of cottontail rabbits and in 66% to 80% of European rabbits.

Diagnosis
The histologic diagnosis is consistent with a squamous papilloma. In contrast to papillomas induced by CRPV, spontaneous nonviral squamous papillomas develop in haired skin. Other causes of skin lesions in rabbits that should be considered in the differential diagnosis include rabbit oral papillomavirus induced conjunctival papilloma and rabbit (Shope) fibroma virus infection. Shope fibromas are typically flattened to

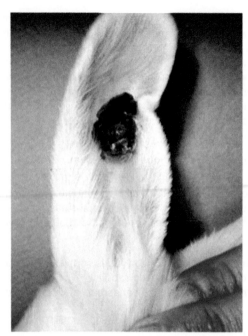

Fig. 4. CRPV-induced papilloma on the ear of a New Zealand white rabbit. Notice how the papilloma shows multiple hornlike masses of firm, protruding keratin.

nodular tumors 0.5 to 6.0 cm in diameter that tend to occur on the forepaws, ears, and head.

Treatment

Intralesional 1% (wt/vol) (0.036 M) cidofovir treatment of rabbit papillomas led to elimination, or "cure" of large papillomas over a 6-week to 8-week treatment period.[133] However, recurrences at periods from 1 to 8 weeks after treatment cessation were observed in approximately 50% of cured sites. Tumor reappearance occurred because of latent virus around the inoculation sites.

Immune stimulation with unmethylated dinucleotides of cytosine and guanine (CpG) have shown efficacy against papillomas as monotherapy, as vaccine adjuvants, and in combination with chemotherapies.[134] Despite the potency of CpG in triggering host immunity, CpG oligodeoxynucleotide has experimentally not shown a therapeutic effect against experimentally induced CRPV papilloma in rabbits.

Surgical excision of papillomas can be attempted, but a wide margin is required. PCR of the edges of excised skin can be used to detect CRPV DNA and determine if all latent infected cells were removed. However, even if one lesion is completely removed, there are likely to be other latent infected inoculation sites in surrounding skin that have the potential to develop into papillomas and eventually carcinomas if E6 and/or E7 oncoproteins are present. If a papilloma occurs on the ear, amputation of the ear is a potential but drastic treatment.

Prognosis and outcome

CRPV papillomas develop into carcinomas 8 to 14 months later in 66% to 80% of infected rabbits. Papillomas undergo immune-mediated regression if they do not progress to carcinomas. Infection is uncommon. Only 2 CRPV papillomas (1.1%) were identified in a 16-year retrospective study of cutaneous neoplasms in pet rabbits from the University of Pennsylvania veterinary school.[93]

Prevention

Keep rabbits indoors or in insect-protected enclosures to avoid transmission of virus from cottontail rabbits. This is an issue only in North America where cottontail rabbits occur naturally.

If a papilloma is identified, and PCR identifies CRPV, advise owners to keep their rabbit out of direct sunlight and not to irritate (eg, removing incrustations) the papilloma or surrounding skin, as it will induce the occurrence of new papillomas.

Rabbit Oral Papillomavirus: Oral Papillomatosis

Introduction

Rabbit oral papillomavirus (Family: Papillomaviridae) (ROPV) occurs naturally in domestic rabbits (see **Table 2**). The causative papillomavirus is distinct from the cottontail rabbit papillomavirus (Shope papillomavirus).

Epidemiology

ROPV is widespread among domestic rabbits in Europe and the Americas, particularly young animals.[135–138] Lesions typically occur in rabbits between 2 and 18 months of age. The oral papillomas are not highly contagious. Lesions are found more frequently in young rabbits whose mothers have papillomas; transmission from the mother to offspring during suckling is common.[139] ROPV can be recovered from the mouth washings of rabbits having no oral papillomas, as it is latent in the mouth, and does not proliferate unless the mucous membrane is injured.

Clinical presentation

Tumors are small, gray-white, filiform or pedunculated nodules (5 mm in diameter and 4 mm in height) and are localized mostly on the underside of the tongue (**Fig. 5**)[140]; however, one report describes a conjunctival papilloma.[141] The papillomas usually

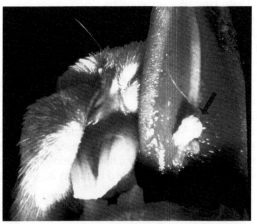

Fig. 5. Rabbit oral papillomavirus tumor presenting as a white pedunculated nodule on the underside of a New Zealand white rabbit tongue (*arrow*). (*Image from* Department of Veterinary Pathology, Armed Forces Institute of Pathology, Washington, DC.)

regress spontaneously within a few weeks to a few months. Most pet rabbit owners do not notice the lesions.

Pathophysiology
ROPV causes papillomas in the oral mucosa of several species of rabbits and hares but fails to cause lesions when inoculated into other rabbit tissues and into the oral mucosa of other species. ROPV differs from the cottontail rabbit papilloma virus (Shope papillomavirus) and homologies between the open reading frames of the 2 viruses vary between 23% and 68%.[142] Rabbits immune to the oral papillomavirus are fully susceptible to cottontail rabbit papilloma virus and vice versa.[142] There is little sequence homology between the genomes of papillomaviruses from different species.[143]

Diagnosis
Lesions are typical squamous papillomas on fibrovascular stalks. Basophilic intranuclear inclusions may be present in the stratum spinosum.[136] Virus particles from lesions may be seen under electron microscopy. Differential diagnosis of oral lesions includes sialoceles.[144]

Treatment and prognosis
Oral papillomas are typically not treated, as they regress spontaneously and show no tendency to malignancy.

Herpes Simplex Virus: Herpes Encephalitis

Introduction
Although rabbits have served as an animal model for herpesvirus encephalitis and keratitis following experimental inoculation with human herpes simplex virus (HSV) (Subfamily: Alphaherpesvirinae; Genus: *simplexvirus*) 4 reports exist of naturally occurring fatal encephalitis in rabbits due to HSV infection.[145–148]

Epidemiology
Owners of rabbits with clinical facial herpesvirus infection are suspected to be the origin of infection. A similar situation has been reported in 2 pet chinchillas (*Chinchilla lanigera*) diagnosed with fatal HSV encephalitis.[149,150]

Viral isolates derived from 2 marmosets and 1 domestic rabbit that died from HSV encephalitis revealed different genotypes, suggesting that certain HSV genotypes with a higher potential of being transmitted to animals do not exist.[147] The infrequency of natural cross-infection between humans and other species has led some researchers to postulate a nonimmunologic protective mechanism against HSV infection in animals.[151]

Clinical presentation
Affected rabbits present with severe signs of central nervous system dysfunction, such as incoordination, intermittent myoclonic seizures, and opisthotonus. In one case, results of hematologic and serum biochemical analyses revealed only lymphopenia, a relative monocytosis, and an increase in serum activity of creatine phosphokinase and serum concentration of total protein.[146]

Diagnosis
All cases described have been diagnosed at necropsy. Histologic evaluation of brain tissue reveals lesions characteristic of severe, diffuse, nonsuppurative meningoencephalitis and a few large, eosinophilic, intranuclear inclusion bodies in neurons and

glial cells. In situ hybridization and/or PCR detect HSV DNA in the nuclei of glial cells, lymphocytes, and neurons.[152]

Treatment
In one case, despite intravenous administration of crystalloid fluids and treatment with antimicrobials, vitamin B complex, nutritional support, and prednisolone, the condition of the rabbit deteriorated and it was euthanized 7 days after admission.[146]

Prognosis and outcome
All cases in rabbits and chinchillas have resulted in death.

Prevention
Owners with active HSV facial lesions should avoid close contact, such as kissing their pet rabbits.

Leporid-4 Herpes Virus: Systemic Herpes Virus Infection

Introduction
A herpes virus designated as leporid herpesvirus 4 (LHV-4) (Subfamily: Alphaherpesvirinae; Genus: *simplexvirus*) that is highly pathogenic for domestic rabbits has been recently described in rabbits in Alaska and Canada.[73,153–155] Analysis of virus samples indicates that the virus is most closely related to bovine herpesvirus-2. The next most closely related viruses are human HSV 1 and 2, and a number of cercopithecine herpesviruses.[156]

Three naturally occurring herpesviruses of rabbits and hares, called leporid herpesviruses 1, 2, and 3 (LHV-1, LHV-2, and LHV-3), have been identified.[156] They have been classified tentatively as belonging to the subfamily Gammaherpesvirus.[156] The best characterized is LHV-3 (*Herpesvirus sylvilagus*), which is endemic in Eastern cottontail rabbits (*S floridanus*) and causes tumorlike lesions in lymph nodes, kidney, spleen, and liver[157]; however, it does not cause disease in domestic rabbits.[156] LHV-2 (*Herpesvirus cuniculi*) causes asymptomatic infections of domestic rabbits.[156] LHV-1 is found in cottontail rabbits[158,159] and no disease has been reported to be associated with it in domestic rabbits.[156] The novel herpes virus identified in Alaska and Canada is referred to as LHV-4.[153]

Epidemiology
Reports to date of LHV-4 infection are limited to commercial rabbitries. Experimental exposure of domestic rabbits to virus isolates results in severe clinical disease and necrosis in the spleen and lymph nodes.[156] Viral DNA has been identified in a variety of tissues by PCR, consistent with a systemic infection.

It is possible that LHV-4 is present in an animal reservoir found in northwestern North America, in which it causes asymptomatic infections and infrequently comes in contact with domestic rabbits. It is also possible that LHV-4 is present in wild rabbit populations but is not often transmitted to domestic rabbits.[158]

Clinical presentation
The primary lesions are conjunctivitis and periocular swelling, multifocal hemorrhagic/ulcerative dermatitis on the face and dorsum.[154] Clinical signs include progressive weakness, anorexia, respiratory distress, and abortion.[73] Frequently animals are found dead with no previous evidence of disease.

Pathophysiology
Death is due to cardiovascular and respiratory failure.[155]

Diagnosis

At necropsy there is massive necrosis and fibrin deposition within red pulp of the spleen.[73] Large eosinophilic, intranuclear inclusion bodies are observed microscopically in tissue sections of skin, spleen, and lung.[154] Hemorrhagic dermatitis and panniculitis are associated with epidermal microvesicular degeneration, dermal and subcutaneous vascular necrosis, and thrombosis. Other findings include hemorrhagic necrosis of the myocardium with rare intranuclear inclusions within stromal cells, multifocal pulmonary hemorrhage, and hemorrhage with sinus erythrophagocytosis in lymph nodes.[73]

VIRAL INFECTIONS OF LABORATORY SIGNIFICANCE
Astrovirus: Probable Factor in Enteritis Complex

A novel astrovirus (Family: Astroviridae; Genus: *mamastrovirus*) was recently identified by screening rabbits with enteritis complex and healthy rabbits.[160] Rabbit astrovirus was found in 10 (43%) of 23 samples from rabbits with enteric disease and in 25 (18%) of 139 samples from healthy rabbits in Italy during 2005 to 2008. The median titers of virus in the rabbits with enteric disease were 10^3 greater than in the healthy rabbits.

Astroviruses are a family of RNA viruses with 2 genera: *mamastrovirus* and *avastrovirus*. The genus *mamastrovirus* is associated with gastroenteritis in most animal species and humans.[161] Astrovirus infections are regarded as the second most common cause of viral diarrhea in children after rotavirus infection, but in animals, their association with enteric diseases is not well documented, with the exception of turkey and mink astrovirus infection.[161]

The multifactorial enteritis complex of juvenile rabbits[103,105,117] can be caused by bacteria, viruses, and parasites. Several different viruses have been isolated from rabbits with diarrhea, such as rotavirus, coronavirus, and now astrovirus. Whether natural outbreaks of enteritis can be caused by these viral agents alone or in conjunction with other pathogens is not clear. Rabbit astroviruses should be included in the diagnostic algorithm of rabbit enteritis complex. Further experiments to increase information about their epidemiology and potential pathogenic role are required.

Bornavirus: Borna Disease

Borna disease virus (Family: Bornaviridae; Genus: *bornavirus*) (BDV) is the cause of a fatal neurologic disease primarily of horses and sheep that occurs sporadically in central Europe. Incidence is highest during spring and summer. Arthropods have been discussed as a potential vector, but BDV has never been isolated from insects in Europe.[162] A definite virus reservoir for BDV has not been found; various rodents most likely represent such a reservoir.[162] Natural infections in other Equidae, ruminants, rabbits, and cats have also been described in Europe, North Africa, and the Middle East[162,163]; however, the virus exists worldwide. The infection can be fatal, but most carriers are persistently infected without showing clinical signs. Recently, avian bornavirus was identified as the cause of proventricular dilatation disease in parrots, and, like Borna disease virus, has been detected worldwide.[164]

BDV is assumed to be transmitted through salivary, nasal, or conjunctival secretions. Animals become infected by direct contact with these secretions or by exposure to contaminated food or water. A minimum incubation period of 4 weeks is estimated for horses and sheep. In rabbits, natural infections have been reported only in Germany.[163] Clinical signs in naturally and experimentally infected rabbits are neurologic. Although Borna disease is rare in rabbits, the worldwide existence of the virus means the infection must be differentiated from rabies virus infection and *Encephalitozoon cuniculi* infection.[165] Histopathologically, Borna disease is characterized by a nonpurulent inflammation of the brain and the spinal cord.[166] The detection of BDV in diseased animals, mainly sheep and horses, is achieved by histologic, immunohistochemical, and serologic approaches and/or PCR-based technologies.[167]

Rabies Virus: Rabies

Rabies virus (Family: Rhabdoviridae; Genus: *lyssavirus*) infection is relatively rare in both pet and feral rabbits. Of the 87,700 cases of animal rabies reported in the United States from 1992 to 2002, only 621 occurred in rodents or lagomorphs.[168,169] The majority (559 cases) occurred in groundhogs (*Marmota monax*) and were most likely because of den contact from infected skunks or raccoons.[169] Despite its rarity, rabies has been reported in pet rabbits in Western Europe and North America.[170–174] All cases have been in outdoor-housed pet rabbits. Most cases have come in contact with wildlife carrying rabies (eg, raccoon in North America, fox in Europe) but the source of infection in some rabbits remains unknown.

Both furious and dumb forms of rabies have been reported in naturally infected rabbits; however, the dumb form seems more common. Unilateral pelvic limb paresis or paralysis has been reported as an early clinical sign in domestic rabbits.[171] The one case of furious rabies described the rabbit biting at inanimate objects.[172]

Currently, there is not a rabies vaccine approved for use in rabbits. The only way to prevent rabies infection in rabbits is to prevent exposure. Veterinarians in rabies-enzootic areas should be familiar with the clinical signs of rabies in rabbits and should caution rabbit owners about the need to protect their pets from contact with wildlife.

Vaccinia Virus: Rabbitpox (Rabbit Plague)

Because of its widespread use as a smallpox vaccination in humans, and its wide host range, vaccinia virus (Subfamily: Chordopoxvirinae; Genus: *orthopoxvirus*) sometimes has caused naturally spreading diseases in domestic animals (eg, teat infections of cattle) and also in laboratory rabbits (rabbitpox). Epidemics of rabbitpox occurring in isolated animal rooms were reported in the United States and Netherlands.[175,176]

The disease is acute and rapidly fatal. Confluent papules on the skin, sometimes accompanied by necrosis and hemorrhage, characterize rabbitpox.[177,178] Papular lesions may occur in the oropharynx, respiratory tract, spleen, and liver.[179] In the so-called "pockless" form, a few pocks were present in the oral cavity, and focal hepatic necrosis, pleuritis, and splenomegaly were observed.[180] The primary site for replication in the naturally occurring disease is the respiratory tract.[181] There is a subsequent viremia with replication in lymphoid tissues and skin.[181]

Now that smallpox vaccination has been discontinued for the civilian populations of all countries, rabbitpox is unlikely to be seen. However, the use of aerosolized rabbitpox infection as an animal model for evaluation of antivirals under development for the therapeutic treatment of human smallpox still continues. Consequently, rabbitpox may be seen in laboratory rabbits if the experimental virus is not confined to the biocontainment research area.[182]

Pleural Effusion Disease Virus (Infectious Cardiomyopathy Virus): Pleural Effusion Disease and Cardiomyopathy

Pleural effusion, right-sided heart enlargement, mesenteric lymphadenopathy, and multifocal necrosis of multiple organs have been associated with infection by a coronavirus referred to as pleural effusion disease virus (PEDV) (Family: Coronaviridae; Genus: *coronavirus*) in laboratory rabbits in North America and Europe.[183] PEDV was discovered as a contaminant of *Treponema pallidum* (the causative agent of syphilis), which is maintained by intratesticular inoculation of laboratory rabbits.[184] PEDV infection is not seen in pet rabbits. Different PEDV isolates vary in pathogenicity and range from subclinical infection to infection causing more than 50% mortality.[185] Lymphoid depletion of splenic follicles, focal degenerative changes in lymph nodes and thymus, proliferative changes in glomerular tufts, and uveitis characterized fatal infections.[183,186] In one infection, multifocal myocardial degeneration and necrosis were seen.[187] Antibodies to 2 human strains of coronavirus have been demonstrated in convalescent rabbit sera and antigen to human 229E coronavirus (one of the 4 human coronaviruses circulating worldwide and a proven common cold virus in healthy adults) was detected in myocardial lesions.[188,189] The evidence suggests that the causative agent is not a natural pathogen of rabbits.

Rabbit Enteric Coronavirus: Coronaviral Enteritis

Rabbit enteric coronavirus (RECV) (Family: Coronaviridae; Genus: *coronavirus*) induces disease in juvenile rabbits that is characterized by intestinal villus attenuation, malabsorption, and diarrhea. Infection may predispose rabbits to, or be obscured by, the enteritis complex. Although RECV has been isolated, it has not been characterized.[190]

Coronavirus-associated enteritis has been reported in commercial rabbitries but generally with low mortality.[191] In one report, an outbreak of fatal enteritis in 3 to 8-week old rabbits occurred in a barrier-maintained breeding colony in Germany.[192] The prevalence of detectable antibody in a serologic survey of North American commercial rabbitries ranged from 3% to 40%.[193] The presence of coronaviral particles in feces of young diarrheic rabbits indicates the virus may play a role in enteritis complex. However, coronaviral particles have also been observed in gastrointestinal contents of healthy rabbits. Differential diagnoses include *E coli* infections, coccidiosis, rotavirus infection, and clostridial enteropathies.

Experimentally and naturally infected young rabbits may be emaciated and dehydrated and show perineal fecal staining.[192,194] The cecum may be distended, with a milky to tan liquid.[192,194] Microscopic changes are confined to the small and large intestines.[194] Distinctive findings include villous blunting, vacuolation and necrosis of enterocytes, mucosal edema, and polymorphonuclear and mononuclear cell infiltration.

Confirmation of diagnosis requires demonstration of coronaviral particles from gastrointestinal contents by electron microscopy.[190] The virus has not been grown in cell culture.

REFERENCES

1. Cooke BD, Fenner F. Rabbit haemorrhagic disease and the biological control of wild rabbits, *Oryctolagus cuniculus*, in Australia and New Zealand. Wildl Res 2002;29(6):689–706.
2. Anonymous, AVMA News. Rabbit calicivirus infection confirmed in Iowa rabbitry. J Am Vet Med Assoc 2000;216(10):1537.
3. Campagnolo ER, Ernst MJ, Berninger ML, et al. Outbreak of rabbit hemorrhagic disease in domestic lagomorphs. J Am Vet Med Assoc 2003;223(8):1151–5, 1128.
4. McIntosh MT, Behan SC, Mohamed FM, et al. A pandemic strain of calicivirus threatens rabbit industries in the Americas. Virol J 2007;4:96.

5. Center for Emerging Issues, USDA. Rabbit hemorrhagic disease, Indiana, June 15, 2005. Impact Worksheet. Available at: http://www.aphis.usda.gov/animal_health/emergingissues/impactworksheets/iw_2005_files/domestic/rhdindiana061505.htm. Accessed December 3, 2012.

6. Capucci L, Fusi P, Lavazza A, et al. Detection and preliminary characterization of a new rabbit calicivirus related to rabbit hemorrhagic disease virus but nonpathogenic. J Virol 1996;70(12):8614–23.

7. Forrester NL, Trout RC, Gould EA. Benign circulation of rabbit haemorrhagic disease virus on Lambay Island, Eire. Virology 2007;358(1):18–22.

8. Strive T, Wright J, Kovaliski J, et al. The non-pathogenic Australian lagovirus RCV-A1 causes a prolonged infection and elicits partial cross-protection to rabbit haemorrhagic disease virus. Virology 2010;398(1):125–34.

9. Strive T, Wright JD, Robinson AJ. Identification and partial characterisation of a new Lagovirus in Australian wild rabbits. Virology 2009;384(1):97–105.

10. Jahnke M, Holmes EC, Kerr PJ, et al. Evolution and phylogeograph of the non-pathogenic calicivirus RCV-A1 in wild rabbits in Australia. J Virol 2010;84(23):12397–404.

11. Bergin IL, Wise AG, Bolin SR, et al. Novel calicivirus identified in rabbits, Michigan, USA. Emerg Infect Dis 2009;15(12):1955–62.

12. Cooke BD, Chapuis JL, Magnet V, et al. Potential use of myxoma virus and rabbit haemorrhagic disease virus to control feral rabbits in the Kerguelen Archipelago. Wildl Res 2004;31(4):415–20.

13. Marchandeau S, Bertagnoli S, Leonard Y, et al. Serological evidence for the presence of non-pathogenic rabbit haemorrhagic disease virus-like strains in rabbits (*Oryctolagus cuniculus*) of the Kerguelen archipelago. Polar Biol 2010; 33(7):985–9.

14. O'Keefe JS, Tempero JE, Motha MX, et al. Serology of rabbit haemorrhagic disease virus in wild rabbits before and after release of the virus in New Zealand. Vet Microbiol 1999;66(1):29–40.

15. Dalton KP, Nicieza I, Balseiro A, et al. Variant rabbit hemorrhagic disease virus in young rabbits, Spain. Emerg Infect Dis 2012;18(2):2009–12.

16. Le Gall-Recule G, Zwingelstein F, Boucher S, et al. Detection of a new variant of rabbit haemorrhagic disease virus in France. Vet Rec 2011;168(5):137–8.

17. Robinson AJ, So PT, Muller WJ, et al. Statistical models for the effect of age and maternal antibodies on the development of rabbit haemorrhagic disease in Australian wild rabbits. Wildl Res 2002;29(6):663–71.

18. McColl KA, Morrissy CJ, Collins BJ, et al. Persistence of rabbit haemorrhagic disease virus in decomposing rabbit carcasses. Aust Vet J 2002;80(5): 298–9.

19. Henning J, Meers J, Davies PR, et al. Survival of rabbit haemorrhagic disease virus (RHDV) in the environment. Epidemiol Infect 2005;133(4):719–30.

20. McColl KA, Merchant JC, Hardy J, et al. Evidence for insect transmission of rabbit haemorrhagic disease virus. Epidemiol Infect 2002;129(3):655–63.

21. Lenghaus C, Westbury H, Collins B, et al. Overview of the RHD project in the Australian Animal Health Laboratory. In: Munro RK, Williams RT, editors. Rabbit haemorrhagic disease: issues in assessment for biological control. Canberra (Australia): Bureau of Resource Sciences; 1994. p. 104–29.

22. Capucci L, Nardin A, Lavazza A. Seroconversion in an industrial unit of rabbits infected with a non-pathogenic rabbit haemorrhagic disease-like virus. Vet Rec 1997;140(25):647–50.

23. Mutze G, Sinclair R, Peacock D, et al. Does a benign calicivirus reduce the effectiveness of rabbit haemorrhagic disease virus (RHDV) in Australia? Experimental evidence from field releases of RHDV on bait. Wildl Res 2010;37(4): 311–9.

24. Parkes JP, Norbury GL, Heyward RP, et al. Epidemiology of rabbit haemorrhagic disease (RHD) in the South Island, New Zealand, 1997-2001. Wildl Res 2002; 29(6):543–55.

25. McPhee SR, Butler KL, Kovaliski J, et al. Antibody status and survival of Australian wild rabbits challenged with rabbit haemorrhagic disease virus. Wildl Res 2009; 36(5):447–56.

26. Marchandeau S, Le Gall-Recule G, Bertagnoli S, et al. Serological evidence for a non-protective RHDV-like virus. Vet Res 2005;36(1):53–62.

27. Teifke JP, Reimann I, Schirrmeier H. Subacute liver necrosis after experimental infection with rabbit haemorrhagic disease virus (RHDV). J Comp Pathol 2002; 126(2–3):231–4.

28. Tunon MJ, Sanchez-Campos S, Garcia-Ferreras J, et al. Rabbit hemorrhagic viral disease: characterization of a new animal model of fulminant liver failure. J Lab Clin Med 2003;141(4):272–8.

29. Ferreira PG, Costa-e-Silva A, Oliveira MJ, et al. Severe leukopenia and liver biochemistry changes in adult rabbits after calicivirus infection. Res Vet Sci 2006;80(2):218–25.

30. Sánchez-Campos S, Alvarez M, Culebras JM, et al. Pathogenic molecular mechanisms in an animal model of fulminant hepatic failure: rabbit hemorrhagic virus disease. J Lab Clin Med 2004;144(4):215–22.

31. Chen SY, Chou CC, Liu CI, et al. Impairment of renal function and electrolyte balance in rabbit hemorrhagic disease. J Vet Med Sci 2008;70(9): 951–8.

32. Chen SY, Shien JH, Ooi HK. Hyperlipidemia in rabbit hemorrhagic disease. Exp Anim 2008;57(5):479–83.

33. Fuchs A, Weissenbock H. Comparative histopathological study of rabbit haemorrhagic disease (RHD) and European brown hare syndrome (EBHS). J Comp Pathol 1992;107(1):103–13.

34. Shien JH, Shieh HK, Lee LH. Experimental infections of rabbits with rabbit haemorrhagic disease virus monitored by polymerase chain reaction. Res Vet Sci 2000;68(3):255–9.

35. Forrester NL, Boag B, Moss SR, et al. Long-term survival of New Zealand rabbit haemorrhagic disease virus RNA in wild rabbits, revealed by RT-PCR and phylogenetic analysis. J Gen Virol 2003;84(Pt 11):3079–86.

36. Gall A, Hoffmann B, Teifke JP, et al. Persistence of viral RNA in rabbits which overcome an experimental RHDV infection detected by a highly sensitive multiplex real-time RT-PCR. Vet Microbiol 2007;120(1–2):17–32.

37. Lavazza A, Capucci L. Rabbit haemorrhagic disease. In: OIE Biological Standards Commission, editor. Manual of Diagnostic Tests and Vaccines for Terrestrial Animals. 7th edition. Paris: Office International des Épizooties; 2012. Section 2:6:2.

38. Liu J, Kerr PJ, Wright JD, et al. Serological assays to discriminate rabbit haemorrhagic disease virus from Australian non-pathogenic rabbit calicivirus. Vet Microbiol 2012;157(3–4):345–54.

39. Crespo I, Miguel BS, Laliena A, et al. Melatonin prevents the decreased activity of antioxidant enzymes and activates nuclear erythroid 2-related factor 2 signaling in an animal model of fulminant hepatic failure of viral origin. J Pineal Res 2010;49(2):193–200.

40. Tuñón MJ, San Miguel B, Crespo I, et al. Melatonin attenuates apoptotic liver damage in fulminant hepatic failure induced by the rabbit haemorrhagic disease virus. J Pineal Res 2011;50(1):38–45.
41. Tunon MJ, San Miguel B, Crespo I, et al. Cardiotrophin-1 promotes a high survival rate in rabbits with lethal fulminant hepatitis of viral origin. J Virol 2011;85(24):13124–32.
42. Laliena A, San Miguel B, Crespo I, et al. Melatonin attenuates inflammation and promotes regeneration in rabbits with fulminant hepatitis of viral origin. J Pineal Res 2012;53(3):270–8.
43. Wang XL, Hao HF, Qiu L, et al. Phylogenetic analysis of rabbit hemorrhagic disease virus in China and the antigenic variation of new strains. Arch Virol 2012;157(8):1523–30.
44. Spibey N, McCabe VJ, Greenwood NM, et al. Novel bivalent vectored vaccine for control of myxomatosis and rabbit haemorrhagic disease. Vet Rec 2012; 170(12):309.
45. Kerr PJ. Myxomatosis in Australia and Europe: a model for emerging infectious diseases. Antiviral Res 2012;93(3):387–415.
46. Fenner F, Ratcliffe FN. Myxomatosis. Cambridge (England): Cambridge University Press; 1965.
47. Fenner F, Marshall ID. Passive immunity in myxomatosis of the European rabbit (*Oryctolagus cuniculus*): the protection conferred on kittens born by immune does. J Hyg (Lond) 1954;52(3):321–36.
48. Day MF, Fenner F, Woodroofe GM, et al. Further studies on the mechanism of mosquito transmission of myxomatosis in the European rabbit. J Hyg (Lond) 1956;54(2):258–83.
49. Marshall ID, Regnery DC. Myxomatosis in a California brush rabbit (*Sylvilagus bachmani*). Nature 1960;188:73–4.
50. Marshall ID, Regnery DC, Grodhaus G. Studies in the epidemiology of myxomatosis in California. I. Observations on two outbreaks of myxomatosis in coastal California and the recovery of myxoma virus from a brush rabbit (*Sylvilagus bachmani*). Am J Hyg 1963;77(2):195–204.
51. Kessel JF, Fisk RT, Prouty CC. Studies with the Californian strain of the virus of infectious myxomatosis. In: Cook SJ, editor. Proceedings of the 5th Pacific Science Congress, Canada, 1933. University of Toronto Press; 1934. p. 2927–39.
52. Patton NM, Holmes HT. Myxomatosis in domestic rabbits in Oregon. J Am Vet Med Assoc 1977;171(6):560–2.
53. Licon Luna RM. First report of myxomatosis in Mexico. J Wildl Dis 2000;36(3): 580–3.
54. Kritas SK, Dovas C, Fortomaris P, et al. A pathogenic myxoma virus in vaccinated and non-vaccinated commercial rabbits. Res Vet Sci 2008;85(3): 622–4.
55. Marlier D, Mainil J, Sulon J, et al. Study of the virulence of five strains of amyxomatous myxoma virus in crossbred New Zealand White/Californian conventional rabbits, with evidence of long-term testicular infection in recovered animals. J Comp Pathol 2000;122(2–3):101–13.
56. Arthur CP, Louzis C. La myxomatose du lapin en France: une revue. Rev Sci Tech 1988;7(4):937–57.
57. Marlier D, Cassart D, Boucraut-Baralon C, et al. Experimental infection of specific pathogen-free New Zealand White rabbits with five strains of amyxomatous myxoma virus. J Comp Pathol 1999;121(4):369–84.

58. Marlier D, Herbots J, Detilleux J, et al. Cross-sectional study of the association between pathological conditions and myxoma virus seroprevalence in intensive rabbit farms in Europe. Prev Vet Med 2001;48(1):55–64.

59. Fenner F, Marshall ID. A comparison of the virulence for European rabbits (*Oryctolagus cuniculus*) of strains of myxoma virus recovered in the field in Australia, Europe and America. J Hyg (Lond) 1957;55(2):149–91.

60. Fenner F. The Florey lecture, 1983. Biological control, as exemplified by smallpox eradication and myxomatosis. Proc R Soc Lond B Biol Sci 1983; 218(1212):259–85.

61. Fountain S, Holland MK, Hinds LA, et al. Interstitial orchitis with impaired steroidogenesis and spermatogenesis in the testes of rabbits infected with an attenuated strain of myxoma virus. J Reprod Fertil 1997;110(1):161–9.

62. Best SM, Collins SV, Kerr PJ. Coevolution of host and virus: cellular localization of virus in myxoma virus infection of resistant and susceptible European rabbits. Virology 2000;277(1):76–91.

63. Fenner F, Woodroofe GM. The pathogenesis of infectious myxomatosis; the mechanism of infection and the immunological response in the European rabbit (*Oryctolagus cuniculus*). Br J Exp Pathol 1953;34(4):400–11.

64. Best SM, Kerr PJ. Coevolution of host and virus: the pathogenesis of virulent and attenuated strains of myxoma virus in resistant and susceptible European rabbits. Virology 2000;267(1):36–48.

65. Mims C. Aspects of the pathogenesis of viral diseases. Bacteriol Rev 1964;28: 30–71.

66. Strayer DS. Determinants of virus-related suppression of immune responses as observed during infection with an oncogenic poxvirus. In: Melnick JL, editor. Progress in medical virology. Basel (Switzerland): Karger; 1992. p. 228–55.

67. Cameron CM, Barrett JW, Liu L, et al. Myxoma virus M141R expresses a viral CD200 (vOX-2) that is responsible for down-regulation of macrophage and T-cell activation in vivo. J Virol 2005;79(10):6052–67.

68. Johnston JB, Barrett JW, Nazarian SH, et al. A poxvirus-encoded pyrin domain protein interacts with ASC-1 to inhibit host inflammatory and apoptotic responses to infection. Immunity 2005;23(6):587–98.

69. Jeklova E, Leva L, Matiasovic J, et al. Characterisation of immunosuppression in rabbits after infection with myxoma virus. Vet Microbiol 2008;129(1–2):117–30.

70. Cameron CM, Barrett JW, Mann M, et al. Myxoma virus M128L is expressed as a cell surface CD47-like virulence factor that contributes to the downregulation of macrophage activation in vivo. Virology 2005;337(1):55–67.

71. Hurst EW. Myxoma and the Shope fibroma. I. The histology of myxoma. Br J Exp Pathol 1937;18(1):1–15.

72. Bertagnoli S. Myxomatosis. In: OIE Biological Standards Commission, editor. Manual of Diagnostic Tests and Vaccines for Terrestrial Animals. 7th edition. Paris: Office International des Épizooties; 2012. Section 2:6.1.

73. Jin L, Valentine BA, Baker RJ, et al. An outbreak of fatal herpesvirus infection in domestic rabbits in Alaska. Vet Pathol 2008;45(3):369–74.

74. Marshall ID. The influence of ambient temperature on the course of myxomatosis in rabbits. J Hyg (Lond) 1959;57:484–97.

75. McKercher DG. Infectious myxomatosis. I. Vaccination. II. Antibiotic therapy. Am J Vet Res 1952;13(48):425–9.

76. Robinson AJ, Muller WJ, Braid AL, et al. The effect of buprenorphine on the course of disease in laboratory rabbits infected with myxoma virus. Lab Anim 1999;33(3):252–7.

77. Adams MM, Rice AD, Moyer RW. Rabbitpox virus and vaccinia virus infection of rabbits as a model for human smallpox. J Virol 2007;81(20):11084–95.
78. Rice AD, Adams MM, Wallace G, et al. Efficacy of CMX001 as a post exposure antiviral in New Zealand white rabbits infected with rabbitpox virus, a model for orthopoxvirus infections of humans. Viruses 2011;3(1):47–62.
79. Marlier D. Vaccination strategies against myxomavirus infections: are we really doing the best? Tijdschr Diergeneeskd 2010;135(5):194–8.
80. Brun A, Godard A, Moreau Y. La vaccination contre la myxomatose. Vaccins heterologues et homologues. Bulletin de la Société des sciences vétérinaires de (Lyon) 1981;83(5):251–4.
81. Vautherot JF, Milon A, Petit F, et al. Vaccines for lagomorphs. In: Pastoret PP, Blancou J, Vannier P, et al, editors. Veterinary vaccinology. Amsterdam (Netherlands): Elsevier; 1997. p. 406–10.
82. Hyde RR, Gardner RE. Transmission experiments with the fibroma (Shope) and myxoma (Sanarelli) viruses. Am J Hyg 1939;30(1/3):57–63.
83. Smith JW, Tevethia SS, Levy BM, et al. Comparative studies on host responses to Shope fibroma virus in adult and newborn rabbits. J Natl Cancer Inst 1973; 50(6):1529–39.
84. Fenner F, Woodroofe GM. Protection of laboratory rabbits against myxomatosis by vaccination with fibroma virus. Aust J Exp Biol Med Sci 1954;32(5):653–68.
85. Shope RE. A transmissible tumor-like condition in rabbits. J Exp Med 1932; 56(6):793–802.
86. Kilham L, Dalmat HT. Host-virus-mosquito relations of Shope fibromas in cotton-tail rabbits. Am J Hyg 1955;61(1):45–54.
87. Kilham L, Woke PA. Laboratory transmission of fibromas (Shope) in cottontail rabbits by means of fleas and mosquitoes. Proc Soc Exp Biol Med 1953; 83(2):296–301.
88. Joiner GN, Jardine JH, Gleiser CA. An epizootic of shope fibromatosis in a commercial rabbitry. J Am Vet Med Assoc 1971;159(11):1583–7.
89. Dalmat HT. Arthropod transmission of rabbit fibromatosis (Shope). J Hyg (Lond) 1959;57(1):1–30.
90. Dalmat HT, Stanton MF. A comparative study of the Shope fibroma in rabbits in relation to transmissibility by mosquitoes. J Natl Cancer Inst 1959;22(3): 593–615.
91. Dalmat HT. Effects of x-rays and chemical carcinogens on infectivity of domestic rabbit fibromas for arthropods. J Infect Dis 1958;102(2):153–7.
92. Raflo CP, Olsen RG, Pakes SP, et al. Characterization of a fibroma virus isolated from naturally-occurring skin tumors in domestic rabbits. Lab Anim Sci 1973; 23(4):525–32.
93. von Bomhard W, Goldschmidt MH, Shofer FS, et al. Cutaneous neoplasms in pet rabbits: a retrospective study. Vet Pathol 2007;44(5):579–88.
94. Hurst EW. Myxoma and the Shope fibroma. IV. The histology of Shope fibroma. Aust J Exp Biol Med Sci 1938;16(1):53–64.
95. Sell S, Scott CB. An immunohistologic study of Shope fibroma virus in rabbits: tumor rejection by cellular reaction in adults and progressive systemic reticulo-endothelial infection in neonates. J Natl Cancer Inst 1981;66(2):363–73.
96. Rizzi V, Legrottaglie R, Cini A, et al. Electrophoretic typing of some strains of enteric viruses isolated in rabbits suffering from diarrhoea. New Microbiol 1995;18(1):77–81.
97. Tanaka TN, Conner ME, Graham DY, et al. Molecular characterization of three rabbit rotavirus strains. Arch Virol 1988;98(3):253–65.

98. Thouless ME, DiGiacomo RF, Neuman DS. Isolation of two lapine rotaviruses: characterization of their subgroup, serotype and RNA electropherotypes. Arch Virol 1986;89(1):161–70.

99. Martella V, Ciarlet M, Camarda A, et al. Molecular characterization of the VP4, VP6, VP7, and NSP4 genes of lapine rotaviruses identified in Italy: emergence of a novel VP4 genotype. Virology 2003;314(1):358–70.

100. Endre K, Iren H, Arpad A, et al. Occurrence of rotavirus infection of rabbits in Hungary. Magy Allatorvosok Lapja 1982;37(4):248–54.

101. Bányai K, Forgách P, Erdélyi K, et al. Identification of the novel lapine rotavirus genotype P[22] from an outbreak of enteritis in a Hungarian rabbitry. Virus Res 2005;113(2):73–80.

102. Martella V, Ciarlet M, Lavazza A, et al. Lapine rotaviruses of the genotype P[22] are widespread in Italian rabbitries. Vet Microbiol 2005;111(1–2): 117–24.

103. Badagliacca P, Letizia A, Candeloro L, et al. Clinical, pathological and microbiological profiles of spontaneous enteropathies in growing rabbits. World Rabbit Sci 2010;18(4):187–98.

104. Marlier D, Vindevogel H. Les maladies virales chez le lapin Européen (*Oryctolagus cuniculus*). Ann Med Vet 1996;140(6):393–403.

105. Percy DH, Muckle CA, Hampson RJ, et al. The enteritis complex in domestic rabbits: a field study. Can Vet J 1993;34(2):95–102.

106. Schoeb TR, Casebolt DB, Walker VE, et al. Rotavirus-associated diarrhea in a commercial rabbitry. Lab Anim Sci 1986;36(2):149–52.

107. Iwai H, Machii K, Ohtsuka Y, et al. Prevalence of antibodies to Sendai virus and rotavirus in laboratory rabbits. Jikken Dobutsu 1986;35(4):491–4

108. Petric M, Middleton PJ, Grant C, et al. Lapine rotavirus: preliminary studies on epizoology and transmission. Can J Comp Med 1978;42(1):143–7.

109. Legrottaglie R, Mannelli A, Rizzi V, et al. Isolation and characterization of cytopathic strains of rotavirus from hares (*Lepus europaeus*). New Microbiol 1997; 20(2):135–40.

110. Thouless ME, DiGiacomo RF, Deeb BJ, et al. Pathogenicity of rotavirus in rabbits. J Clin Microbiol 1988;26(5):943–7.

111. Li D, Gu AZ, Zeng S, et al. Evaluation of the infectivity, gene and antigenicity persistence of rotaviruses by free chlorine disinfection. J Environ Sci (China) 2011;23(10):1691–8.

112. Saif LJ. Reoviridae. In: Maclachlan NJ, Dubovi EJ, editors. Fenner's veterinary virology. 4th edition. San Diego (CA): Academic Press; 2011. p. 275–91.

113. Ciarlet M, Gilger MA, Barone C, et al. Rotavirus disease, but not infection and development of intestinal histopathological lesions, is age restricted in rabbits. Virology 1998;251(2):343–60.

114. DiGiacomo RF, Thouless ME. Epidemiology of naturally occurring rotavirus infection in rabbits. Lab Anim Sci 1986;36(2):153–6.

115. Lorrot M, Martin S, Vasseur M. Rotavirus infection stimulates the Cl- reabsorption process across the intestinal brush-border membrane of young rabbits. J Virol 2003;77(17):9305–11.

116. Halaihel N, Lievin V, Alvarado F, et al. Rotavirus infection impairs intestinal brush-border membrane Na(+)-solute cotransport activities in young rabbits. Am J Physiol Gastrointest Liver Physiol 2000;279(3):G587–96.

117. Thouless ME, DiGiacomo RF, Deeb BJ. The effect of combined rotavirus and *Escherichia coli* infections in rabbits. Lab Anim Sci 1996;46(4):381–5.

118. Fushuku S, Fukuda K. Examination of the applicability of a commercial human rotavirus antigen detection kit for use in laboratory rabbits. Exp Anim 2006; 55(1):71–4.

119. Sato K, Inaba Y, Miura Y, et al. Isolation of lapine rotavirus in cell cultures. Arch Virol 1982;71(3):267–71.

120. Conner ME, Estes MK, Graham DY. Rabbit model of rotavirus infection. J Virol 1988;62(5):1625–33.

121. Ciarlet M, Crawford SE, Barone C, et al. Subunit rotavirus vaccine administered parenterally to rabbits induces active protective immunity. J Virol 1998;72(11): 9233–46.

122. Rous P, Kidd JG. The carcinogenic effect of a papilloma virus on the tarred skin of rabbits: I. Description of the phenomenon. J Exp Med 1938;67(3): 399–428.

123. Shope RE. Immunization of rabbits to infectious papillomatosis. J Exp Med 1937;65(2):219–31.

124. Shope RE, Hurst EW. Infectious papillomatosis of rabbits: with a note on the histopathology. J Exp Med 1933;58(5):607–24.

125. Weiner CM, Rosenbaum MD, Fox K, et al. Cottontail rabbit papillomavirus in Langerhans cells in Sylvilagus spp. J Vet Diagn Invest 2010;22(3):451–4.

126. Griem W. Kaninchen Papillomatose: einen Bericht über drei spontane Fälle unter den Versuchstieren. Z Versuchstierkd 1982;24(1/2):36.

127. Hagen KW. Spontaneous papillomatosis in domestic rabbits. Bull Wildl Dis Ass 1966;2(4):108–10.

128. Watts SL, Ostrow RS, Phelps WC, et al. Free cottontail rabbit papillomavirus DNA persists in warts and carcinomas of infected rabbits and in cells in culture transformed with virus or viral DNA. Virology 1983;125(1):127–38.

129. Hu J, Budgeon LR, Cladel NM, et al. Detection of L1, infectious virions and anti-L1 antibody in domestic rabbits infected with cottontail rabbit papillomavirus. J Gen Virol 2007;88(Pt 12):3286–93.

130. Amella CA, Lofgren LA, Ronn AM, et al. Latent infection induced with cottontail rabbit papillomavirus. A model for human papillomavirus latency. Am J Pathol 1994;144(6):1167–71.

131. Zhang P, Nouri M, Brandsma JL, et al. Induction of E6/E7 expression in cottontail rabbit papillomavirus latency following UV activation. Virology 1999;263(2): 388–94.

132. Zeltner R, Borenstein LA, Wettstein FO, et al. Changes in RNA expression pattern during the malignant progression of cottontail rabbit papillomavirus-induced tumors in rabbits. J Virol 1994;68(6):3620–30.

133. Christensen ND, Han R, Cladel NM, et al. Combination treatment with intralesional cidofovir and viral-DNA vaccination cures large cottontail rabbit papillomavirus-induced papillomas and reduces recurrences. Antimicrob Agents Chemother 2001;45(4):1201–9.

134. Poetker DM, Kerschner JE, Patel NJ, et al. Immune stimulation for the treatment of papilloma. Ann Otol Rhinol Laryngol 2005;114(9):657–61.

135. Sundberg JP, Junge RE, el Shazly MO. Oral papillomatosis in New Zealand white rabbits. Am J Vet Res 1985;46(3):664–8.

136. Mews AR, Ritchie JS, Romero-Mercado CH, et al. Detection of oral papillomatosis in a British rabbit colony. Lab Anim 1972;6(2):141–5.

137. Weisbroth SH, Scher S. Spontaneous oral papillomatosis in rabbits. J Am Vet Med Assoc 1970;157(11):1940–4.

138. Dominguez JA, Corella EL, Auro A. Oral papillomatosis in two laboratory rabbits in Mexico. Lab Anim Sci 1981;31(1):71–3.

139. Parsons RJ, Kidd JG. Oral papillomatosis of rabbits: a virus disease. J Exp Med 1943;77(3):233–50.

140. Rdzok EJ, Shipkowitz NL, Richter WR. Rabbit oral papillomatosis: ultrastructure of experimental infection. Cancer Res 1966;26(1):160–5.

141. Munday JS, Aberdein D, Squires RA, et al. Persistent conjunctival papilloma due to oral papillomavirus infection in a rabbit in New Zealand. J Am Assoc Lab Anim Sci 2007;46(5):69–71.

142. Christensen ND, Cladel NM, Reed CA, et al. Rabbit oral papillomavirus complete genome sequence and immunity following genital infection. Virology 2000;269(2):451–61.

143. Parrish CR, Papillomaviridae and Polyomaviridae. In: Maclachlan NJ, Dubovi EJ, editors. Fenner's veterinary virology. 4th edition. San Diego (CA): Academic Press; 2011. p. 213–23.

144. Weisbroth SH. Sialocele (ranula) simulating oral papillomatosis in a domestic (*Oryctolagus*) rabbit. Lab Anim Sci 1975;25(3):321–2.

145. Grest P, Albicker P, Hoelzle L, et al. Herpes simplex encephalitis in a domestic rabbit (*Oryctolagus cuniculus*). J Comp Pathol 2002;126(4):308–11.

146. Muller K, Fuchs W, Heblinski N, et al. Encephalitis in a rabbit caused by human herpesvirus-1. J Am Vet Med Assoc 2009;235(1):66–9.

147. Sekulin K, Jankova J, Kolodziejek J, et al. Natural zoonotic infections of two marmosets and one domestic rabbit with herpes simplex virus type 1 did not reveal a correlation with a certain gG-, gI- or gE genotype. Clin Microbiol Infect 2010;16(11):1669–72.

148. Weissenböck H, Hainfellner JA, Berger J, et al. Naturally occurring herpes simplex encephalitis in a domestic rabbit (*Oryctolagus cuniculus*). Vet Pathol 1997;34(1):44–7.

149. Wohlsein P, Thiele A, Fehr M, et al. Spontaneous human herpes virus type 1 infection in a chinchilla (*Chinchilla lanigera* f. dom.). Acta Neuropathol 2002; 104(6):674–8.

150. Goudas P, Giltoy JS. Spontaneous herpes-like viral infection in a chinchilla (Chinchilla laniger). J Wildl Dis 1970;6(3):175–9.

151. Skinner GR, Ahmad A, Davies JA. The infrequency of transmission of herpesviruses between humans and animals; postulation of an unrecognised protective host mechanism. Comp Immunol Microbiol Infect Dis 2001;24(4): 255–69.

152. Gruber A, Pakozdy A, Weissenbock H, et al. A retrospective study of neurological disease in 118 rabbits. J Comp Pathol 2009;140(1):31–7.

153. Brash ML, Nagy E, Pei Y, et al. Acute hemorrhagic and necrotizing pneumonia, splenitis, and dermatitis in a pet rabbit caused by a novel herpesvirus (leporid herpesvirus-4). Can Vet J 2010;51(12):1383–6.

154. Onderka DK, Papp-Vid G, Perry AW. Fatal herpesvirus infection in commercial rabbits. Can Vet J 1992;33(8):539–43.

155. Swan C, Perry A, Papp-Vid G. Alberta. Herpesvirus-like viral infection in a rabbit. Can Vet J 1991;32(10):627–8.

156. Jin L, Lohr CV, Vanarsdall AL, et al. Characterization of a novel alphaherpesvirus associated with fatal infections of domestic rabbits. Virology 2008;378(1):13–20.

157. Medveczky PG. Herpesvirus sylvilagus (Herpesviridae). In: Allan G, Robert GW, editors. Encyclopedia of virology. Oxford (United Kingdom): Elsevier; 1999. p. 703–6.

158. Schmidt SP, Bates GN, Lewandoski PJ. Probable herpesvirus-infection in an eastern cottontail (*Sylvilagus floridanus*). J Wildl Dis 1992;28(4):618–22.
159. Hesselton RM, Yang WC, Medveczky P, et al. Pathogenesis of herpesvirus sylvilagus infection in cottontail rabbits. Am J Pathol 1988;133(3):639–47.
160. Martella V, Moschidou P, Pinto P, et al. Astroviruses in rabbits. Emerg Infect Dis 2011;17(12):2287–93.
161. De Benedictis P, Schultz-Cherry S, Burnham A, et al. Astrovirus infections in humans and animals—molecular biology, genetic diversity, and interspecies transmissions. Infect Genet Evol 2011;11(7):1529–44.
162. Richt JA, Pfeuffer I, Christ M, et al. Borna disease virus infection in animals and humans. Emerg Infect Dis 1997;3(3):343–52.
163. Metzler A, Ehrensperger F, Wyler R. Naturliche Bornavirus-Infektion bei Kaninchen. Zentralbl Veterinarmed B 1978;25(2):161–4.
164. Staeheli P, Rinder M, Kaspers B. Avian bornavirus associated with fatal disease in psittacine birds. J Virol 2010;84(13):6269–75.
165. Gosztonyi G, Dietzschold B, Kao M, et al. Rabies and borna disease. A comparative pathogenetic study of two neurovirulent agents. Lab Invest 1993;68(3):285–95.
166. Ludwig H, Kraft W, Kao M, et al. Borna-Virus-Infektion (Borna-Krankheit) bei naturlich und experimentell infizierten Tieren: ihre Bedeutung fur Forschung und Praxis. Tierarztl Prax 1985;13(4):421–53.
167. Schindler AR, Vogtlin A, Hilbe M, et al. Reverse transcription real-time PCR assays for detection and quantification of Borna disease virus in diseased hosts. Mol Cell Probes 2007;21(1):47–55.
168. Krebs JW, Wheeling JT, Childs JE. Rabies surveillance in the United States during 2002. J Am Vet Med Assoc 2003;223(12):1736–48.
169. Childs JE, Colby L, Krebs JW, et al. Surveillance and spatiotemporal associations of rabies in rodents and lagomorphs in the United States, 1985–1994. J Wildl Dis 1997;33(1):20–7.
170. Eidson M, Matthews SD, Willsey AL, et al. Rabies virus infection in a pet guinea pig and seven pet rabbits. J Am Vet Med Assoc 2005;227(6):932–5.
171. Karp BE, Ball NE, Scott CR, et al. Rabies in two privately owned domestic rabbits. J Am Vet Med Assoc 1999;215(12):1824–7.
172. Forest E. Un cas de rage chez un lapin a Montreal. Med Vet Quebec 1990; 20(1):33.
173. Weyhe D. Tollwut beim Hauskaninchen. Monatsh Veterinarmed 1979;34(9): 336–7.
174. Hohner L, Klotzer HH, Heucke H. Zwei Falle von Lyssa beim Hauskaninchen. Monatsh Veterinarmed 1978;33(14):550–1.
175. Rosahn PD, Hu CK. Rabbit pox: report of an epidemic. J Exp Med 1935;62(3): 331–47.
176. Verlinde JD, Wensinck F. Manifestation of a laboratory epizootic of rabbit pox by non-specific stimuli. Antonie Van Leeuwenhoek 1951;17(4):232–6.
177. Greene HS. Rabbit pox: I. Clinical manifestations and course of disease. J Exp Med 1934;60(4):427–40.
178. Rosahn PD, Hu CK, Pearce L. Studies on the etiology of rabbit pox: II. Clinical characteristics of the experimentally induced disease. J Exp Med 1936;63(2): 259–76.
179. Greene HS. Rabbit pox: II. Pathology of the epidemic disease. J Exp Med 1934; 60(4):441–55.
180. Christensen LR, Bond E, Matanic B. "Pock-less" rabbit pox. Lab Anim Care 1967;17(3):281–96.

181. Bedson HS, Duckworth MJ. Rabbit pox: an experimental study of the pathways of infection in rabbits. J Pathol Bacteriol 1963;85:1–20.

182. Roy CJ, Voss TG. Use of the aerosol rabbitpox virus model for evaluation of anti-poxvirus agents. Viruses 2010;2(9):2096–107.

183. Christensen N, Fennestad KL, Bruun L. Pleural effusion disease in rabbits. Histo-pathological observations. Acta Pathol Microbiol Scand A 1978;86(3):251–6.

184. Fennestad KL, Bruun L, Wedo E. Pleural effusion disease agent as passenger of *Treponema pallidum* suspensions from rabbits. Survey of laboratories. Br J Vener Dis 1980;56(4):198–203.

185. Fennestad KL, Mansa B, Christensen N, et al. Pathogenicity and persistence of pleural effusion disease virus isolates in rabbits. J Gen Virol 1986;67(Pt 6): 993–1000.

186. Fledelius H, Bruun L, Fennestad KL, et al. Uveitis in rabbits with pleural effusion disease. Clinical and histopathological observations. Acta Ophthalmol (Copenh) 1978;56(4):599–606.

187. Osterhaus AD, Teppema JS, van Steenis G. Coronavirus-like particles in labora-tory rabbits with different syndromes in the Netherlands. Lab Anim Sci 1982; 32(6):663–5.

188. Small JD, Aurelian L, Squire RA, et al. Rabbit cardiomyopathy associated with a virus antigenically related to human coronavirus strain 229E. Am J Pathol 1979;95(3):709–29.

189. Small JD, Woods RD. Relatedness of rabbit coronavirus to other coronaviruses. Adv Exp Med Biol 1987;218:521–7.

190. Descoteaux JP, Lussier G, Berthiaume L, et al. An enteric coronavirus of the rabbit: detection by immunoelectron microscopy and identification of structural polypeptides. Arch Virol 1985;84(3–4):241–50.

191. Peeters JE, Pohl P, Charlier G. Infectious agents associated with diarrhoea in commercial rabbits: a field study. Ann Rech Vet 1984;15(3):335–40.

192. Eaton P. Preliminary observations on enteritis associated with a coronavirus-like agent in rabbits. Lab Anim 1984;18(1):71–4.

193. Deeb BJ, DiGiacomo RF, Evermann JF, et al. Prevalence of coronavirus anti-bodies in rabbits. Lab Anim Sci 1993;43(5):431–3.

194. Descoteaux JP, Lussier G. Experimental infection of young rabbits with a rabbit enteric coronavirus. Can J Vet Res 1990;54(4):473–6.

Selected Emerging Diseases in Ferrets

Nicole R. Wyre, DVM, DABVP (Avian)[a],*, Dennis Michels, VMD[b],
Sue Chen, DVM, DABVP (Avian)[b]

KEYWORDS

- Ferrets • Cryptococcosis • Hypothyroidism • Influenza • Pure red cell aplasia

KEY POINTS

- Cryptococcosis has been described in 17 ferrets worldwide, with 12 of these cases being reported since 2002, and has only recently been reported in the United States and Europe.
- Influenza is both a zoonotic and anthroponotic disease; therefore, recognition of influenza infection in ferrets by veterinarians can aid in increased surveillance in humans, as was seen in the 2009 pandemic H1N1.
- Although treatment of hypothyroidism in ferrets is simple and similar to that for dogs and cats, the clinical signs are ambiguous and include obesity, lethargy, decreased activity, excessive sleeping, and in some ferrets hind-end weakness.
- Pure red cell aplasia (PRCA) is a nonregenerative anemia that should be considered when presented with an anemic ferret. Prompt and aggressive therapy with long-term immunosuppressive medications and blood transfusions as needed are vital in the successful treatment of this condition.

Several emerging diseases have been recently reviewed, with little to no new information arising since the publication of these comprehensive reviews. The reader is encouraged to seek the following resources for additional information on those emerging conditions in previous editions of *Veterinary Clinics of North America— Exotic Animal Practice*:

- Disseminated idiopathic myofasciitis:
  Ramsell KD, Garner MM. Disseminated idiopathic myofasciitis in ferrets. Vet Clin North Am Exot Anim Pract 2010;13(3):561–75.
- Mycobacteriosis:
  Pollock C. Mycobacterial infection in the ferret. Vet Clin North Am Exot Anim Pract 2012;15(1):121–9.

[a] Section of Exotic Companion Animal Medicine and Surgery, Department of Clinical Studies, School of Veterinary Medicine, University of Pennsylvania, 3900 Delancey Street, Philadelphia, PA 19104, USA; [b] Gulf Coast Avian and Exotics, Gulf Coast Veterinary Specialists, 1111 West Loop South, Suite 110, Houston, TX 77027, USA
* Corresponding author.
E-mail address: wyredvm@gmail.com

Vet Clin Exot Anim 16 (2013) 469–493
http://dx.doi.org/10.1016/j.cvex.2013.02.003
vetexotic.theclinics.com
1094-9194/13/$ – see front matter © 2013 Elsevier Inc. All rights reserved.

- Systemic coronavirus:
    Murray J, Kiupel M, Maes RK. Ferret coronavirus-associated diseases. Vet Clin North Am Exot Anim Pract 2010;13(3):543–60.

CRYPTOCOCCOSIS
Etiology and Epidemiology

Cryptococcus spp are capsulated, dimorphic, basidiomycetous fungi that are found in soil, air, and trees.[1] Although there are 39 recognized species, only a few species are found to cause disease in humans and animals.[2] The most medically relevant species are *Cryptococcus neoformans* and *Cryptococcus gattii*. *C neoformans* is split into 2 distinct variants: var. *neoformans* (previously called serotype D) and var. *grubii* (previously called serotype A).[3] This species is classically identified as causing meningitis and meningoencephalitis in immunosuppressed people, has a worldwide distribution, and is found in pigeon droppings.[1] *C gattii* (previously called *Cryptococcus neoformans* var. *gattii*) is also synonymously called *Cryptococcus bacillisporus* in some texts. It is endemic in tropical and subtropical climates, although it is being found in more areas, and is an emerging pathogen in immunocompetent humans in North America.[2,4] Additional species that can cause disease in immunosuppressed humans include *Cryptococcus albidus* and *Cryptococcus laurentii*, but to date these species have not been documented to cause disease in ferrets.

This fungus has a special life cycle that involves a yeast form and a filamentous form. The most medically relevant form is the basiospore, which is the infectious form in mammals. The natural route of infection is via inhalation of the basiospores or actual yeast cells. In the host, the yeast appears as round-ovoid structures with a polysaccharide capsule.[1] This thick capsule helps prevent desiccation[1] and, in the correct environment, allows the organism to stay viable for up to 2 years.[2] In addition, this capsule in *C neoformans* also functions as its major virulence factor because it helps to evade the host's immune system.[2,5] Because entry is via inhalation, the nasal cavity and lungs can be infected first, followed by hematogenous spread to the central nervous system (CNS).[2]

Cryptococcosis in ferrets

Since it was first reported in the literature in the United Kingdom in 1954,[6] there have been 16 reported cases of cryptococcosis in ferrets. Before 2000 there had been 4 reported cases: 1 in the United Kingdom, 1 in Australia, and 2 in North America. Since 2000 there have been several cases in Australia, 3 in North America, and 1 in Spain.

As with cryptococcosis in humans, cats, and dogs,[2,5,7] the 2 most common species reported in ferrets is *C neoformans* and *C gattii* (**Table 1**). Of the 13 cases that reported the infectious species, 6 ferrets were infected with *C neoformans*[6–11] and 6 were infected with *C gatti*.[7,12–14] In the 3 cases that the variant was listed for *C neoformans*, it was always var. *grubii*.[7,10,11] The infectious species was not explicitly listed in 2 ferrets[15]; they were included in a report of a 2003 outbreak of *Cryptococcus* in Canada, where other animals and humans were infected with both *C neoformans* and *C gattii* (see **Table 1**).

Age and sex

Of the 16 reported cases of cryptococcosis, the sex was reported in 14 cases. There were more cases reported in male ferrets: 12 males[6,7,9–14,16] and only 2 females.[7,16] In addition, there are more cases reported in spayed/castrated ferrets[7,10–14,16] than in intact ferrets.[6–8] The ages of these ferrets were reported in 13 cases and ranged from 17 months to 6 years.[6–11,13,14,16]

Table 1
Cryptococcal species and variant, country of infection, and patient signalment in 16 ferrets with cryptococcosis

	Signalment	*Cryptococcus* Species and Variant	Country	Ref.
1.	Mature M	*C neoformans*	UK	6
2.	3-y-old MI	*C neoformans*	Australia	8
3.	6-y-old FS	Not stated	USA	16
4.	3-y-old M	*C neoformans*	USA (NY)	9
5.	5-y-old MC	*C gattii*[a]	Australia	7,12
6.	6-y-old MC	*C gattii*[a]	Australia	7
7.	2-y-old MC	*C gattii*[a]	Australia	7
8.	2–3-y-old FS	*C neoformans* var. *grubii*	Australia	7
9.	3.5-y-old MC	Not stated	Australia	7
10.	1.75-y-old MC	*C gattii* VGII[b]	Canada	7
11.	3-y-old MI	*C gattii* VGII[b]	Canada	7
12.	Not stated	Not stated	Canada	15
13.	Not stated	Not stated	Canada	15
14.	1.5-y-old MC	*C neoformans* var. *grubii*	USA	10
15.	4-y-old MC	*C neoformans* var. *grubii*	USA	11
16.	17-mo-old MC	*C gattii* serotype B VGI/AFLP4	Spain	13,14

Abbreviations: FS, female spayed; M, male; MC, male castrated; MI, male intact.
[a] Called *C bacillisporus* in publication, which is synonymous with *C gattii*.
[b] Although the original publication (Malik, 2002) states both cases from Canada as *C neoformans* var. *grubii*, a more recent publication[15] and personal communication with Malik indicate that these cases were incorrectly speciated and actually had *C gattii* VGII, not *C neoformans* var. *grubii*. This table reflects the most updated information.

Risk factors

In humans, it has been well documented that immunosuppression is a risk factor for the development of cryptococcosis associated with *C neoformans*.[5] In cats, however, underlying immunosuppressive disease is not commonly found.[2] In the reported cases of ferrets there was one with concurrent lymphosarcoma,[16] potentially causing immunosuppression. Three ferrets were also treated with systemic steroids that may have caused an altered immune status. In one case, dexamethasone SP was used to manage hind-end paresis.[9] When the ferret was euthanized 5 weeks later, it had systemic cryptococcosis. In a case of chorioretinitis, the ferret was treated with oral prednisone.[13,14] This ferret was also treated with fluconazole at the same time, but when he was euthanized 7 months after treatment he had signs of systemic cryptococcosis.

Because *Cryptococcus* is found in soil, bird droppings, and trees, ferrets with outdoor access are at additional risk. Reported exposures include living outdoors in a hutch,[6,8] contact with pigeons and finches,[8] digging outside,[7] leash walks outside,[15] and outdoor play areas.[13,14] The incubation period can range from 2 to 13 months, so previous travel to an endemic area is another potential risk factor.[2]

There are 3 cases of ferrets with cryptococcosis living with other ferrets or humans that had the same species of *Cryptococcus*, either as asymptomatic carriers or with disease themselves. In Australia, two ferrets were infected with the same species of *Cryptococcus*: one with a nasal infection and the other with a retropharyngeal infection.[7,12] A ferret in Spain that died of disseminated cryptococcosis lived with ferrets and humans who were asymptomatic carriers of the same strain of *Cryptococcus* (based on nasal swabs).[13] It is likely that the ferrets and humans in the household were exposed to the same source of *Cryptococcus*. *Cryptococcus* is not a zoonotic disease because the organism does not aerosolize from infected tissue, and therefore does not spread between humans and animals.[2]

Clinical Findings

Presenting complaints and physical examination findings for ferrets with cryptococcosis vary depending on the organ system affected. In cats, upper respiratory tract signs are most common, whereas in dogs disseminated disease affecting the CNS, eyes, urinary system, and nasal cavity are common. Clinical signs similar those found in cats and dogs and reported in ferrets include respiratory,[7,11,12,15] ocular,[13,14] neurologic,[9] musculoskeletal,[7] lymphatic,[7,10,13,14] and gastrointestinal signs[10,11] as well as acute death (**Table 2**).[6,8]

Diagnostic Testing

Clinical laboratory

As with other species, changes in the complete blood count (CBC) and chemistry panel in ferrets with cryptococcosis is generally nonspecific but is an important first step toward finding underlying disease.[2,11] In dogs and cats a mild to moderate regenerative anemia, leukocytosis with a monocytosis, and eosinophilia can be seen, as well as changes in the chemistry panel reflecting specific organs infected.[2] In the literature only 3 ferrets had CBCs and serum biochemistries performed. Reported abnormalities have included monocytosis,[10] lymphopenia,[11] lactic acidosis,[11] hypoglycemia,[11] hypocalcemia,[10,11] hypophosphatemia,[10] hypoalbuminemia,[10,11] and hyperglobulinemia,[11] although in one ferret the CBC and serum biochemistry was within the normal range.[13,14] This ferret had an additional protein electrophoresis run, which indicated an elevation in the α- and β-globulins.[13]

Diagnostic imaging

Depending on the organ system affected, radiographs, ultrasonography, and/or magnetic resonance imaging (MRI) can be helpful diagnostic tools. A pulmonary bronchointerstitial pattern,[11] diffuse alveolar disease,[7] and/or pleural effusion[7] were noted on thoracic radiographs in ferrets that presented for coughing and dyspnea. Cryptococcal infections were found in the lungs at necropsy.[7,11] A cylindrical intra-abdominal mass was noted on abdominal radiographs in one ferret that was found to have an infected jejunum and mesenteric lymph node on necropsy.[7] Another ferret had an abdominal ultrasonogram indicating mesenteric lymphadenopathy, which was found

Table 2	
Clinical signs and physical examination findings by system in 16 ferrets with cryptococcosis	
System	**Clinical Signs and Physical Examination Findings**
Musculoskeletal	Swollen limbs or digits[7]
Respiratory	Nasal discharge, coughing, sneezing, dyspnea, swelling over nasal bridge[7,11,12,15]
Ocular	Chorioretinitis, acute bilateral blindness[13,14]
Gastrointestinal	Regurgitation, retching, gagging[7,10,11]
Neurologic	Posterior paresis[9]
Lymphadenopathy	Popliteal, cervical, submandibular[7,10,13,14]

to be an infected portal lymph node on biopsy.[11] One ferret that presented for acute blindness developed neurologic signs of incontinence and pain 7 months into the treatment regimen and had MRI performed. This animal had a mass compressing the thoracic region of the spinal cord and had cryptococcal infection in the spinal cord on necropsy.[13,14] When indicated by clinical signs or physical examination findings, diagnostic imaging was helpful in pointing to a diagnosis of cryptococcosis.

Serologic and cerebrospinal fluid testing

The latex cryptococcal antigen agglutination test (LCAT) detects the polysaccharide capsular antigen, and can be used on cerebrospinal fluid (CSF) and serum.[17] This test detects all known cryptococcal serotypes.[2] In humans, commercial kits have high sensitivity and specificity, but false-negative results can occur when disease is localized.[2] Antigen was detected in the CSF of one ferret that had chorioretinitis, but it could not be titrated.[13] Serum LCAT was positive in 4 ferrets in which the test was used,[7,10,12,13] and this was used to monitor response to treatment in cryptococcal infections of the left forelimb[7] and mandibular lymph nodes.[10] Because titer results from different LCAT kits can vary, it is important to use the same kit when monitoring response to treatment.[2]

Cytology

Cytology of affected tissue can lead to a quick presumptive diagnosis of *Cryptococcus*. Diff Quick, Giemsa, Wright, new methylene blue, and Gram stain can all be used, and visualization at low power is usually the best. The presence of spherical capsulate yeast on aspirates or impression smears of enlarged lymph nodes, masses, or draining tracts has been seen in several ferrets.[7,10,12,13] In addition to the presence of the yeast, pyogranulomatous inflammation can also be seen in animals with an intact immune system.

Biopsy

If possible, collection of a piece of affected tissue for biopsy is the most important diagnostic step. If tissue is collected, impression smears should be made for cytologic analysis, part of the sample should be used for culture, and the rest should be submitted for histopathology.[2] In the reported ferret cases, identification of the yeast was made on the biopsy of an enlarged lymph node in several cases,[7,11,13,14] as well as a biopsy of an infected digit[7] and a nasal biopsy.[12]

Immunohistochemistry

If tissue is not available for fungal culture and routine histopathology is unable to confirm the presence of cryptococci, immunohistochemistry staining of tissue is available.[2,18] Caution should be exercised if this is the sole method being used to determine the infective species. Previous immunohistochemical testing methods performed in ferrets have been reported to be inaccurate, leading to an improper identification of the cryptococcal species.[11]

Fungal culture

Culturing for *Cryptococcus* is important because it can lead to correct identification of the infectious species and variant. Culture also has the benefit of a sensitivity spectrum, which can aid in choosing an appropriate antimicrobial agent.[12,13] *Cryptococcus* is cultured on a medium of Sabouraud dextrose agar.[2] Cultures have been performed on aspirates of enlarged lymph nodes[10,13] and a nasal swelling in ferrets.[12] Therefore, if *Cryptococcus* is suspected and aspirates or tissue is obtained for cytology or biopsy, a sample should also be submitted for culture.

Polymerase chain reaction

More recently, DNA-based methods have been used to correctly identify the cryptococcal species and variant. DNA polymerase chain reaction (PCR) testing has been used to confirm the diagnosis and identify the infective species and variant in 2 ferrets. PCR extraction was successful on infected lung tissue via necropsy[11] and a lymph node[13,14] collected via biopsy. In addition, PCR confirmed identical strains in 2 ferrets with cryptococcosis from the same household.[7]

Pathology

Granulomatous or pyogranulomatous inflammation is typically seen in animals with cryptococcosis that have intact immune systems. In cats, the nose, lungs, spinal cord, and eyes are often affected, whereas dogs commonly have disseminated disease and/or infection in the CNS and eyes.[2] Necropsy results were available for 8 ferrets. Four of these animals had evidence of disseminated disease.[6,7,11,13,14] Six ferrets had infected lymph nodes[6,7,11,16] and, as expected owing to its entry via inhalation, 5 ferrets had evidence of disease in their lungs.[7,8,11,13] Cryptococcus has a predilection for the CNS, and infection was noted in 3 ferrets.[9,11,13,14] Two ferrets each had disease in their liver[6,7] and spleen,[6,11] whereas 1 ferret each had signs of disease in the intestine,[7] thymus,[13] eyes,[13] mediastinum,[7] and peritoneum.[6]

Treatment

Managing immunosuppression

Identification and treatment of any underlying disease causing immunosuppression is important in managing cryptococcosis. Successful treatment is limited if the cause of immunosuppression cannot be controlled.[5] In humans, cancer and high-dose corticosteroid treatment have been linked with cryptococcosis.[5] Concurrent neoplasia may have played a role in the one ferret that was reported to have both cryptococcosis and lymphosarcoma.[9]

Surgical debulking

If possible, surgical debulking or removal of the affected area can be an effective treatment. This approach was used successfully in one ferret with a digit infection[7] and in one with a nasal infection.[12]

Antifungal agents

In humans with cryptococcosis, most initial isolates are susceptible to the major classes of antifungal agents including amphotericin B, flucytosine, and the azoles.[5] Different antifungal medications are warranted depending on the severity of disease and the organ system affected. A variety of antifungal agents, doses, and frequencies have been used to treat cryptococcosis in ferrets, with variable success (**Table 3**).

Amphotericin B (AMB) acts by binding to sterols (primarily ergosterol) in the cell membrane of fungal organisms, and alters the permeability of this membrane.[19] In humans AMB has cured countless cases of disseminated cryptococcosis that would have been fatal before the advent of its use.[5] This medication can be expensive, must be administered parenterally, and can cause nephrotoxicity.[19] Newer, lipid-based products are less nephrotoxic and penetrate better into tissues.[19] AMB in combination with itraconazole has been used in one ferret with disseminated cryptococcosis, but the ferret succumbed to disease 4 days after initiating treatment.[11]

Flucytosine inhibits protein, RNA, and DNA synthesis in fungal cells, and is useful against strains of Cryptococcus and Candida.[20] This medication reaches high levels in the CNS, but there is a high incidence of resistance, so it must be used with another antifungal agent such as AMB.[5] This combination is used in humans,[5] dogs, and cats.[2]

Side effects of this medication can include bone marrow suppression and gastrointestinal (GI) disease in humans and animals.[2,20] There are no reports on the use of flucytosine in the treatment of cryptococcosis in ferrets.

The azole antifungal agents include both imidazoles (ketoconazole, miconazole) and triazoles (fluconazole and itraconazole). These agents work by altering the cellular membranes of susceptible fungi.[21] Azoles are fungistatic and rely on an intact immune system to remove the infectious agent, so they may not be effective as a single modality in immunosuppressed patients.[2] In human cases of cryptococcal meningitis, ketoconazole was found to be ineffective, and miconazole is no longer used owing to its toxicity.[5] There are no reports of the use of ketoconazole or miconazole in the treatment of cryptococcosis in ferrets.

Itraconazole is effective against *Cryptococcus*, but has poor penetration into the CSF and the aqueous humor.[21] However, it has been used successfully in the management of meningeal and ocular cryptococcosis in humans, dogs, and cats, potentially because of the compromised blood-brain or blood-aqueous barriers during infection.[2,5] Itraconazole has good bioavailability if administered with food, and in most species has the additional benefit of once-daily dosing.[21] Side effects seem to be dose related, and include hepatotoxicity, GI disturbances, and vasculitis.[21] Fluconazole is effective against *Cryptococcus* and has good penetration into the CSF, eye, and peritoneal fluid.[22] It is has a high bioavailability and rapid absorption when administered orally, and has minimal side effects that can include anorexia and, rarely, hepatotoxicity.[22] However, resistance to fluconazole has recently been reported in *C gattii* in North America.[2] Both itraconazole and fluconazole have been used singly in cats with mild to moderate cryptococcosis (without CNS involvement) and in dogs with localized disease. Combination use with AMB is still recommended for disseminated disease or CNS involvement.[2] Itraconazole has been used in the treatment of 4 ferrets with localized disease[7,10,12] and 1 with disseminated systemic disease.[11] Fluconazole has been used in the treatment of 1 ferret with ocular cryptococcosis[13,14] and 1 that had localized disease to the hind limb (see **Table 3**).[7]

Monitoring

Definitive treatment of cryptococcosis can be difficult to determine. It is not uncommon for animals and humans to remain on long-term antifungals, sometimes for the lifetime of the patient.[5] Malik, who has written numerous articles about cryptococcosis in veterinary patients (including ferrets), has seen recurrence 10 years after successful therapy, and therefore recommends antifungal administration until cryptococcal antigen titers reach zero.[2] This monitoring plan was used in the successful treatment of a 1.5-year-old ferret that was treated with itraconazole for a total of 43 weeks until his LCAT reached zero.[10] Malik additionally recommends monitoring titers every 3 to 6 months after the titer reaches zero, to catch recurrence early.

If patients are on potentially nephrotoxic (ie, AMB) or hepatotoxic (ie, itraconazole) antifungal agents, routine monitoring of kidney and/or liver values is recommended.

Prognosis

In humans, prognosis depends on the ability to control the patient's underlying disease.[5] Similarly, in cats, feline leukemia virus (FeLV)-positive status is associated with a poor long-term prognosis.[2] In cats there also seems to be a negative outcome with CNS disease, whereas in dogs the outcome may depend on where they live.[2] Because of the paucity of reported cases of cryptococcosis in ferrets, risk factors associated with prognosis cannot be assessed, but those ferrets with localized disease have had a more favorable outcome than those with disseminated disease.

Table 3
Treatments and outcomes in 16 ferrets with cryptococcosis

	Treatment	Route, Dose, Interval	Duration	Outcome	Ref.
1.	None			Presented deceased	6
2.	None			Presented deceased	8
3.	None			<3 mo died of lymphosarcoma	16
4.	Dexamethasone SP	0.15–0.5 mg/kg q 8–48 h	Tapered over 30 d	4 wk PT: improved CS 5 wk PT: euthanized because of cardiac disease; post mortem indicated CNS cryptococcosis	9
5.	Surgical debulking Itraconazole	25 mg PO every 24 h 33 mg PO every 24 h 25 mg PO every 24 h	21 d 21–171 d 171 d to 3 y	171 d PT: nasal disease resolved 3 y PT: euthanized because of abdominal mass; post mortem showed no signs of cryptococcosis	7,12
6.	Itraconazole	33 mg PO every 24 h	Unknown	Initial improvement Euthanized Post mortem: cryptococcus in enlarged and contralateral LN	7
7.	None			Died after sedation	7
8.	None			Died during induction	7

#	Treatment	Dose	Duration	Outcome	Ref
9.	Itraconazole	25 mg/kg PO every 24 h	6 mo	5 wk PT improved 6 mo PT antigen titer 0	7
10.	Surgical excision affected digit			4 mo PT no disease recurrence	7
11.	Fluconazole	12 mg PO every 12 h	≥4 mo	4 mo PT doing well but dragging limb	7
12.	None			Not reported	15
13.	None			Not reported	15
14.	Itraconazole	15 mg/kg PO every 24 h	43 wk	3 wk PT decreased size of LN, stopped regurgitating 6 wk PT normal sized LN 40 wk PT antigen titer 0	10
15.	Itraconazole Amphotericin B	10 mg/kg PO every 12 h 0.25 mg/kg IV every 24 h	4 d 4 d	Died 4 d PT Post mortem showed disseminated cryptococcosis	11
16.	Fluconazole Prednisone Diclofenac	10 mg/kg PO every 24 h 0.5 mg/kg PO every 24 h OU every 4–8 h	6 mo 6 mo 5.5 mo	4 mo PT clinical signs improved but antigen titer unchanged 7 mo PT euthanized because of CNS signs Post mortem showed disseminated cryptococcosis	13,14

Abbreviations: CNS, central nervous system; CS, clinical signs; IV, intravenously; LN, lymph nodes; OU, in both eyes; PO, by mouth; PT, post treatment.

Of the 16 reported cases of ferrets with cryptococcosis, 2 presented deceased,[6,8] 2 did not have the outcome reported,[15] 2 died before treatments could be administered,[7] and 1 died of lymphosarcoma with *Cryptococcus* as an incidental finding on postmortem examination.[16] In addition, 1 ferret was treated with dexamethasone for neurologic disease, only for cryptococcosis to be found on postmortem examination.[9]

A total of 8 ferrets received treatment for cryptococcosis. One ferret with localized disease was treated successfully with only surgical excision of the affected digit.[7] Another ferret with localized nasal cryptococcosis was successfully treated with surgical excision and oral itraconazole for 3 years postoperatively.[12] When he died 3 years after his initial diagnosis, he had no signs of cryptococcosis.

Three ferrets with localized disease were successfully treated with medical management alone. One ferret with localized infection of the forelimb was treated with oral itraconazole and showed improvement 5 weeks into treatment. He was treated for a total of 6 months, at which time LCAT was negative.[7] One ferret with localized disease of the hind leg was treated with oral fluconazole for 4 months until he was systemically well but still dragging his hind leg.[7] The final ferret with localized disease to a submandibular lymph node was treated with oral itraconazole, and showed clinical improvement after 3 weeks. He was treated for a total of 43 weeks and his LCAT titer was negative after 40 weeks.[10]

Three ferrets with cryptococcosis were treated medically but died or were euthanized because of their disease. One ferret with cryptococcosis of the right retropharyngeal lymph node was treated with oral itraconazole, and although he improved initially he was euthanized because of skin disease. On postmortem examination this animal had evidence of *Cryptococcus* in both retropharyngeal lymph nodes.[7] A ferret that presented for respiratory disease was treated with intravenous AMB and oral itraconazole for 4 days before he died. Postmortem examination revealed disseminated cryptococcosis.[11] One ferret with cryptococcal associated chorioretinitis was treated with oral fluconazole and prednisone. This animal showed some initial improvement in his overall health, but remained blind and was euthanized when he developed signs of CNS disease 7 months after treatment. On postmortem examination the ferret had disseminated cryptococcosis.[13,14]

INFLUENZA

Etiology and Epidemiology

Influenza is a contagious respiratory illness caused by influenza viruses.[23] These RNA viruses are in the Orthomyxoviridae family and are classified into 3 species termed A, B, and C, with species A being the most medically relevant to ferrets.[24] Influenza type A viruses are further divided into subtypes, based on 2 proteins that exist on the surface of the virus: hemagglutinin (HA) and neuraminidase (NA). There are 17 known HA subtypes and 10 known NA subtypes. Many different combinations of HA and NA proteins are possible.[25] For the purposes of this article, the focus is on the H1N1 subtype during the influenza season 2009 to 2010. This virus was also called "novel H1N1" or "swine flu," which emerged in the spring of 2009 and caused the first global outbreak of disease caused by a novel influenza virus (influenza pandemic) in more than 40 years.[26] H1N1 was first seen in humans in March 2009 and then became a pandemic by June 2009. As of April 2011, this virus has caused natural disease in at least 10 animal species.[27]

Geographic distribution and age

During 2009 to 2010 there were several reports of influenza in ferrets. There were 2 reports of naturally occurring influenza in pet ferrets in Pennsylvania,[28] Nebraska, and Oregon[29] and one report in a colony of ferrets[30] in Iowa. In addition, there was one black-footed ferret with influenza in a California zoologic setting.[27] During this pandemic, the youngest ferrets affected were 1 year of age while the oldest was 8 years.[29]

Zoonosis and anthroponosis

Influenza is both a zoonotic and anthroponotic disease. In the 1930s the zoonotic spread of influenza from ferrets was first reported.[31] More recently, ferrets have been instrumental in influenza research and as sentinels for this viral infection in humans. Ferrets are used as animal models for influenza infection because they display flulike symptoms and immune responses similar to those of humans.[32] In Pennsylvania in 2009, the diagnosis of influenza in several pet ferrets led to enhanced surveillance for pandemic H1N1 in the region. This vigilance helped to increase the identification of humans infected with this same strain.[28] Experimentally, reassortment of different strains of influenza in ferrets has been proved via coinfection with both a human and avian strain of the virus. Therefore, a ferret exposed to both a pathogenic and seasonal strain of influenza could act as mediator for the formation of a pathogenic form of the seasonal influenza.[33]

Anthroponosis was suspected in several cases of influenza in ferrets in 2009. In a group of ferrets with pandemic H1N1, the owners reported flulike symptoms from 6 to 9 days before clinical signs in the ferrets.[29] In a California zoo 3 animals contracted influenza A H1N1, including a black-footed ferret. It was suspected but not confirmed that the virus was contracted from humans interacting with the animals.[28]

Risk factors

Influenza infection in older people, young children, and those with immunosuppressive conditions are at high risk for serious flu complications,[24] and this may also be true for ferrets because in a report of influenza in 13 ferrets, the 1 ferret that died during the outbreak was 8 years old.[29]

Exposure to swine and birds has been associated with influenza infections in humans. Influenza viruses that normally circulate in pigs are called variant viruses when they are found in people. In humans, certain influenza strains have been associated with prolonged exposure to pigs at agricultural fairs.[34] Avian influenza occurs naturally among anseriformes and domestic poultry, but can infect other avian and animal species, including sporadic human infections.[35] During an outbreak of influenza in a colony of ferrets living on a farm in Iowa, investigation of their housing revealed that they were 0.25 miles away from a swine operation and were exposed to multiple avian species. There was concern for aerosol transmission from the swine farm or locally housed birds.[30]

Clinical Presentation

In humans and animals, influenza is characterized by respiratory signs and a fever. In the naturally occurring cases of influenza in 2009 to 2010, the most common presenting complaints were coughing, sneezing, oculonasal discharge, and lethargy.[27–30] The physical examination findings included dyspnea, oculonasal discharge, and a fever between 104° and 105°F (40°–40.6°C).[28,29]

Ferrets are used frequently in a research setting for influenza investigation. Therefore, a more complete picture of the clinical disease has been described in the laboratory setting. In one study that compared the clinical signs and recovery period of ferrets experimentally infected with the pandemic H1N1 influenza versus other strains of this virus, they found that weight loss could be found as early as the first day of infection.[24] In comparison with other strains, ferrets infected with the pandemic H1N1 had the longest period of weight loss, the longest duration of fever, the most profound lethargy, and the most prominent sneezing and nasal discharge. The more intense clinical signs were thought to be due to the profound cytokine production and broader tissue tropism of this pandemic strain.[24]

Diagnostic Testing

In ferrets with suspected influenza, the initial database included a CBC, serum biochemistry, and diagnostic imaging. Of the ferrets reported during the 2009 to 2010 pandemic, CBC changes included anemia[28] and biochemistry changes included an increased alanine aminotransferase, increased alkaline phosphatase, and a low total protein, potassium, and chloride.[28] Thoracic radiographs were only performed in a few ferrets, and were mostly unremarkable.[28]

Influenza is both an anthroponotic and zoonotic disease. Therefore, identification of the influenza strain is very important. Suspected cases should have samples collected for confirmation and speciation via PCR and/or immunohistochemical staining. Samples for real-time reverse transcriptase (rRT)-PCR submission include nasal, pharyngeal, and conjunctival swabs, bronchoalveolar lavage fluid, and swabs from the lungs on postmortem specimens. Depending on the ferret's location, samples may be submitted to the state animal health laboratory. During the pandemic, rRT-PCR samples were helpful in identifying the influenza species in pet, farm, and zoologic ferrets.[27,28,30] Because this is a noninvasive test, it can easily be used on humans and other ferrets in contact with the ill ferret.

If postmortem samples are available, immunohistochemical (IHC) staining can assist in species identification. IHC was particularly helpful in the outbreak of naturally occurring influenza in a farm setting where 8% of the ferrets became clinically ill with influenza.[30] Postmortem samples showed bronchointerstitial pneumonia with necrosuppurative bronchiolitis, and through IHC the investigators were able to identify the influenza as the pandemic H1N1 strain that was of swine lineage in origin.[30]

Additional diagnostic testing includes serum collection for antibody detection. In ferrets that were experimentally infected with H1N1, antibody responses correlated with the severity of the influenza infections.[24] During the outbreak of natural influenza in a colony of farm ferrets, hemagglutination inhibition antibody was high in infected ferrets.[30]

Treatment and Monitoring

The basis of influenza treatment involves supportive care and prevention of secondary bacterial infection. Supportive care includes fluid therapy, either subcutaneously or intravenously, if severely dehydrated or febrile. Weight loss was a common clinical sign noted in ferrets experimentally infected with influenza, so support feeding is also important.[24] Ferrets are strict carnivores with a rapid GI transit time, so a convalescent diet should include a meal that is palatable, and high in fat and protein. Many recovery diets for feline patients are suitable, such as Hill's A/D, Oxbow's Carnivore Care, or Lafeber's Emeraid Carnivore. Coverage with a broad-spectrum antibiotic is warranted if a secondary bacterial infection is suspected. Parenteral antibiotics can be used in ferrets that are too sick or nauseated for oral antibiotics. The use of antiviral drugs in the treatment of influenza is difficult, because this virus mutates and resistance is common.[36] There are variable results in the use of antiviral drugs in experimentally induced influenza in ferrets, which seem to depend on the strain of the virus and the time of administration after infection.[36,37] In the ferrets with pandemic H1N1 influenza, many were successfully treated with subcutaneous fluids, parenteral antibiotics, and support feeding.[27,29,30] It must be noted that influenza is zoonotic and contagious to other ferrets, so appropriate precautions must be taken for all staff and owners involved in treating the ill ferret.

In most cases, monitoring is straightforward during the treatment period. Response to initial supportive care including monitoring of weight gain, hydration status, and temperature are important. In the case of the black-footed ferret with H1N1, he was in a zoologic park setting with exposure to humans. Therefore, his influenza status was monitored via PCR testing. When his clinical signs resolved after treatment with parenteral antibiotics, his influenza PCR was negative.[27]

Prognosis

Depending on the viral strain and concurrent disease, the prognosis for ferrets with influenza is favorable. The ferrets experimentally infected with pandemic H1N1 had severe illness, but the strains were cleared from the ferrets within 7 days after infection. This same clearance was noted in other strains of the more common seasonal influenza strains.[24] During an outbreak in Nebraska and Oregon, only 1 ferret died and 12 others recovered with supportive care. The ferret that died was 8 years old and may have had concurrent disease.[29] In an influenza outbreak in a colony of 1000 ferrets, there was a morbidity rate of 8% and a mortality rate of 0.6%.[30]

HYPOTHYROIDISM

Although one of the most common endocrinopathies seen in dogs, hypothyroidism has only recently been described in 7 ferrets.[38] Impaired production or secretion by the thyroid results in a deficiency of circulating thyroid hormone and associated clinical signs.

Etiology and Pathogenesis

At present, the pathogenesis of hypothyroidism in ferrets is not known. In dogs, primary hypothyroidism is most common, with 2 abnormalities observed that affect the thyroid gland with approximately equal occurrence: lymphocytic thyroiditis and idiopathic thyroid atrophy. Lymphocytic thyroiditis involves infiltration and destruction of the glandular parenchyma by lymphocytes, plasma cells, and macrophages. This condition is believed to be immune mediated, but the exact pathogenesis has not been elucidated. The presence of antithyroglobulin varies between breeds, and whether it occurs before or as a result of follicular damage is unknown. Idiopathic thyroid atrophy is characterized by the loss of the thyroid parenchyma and replacement with adipose connective tissue, with no observable inflammation or fibrosis. Primary and metastatic neoplasia can uncommonly also cause hypothyroidism.[39] In cats, acquired hypothyroidism is almost always the result of treatment for hyperthyroidism. Only one published case of feline hypothyroidism currently exists, which was confirmed to be lymphocytic thyroiditis using histopathology.[40]

Clinical Signs

Clinical signs are often vague, but the most consistent ones are obesity, lethargy, decreased activity, and excessive sleeping. Rear-leg weakness has also been noted in some ferrets. Common clinical signs noted in dogs (eg, hair loss, hypercholesterolemia) were not consistently noted in the 7 ferrets diagnosed with hypothyroidism. Hypoglycemia was also not noted unless associated with a concurrent insulinoma.[38]

Differential Diagnoses

The vague, nonspecific signs of lethargy and decreased activity are present in any myriad of diseases seen in ferrets, especially their most common endocrinopathies, insulinomas, and hyperadrenocorticism. Owners may also mistake the decreased activity as normal changes associated with aging. Ferrets that are on long-term steroid therapy to manage their insulinoma-induced hypoglycemia will often become obese and have a pot-bellied appearance. Rear-leg weakness may be associated with hypoglycemia, myasthenia gravis, or thromboembolic disease.

Diagnostic Testing

As in dogs and cats, eliminating the possibility of sick euthyroid syndrome is essential to diagnosing hypothyroidism. Diagnostic testing to rule out concurrent disease should be performed along with evaluation of the thyroid.

Experimentally, intravenous injection of 1 IU of thyroid-stimulating hormone (TSH) (Dermathycin) per ferret was sufficient to evaluate thyroid function in adult male ferrets, and showed significant increase in circulating thyroxine (T4) after 2 hours. Measured tri-iodothyronine (T3) values did not change for at least 6 hours, making measurement of circulating T4 an easier and more feasible parameter to measure in clinical practice.[41]

Unfortunately, Dermathycin is no longer available for purchase in the United States. More recently, however, T4 levels were measured using human recombinant TSH (Thyrogen) in 11 neutered ferrets, and successful stimulation of the thyroid axis was achieved. Prestimulation values for T4 in neutered male and female ferrets were determined to be 29.9 ± 5.8 ng/mL and 21.8 ± 3.3 ng/mL, respectively. Ferrets were stimulated using 100 µg Thyrogen intramuscularly, and euthyroid ferrets were found to have an increase of 1.4 times basal levels after 4 hours.[38] A concurrent study involving 25 laboratory and pet neutered ferrets using the same protocol was also released in 2012. The investigators noted a median poststimulation T4 level at 34.8% above prestimulatory levels, and found the mean plasma T4 of euthyroid ferrets to be 21.3 nmol/L.[42]

Treatment

Oral levothyroxine at 50 to 100 µg every 12 hours was able to return serum T4 to normal resting levels in test studies. Treatment also led to increased activity, weight loss, and increased rear-leg function. Ferrets with sick euthyroid syndrome were not responsive to levothyroxine therapy.[38]

Prognosis

Prognosis with T4 supplementation has thus far been excellent for the 7 animals studied.[38] As the pathogenesis of hypothyroidism in ferrets is unknown, the long-term prognosis has yet to be determined, as has whether adjustments to the dose of levothyroxine will need to be adjusted over time.

PURE RED CELL APLASIA

Pure red cell aplasia (PRCA) is a nonregenerative anemia characterized by a marked deficiency of erythroid precursors despite normal numbers of granulocytes and megakaryocytes in the bone marrow.[43] Though a rare condition, PRCA may be underreported in ferrets because other more common causes of anemia, such as hyperestrogenism and lymphoma, carry a guarded prognosis. Therefore owners may elect to provide palliative symptomatic care or euthanize the animal rather than have the anemia fully worked up.

Etiology and Pathogenesis

Variable mechanisms have been implicated in the causes of the bone marrow hypoplasia, including the production of antibodies against the erythroid precursors, inhibition of erythropoiesis owing to alterations in cytokine production, production of antibodies against erythropoietin, and induction of antibodies during an infection against antigens that cross-react with an epitope on erythroid precursors.[44]

Congenital and acquired types of PRCA have been described, with the majority of cases being acquired. Congenital PRCA, also known as Diamond-Blackfan anemia, is a heritable disease that develops during early infancy in humans and is often associated with other various congenital abnormalities such as craniofacial dysmorphism, cardiac defects, urogenital malformations, cleft palate, neck and thumb abnormalities, and generalized growth failure.[44,45] A congenital case of PRCA has also been described in a 3-month-old dog based on the criteria of a progressive normochromic and normocytic anemia in infancy and an absence of erythroid maturation in the bone marrow.[46] In the author's (S.C.) practice, a 5-month-old ferret (See **Table 4** - Case A) was presented for a severe and progressive anemia with confirmed erythroid hypoplasia of the bone marrow. This ferret may possibly represent a case of congenital PRCA; however, the ferret had been vaccinated just 3 weeks before presentation, and it is unknown if this animal had an inherited condition or if the PRCA developed as a consequence of the vaccination.

Of those cases of acquired PRCA, primary and secondary forms of PRCA have been documented in dogs,[47–49] cats,[48,50] and humans.[44,51] Primary PRCA is an autoimmune disorder, and is thought to be a variant form of immune-mediated hemolytic anemia (IMHA) whereby antibodies destroy erythroblasts in the bone marrow.[48,49] In these cases, the cause of antibody production is often idiopathic.

Secondary PRCA occurs after a systemic disease (eg, viral infections, various neoplasms) or treatment with certain drugs or vaccines.[44,47–51] Cats infected with FeLV subgroup C can develop a progressive, fatal PRCA,[50] and parvoviral infections in dogs[48,49] have been associated with cases of PRCA. In humans, parvovirus B19 directly infects the erythroid precursors, resulting in premature apoptosis.[44] Aleutian disease is a parvovirus that affects ferrets; however, to date it has not been implicated in the development of PRCA. Formation of antibodies against erythropoietin after treatment with recombinant human erythropoietin is thought to be the cause of some cases of PRCA in dogs.[49,52]

In the published case of an 8-month-old ferret, extensive testing was performed to find an underlying cause of the erythroid hyperplasia, but none was found.[53] Based on the response to immunosuppressive medications, an immune-mediated mechanism was thought to be involved, and the conclusion was made that this was a case of primary PRCA. In the author's (S.C.) practice, 4 additional ferrets have been diagnosed with PRCA based on erythroid hypoplasia of the bone marrow. The previously described 5-month-old ferret (Case A) had been vaccinated for canine distemper just 3 weeks before presentation, and it is unknown whether erythroid hypoplasia in the bone marrow was an idiosyncratic reaction to the vaccine or if this ferret had a primary or congenital form of PRCA. The other 3 ferrets diagnosed with PRCA were mature (older than 4 years) and had other systemic illness preceding or concurrent with their severe anemia, including chronic episodes of diarrhea in one ferret (Case C), insulinoma and hyperadrenocorticism in the second (Case D), and severe leukocytosis and generalized weight loss of unknown cause in the third (Case B) (**Table 4**).

Table 4
PRCA signalment, treatment, and outcome

Signalment	Initial PCV (%)	Concurrent Disease	Treatment	Response to Treatment/Outcome	Ref./Year
8-mo-old female	8		Multiple blood transfusions		[53]
			Prednisolone 2 mg/kg PO every 12 h	No evidence of regeneration noted after 2 wk	
			Cyclosporine 4 mg/kg PO every 12 h (added on 2 wk later)	Marked regenerative response. PCV increased to 25% and increase in reticulocytes within 2 wk.	
			Cyclosporine 6 mg/kg PO every 12 h (dose increased after recurrence of clinical signs on day 86 of treatment)	PCV increased to 37% and reticulocytosis noted within 5 d	
			Azathioprine 1 mg/kg PO every 24 h (given for less than a week)	Likely did not contribute to increase in PCV	
			Erythropoietin 40 U SC every 48 h × 3 injections	Likely did not contribute to increase in PCV	
5-mo-old male (Case A)	18	Vaccinated with distemper 3 wk before presentation[a]	Multiple blood transfusions		2004
			Prednisolone 1 mg/kg PO every 12 h	PCV continued to drop to 10% over 15 d	
			Cyclosporine 2.2 mg/kg PO every 12 h (added on as second immunosuppressive drug owing to lack of response to prednisolone)	Patient was on medication for less than a week before passing away	
			Cyclophosphamide 10 mg/kg PO	Patient passed away 5 d after receiving single dose	

Signalment		Clinical History	Treatment	Outcome	Year
4-y-old male (Case B)	26	Severe lymphocytic leukocytosis 3 wk prior with a PCV of 38%. Leukocytosis improved with a three week course of Clavamox 12.5 mg/kg PO 12 h (suspected to be reactive lymphocytes due to immune stimulation)	Prednisolone 2 mg/kg PO every 12 h Tapered prednisolone in 4-wk increments down to 1 mg/kg PO every 24 h Cyclophosphamide 5 mg/kg PO every 12 h (added on, in addition to increasing prednisolone back to 2 mg/kg PO every 12 h)	PCV increased to 41% within 4 wk Patient became anemic again (32%) 10 wk into treatment (week 6 of taper) Patient euthanized 6 d later when patient presented in lateral recumbency. Biliary hyperplasia and hepatocellular degeneration noted on necropsy. Numerous hemosiderin laden macrophages noted in the bone marrow and all cell lines were present at the time of death	2009
6 y-old female (Case C)	27	Normal PCV just 6 wk prior. Month-long history of diarrhea, mild fever, and splenomegaly	Prednisolone 2 mg/kg PO every 12 h	PCV 46% within 4 wk. Complete remission Patient became diabetic 5 mo later; was tapered off the prednisolone and started on insulin. No recurrence of anemia	2012
6-y-old male (Case D)[b]	17	Insulinoma and hyperadrenocorticism (confirmed with adrenal panel). Was 38% on preoperative blood work just 4 d prior	Multiple blood transfusions Was already on Prednisolone 0.75 mg/kg PO every 12 h for management of hypoglycemia. Unable to wean off prednisolone because of persistent hypoglycemia after surgery	Adrenalectomy and insulinoma nodulectomy performed because hyperestrogenism was the suspected cause for the anemia and thrombocytopenia. Patient's PCV increased to 51% after 4 wk PCV remained normal for 9 wk	2012
	11	Insulinoma; cachexia of unknown cause. No recurrence of hyperestrogenism based on repeated adrenal panel just 2 wk prior	Multiple blood transfusions Patient passed away before immunosuppressive therapy could be initiated	Presented 13 wk after surgery. Patient arrested during sedation to collect bone marrow aspirate and core biopsy	

Cases A–D are ferrets that presented to the author's (S.C.) clinic. All ferrets had erythroid hypoplasia on cytologic analysis of the bone marrow.

Abbreviations: PCV, packed cell volume; PO, by mouth; PRCA, pure red cell aplasia; SC, subcutaneously.

a It is unknown whether vaccination was the trigger for this ferret's PRCA.

b Initial presentation of anemia believed to be caused by hyperestrogenism secondary to hyperadrenocorticism because the ferret had a concurrent thrombocytopenia and the PCV improved several weeks after adrenalectomy. Recurrence of anemia noted 13 weeks later was believed to be caused by PRCA, because no evidence of hyperestrogenism was noted 2 weeks prior on an adrenal sex hormone panel and normal numbers of megakaryocytes and granulocytes were noted in the bone marrow.

Clinical Signs

Similar to cases seen in dogs[47,49] and cats,[50] ferrets with PCRA usually present for a progressive weakness and lethargy ranging from several days to a few months in duration, although some were alert and responsive on admission despite their moderate to severe anemia. On physical examination, extreme pallor of the mucous membranes is the primary abnormality noted, just as seen in canine[49] and feline[50] cases. Cardiac murmurs have been reported in both dogs[49] and cats,[50] but were not noted in the published ferret case[53] or in any of the ferrets in the author's (S.C.) practice. The 3 older ferrets presented to this clinic were in fair to poor body condition, presumably resulting from their concurrent illnesses.

Differential Diagnoses

Differentials for PRCA encompass other more common causes of anemia. Anemia due to blood loss, secondary to trauma and gastric ulceration, is a common occurrence in ferrets. Gastric ulceration induced by stress and Helicobacter mustelidae can lead to significant melena and chronic anemia. Coagulopathies can also result in significant blood loss, and include certain types of rodenticide toxicities, disseminated intravascular coagulation, thrombocytopenia, and severe hepatic failure, resulting in deficits of coagulation factors. Anemia can also be a result of decreased red cell production, with lymphoma and renal disease as possible causes. Although anemia of chronic disease was considered as a possible differential for the ferrets with concurrent disease, the progressive decline in the packed cell volume (PCV) despite improvement or resolution of their underlying condition makes this less likely.

Hyperestrogenemia can result in a life-threatening anemia attributable to a pancytopenia. The anemia is a result of decreased production of red blood cells and increased blood loss secondary to thrombocytopenia. Bone marrow suppression from hyperestrogenism has been documented in intact females in prolonged estrus, spayed females with an ovarian remnant, and rarely in neutered males and females with hyperadrenocorticism.[54,55]

Anecdotally, immune-mediated hemolytic anemia (IMHA) has been noted in ferrets, although there are no published cases in the literature.[54] Dogs and cats with IMHA typically have a strong regenerative response, indicating that the destruction is targeted at mature red cells rather than the erythroblasts in the bone marrow.[47] Although a strong regenerative response is noted in most cases of IMHA, a nonregenerative IMHA characterized by erythroid maturation arrest and pathologic changes in the bone marrow (eg, dysmyelopoiesis, myelonecrosis, myelofibrosis) has been described in dogs and cats.[48]

Diagnostic Testing

A severe anemia without leukopenia or thrombocytopenia is the primary clinical finding in animals with PRCA. The normal hematocrit of ferrets is 46% to 61% and is higher than in other species, so a mild or moderate anemia may go unrecognized unless a clinician is aware of this difference.[54] The anemia is typically normocytic and normochromic with a poor reticulocyte response to the anemia, indicating that the anemia is nonregenerative.[43] In ferrets, normal reticulocyte counts can be as high as 10%, with counts higher than 12% during a regenerative response.[54]

Severe anemia (<18%) was noted in 2 of the ferrets (see **Table 4**, Cases A and D) in the author's (S.C.) practice and in the one published case report.[53] The number of leukocytes and platelets were not affected except in one patient that had a lymphocytic leukocytosis three weeks prior suggestive of immune stimulation (Case B - see **Table 4**).

For those ferrets that were severely anemic, serum biochemistries were not performed. Serum biochemistries performed on the ferrets that were only moderately anemic on initial presentation had no significant abnormalities, other than hypoglycemia in one ferret that had an insulinoma.

A bone marrow aspirate or bone core biopsy is indicated in any nonregenerative anemia.[54] Ideally both are performed, because aspirates are ideal for evaluating cell morphology, whereas core biopsies are preferred for evaluating marrow cellularity.[56] A CBC should also be performed at the same time as sample collection for an accurate interpretation of the bone marrow (**Fig. 1**).[56] Samples can be collected in ferrets from the proximal femur, humerus, and iliac crest.[57] Analysis of the bone marrow reveals extreme depletion of the erythroid precursors in the presence of normal granulopoiesis and thrombopoiesis.[49,50,53] This selective hypoplasia is believed to be a result of immune-mediated destruction of erythroblasts. This disease differs from the typical appearance of IMHA, whereby there are normal to increased numbers of erythroblasts in the bone marrow. The singular loss of only the erythroid cell line and no changes in the myeloid or megakaryocytic cell lines results in a marked increase in the myeloid-to-erythroid ratio. The myeloid-to-erythroid ratio in ferrets has been reported to range from 1:3 to 3:1.5.[58] In the one published case report, the ferret had a myeloid-to-erythroid ratio of 4.6:1.[53]

An antinuclear antibody test (ANA) can be performed to assess for autoantibodies as part of the diagnostic workup of certain autoimmune diseases. However, it is uncertain whether this test is effective in ferrets because ANA titers were negative in the one published case study.[53]

Treatment

The mainstay of treatment is to provide whole blood transfusions to support the ferret while using immunosuppressive drug therapy to cease the destruction of the immature red blood cells.

Blood transfusion

For ferrets that are clinical for their anemia, blood transfusions are indicated to provide symptomatic support so that immunosuppressive therapy has an opportunity to take effect. There are no known blood types in ferrets, so risk from transfusion reaction is

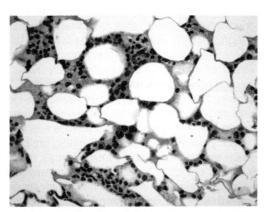

Fig. 1. Ferret bone marrow with erythroid hypoplasia. (original magnification ×40). (*Courtesy of* Catherine Pfent, DVM, Texas A&M College of Veterinary Medicine, College Station, TX.)

lower than for other species.[59] In the published case report, the anemic ferret received multiple transfusions over the course of treatment, including blood from 3 different donors for the third transfusion.[53] Multiple blood transfusions from different individuals have also been administered to anemic ferrets in the author's (S.C.) practice, with no observed adverse effects. However, the recipient is always closely monitored during a transfusion for adverse reactions, such as spikes in temperature, tachycardia, tachypnea, pruritus, and vomiting. If noted, administration of the blood is temporarily stopped or given more slowly. The recipient can also be premedicated with diphenhydramine (2 mg/kg intramuscularly, intravenously, or orally) as a preventative for a transfusion reaction.[60]

Large healthy males make the best donors, as they are able to donate a larger volume of blood. Approximately 1% of the donor's body weight can be collected safely. Because a relatively large volume is being collected, the donor should be sedated to minimize risks of venipuncture from the anterior vena cava. Isoflurane is commonly used; however, this can cause a significant drop in PCV because of splenic sequestration of red blood cells.[61] In their practice, the authors have sedated donor ferrets with subcutaneous or intramuscular injections of ketamine (10 mg/kg) and midazolam (1 mg/kg) to minimize the reduction in PCV. The neck of the donor ferret is shaved and sterilely prepped before venipuncture. A 23-gauge butterfly catheter is inserted into the thoracic cavity just cranial to the first rib and directed toward the opposite rear limb. The blood is collected into a syringe prefilled with Acid-Citrate-Dextrose (ACD) anticoagulant (1 part ACD to 9 parts blood). Supplemental subcutaneous fluids and an injection of iron dextran (10 mg/kg intramuscularly) are administered to the donor ferret during recovery.

If a donor is not available, oxyglobin (hemoglobin glutamer 200 [bovine]) can be used if the ferret is in an acute crisis from its anemia.[62] However, its use is limited for stable patients with chronic anemia because of oxyglobin's short half-life of approximately 18 to 43 hours.[63] Oxyglobin had been previously withdrawn from the market in 2010, but production has resumed in early 2013 and it is now available in the United Kingdom and Republic of Ireland (http://www.dechra.eu/dechra-news.aspx?PID=199&Action=1&Year=2013&NewsId=1299; accessed January 29, 2013).

Immunosuppressive therapy

Corticosteroids are often given as the first treatment in cases of PRCA for humans,[44,51] dogs,[49] and cats.[50] However, relapse is not uncommon (up to 80% in human cases), especially when the medication is tapered after remission.[51] Prednisolone at immunosuppressive doses (2 mg/kg orally every 12–24 hours) have been used in ferrets. In the published case report, no evidence of regeneration (reticulocyte count of 0 cells/μL) was noted after 2 weeks of prednisolone (2 mg/kg orally every 12 hours) therapy alone.[53] Improvement on prednisolone (2 mg/kg orally every 12 hours) was seen in 2 of the 4 cases (Case B and C) seen in the author's practice. Increases in PCV to near normal levels were noted within 4 to 5 weeks. However, relapse of the anemia was seen in 1 of the ferrets (Case B) while the prednisolone was being tapered. A third ferret (Case D) was already on prednisolone (0.75 mg/kg orally every 12 hours) for management of insulinomas when it presented for its anemia, though not at an immunosuppressive dose. In this particular ferret, his initial presentation of anemia was believed to be caused by hyperestrogenism secondary to confirmed hyperadrenocorticism, because the patient had a concurrent thrombocytopenia and its PCV increased from 18% to 51% within 4 weeks after surgery. The ferret's PCV remained in normal ranges until recurrence of the anemia was noted 13 weeks later. This second incidence was believed to be caused by PRCA, because no evidence of hyperestrogenism was noted 2 weeks prior on an adrenal sex hormone panel. Erythroid hypoplasia of the bone marrow was confirmed at necropsy. The PCV of the final ferret (Case A) continued to drop from 18% down to 10% over 2 weeks while receiving prednisolone, but it was most likely receiving a suboptimal dose (1 mg/kg orally every 12 hours) (see **Table 4**).

Because of the high rate of reoccurrence, prednisolone is rarely used alone for the treatment of PRCA. Response to cyclosporine A is considered excellent in humans.[51] In the published ferret case, a regenerative response and improvement in the anemia were noted 2 weeks after the administration of cyclosporine (4 mg/kg orally every 12 hours) as a second immunosuppressive medication.[53] A recurrence of the nonregenerative anemia was noted on day 86 of treatment, approximately 2 weeks after the trough plasma concentration of cyclosporine had decreased. The cyclosporine dosage was increased (6 mg/kg orally every 12 hours), and a significant increase in both reticulocyte number and trough plasma concentration of cyclosporine was noted within 5 days. Administration of both prednisolone and cyclosporine were continued for a total of 14 months, at which point the ferret appeared to be in complete remission and remained in remission for up to 21 months after cessation of all medications.[53]

In the published report, azathioprine (1 mg/kg orally every 24 hours) was initiated when the ferret came out of remission on day 86. However, because azathioprine has delayed immunosuppressive effects, it most likely did not play a role in the ferret's regenerative response and was discontinued after less than a week.[53] Cyclophosphamide, an alkylating agent used to treat various autoimmune conditions and cancer, has been used in dogs[49] and cats[50] for the treatment of PRCA. Although cyclophosphamide is used in chemotherapeutic protocols for lymphoma in ferrets,[64] its use for treatment of PRCA in ferrets has not been documented. Antithymocyte globulin, alemtuzumab, rituximab, and intravenous immunoglobulin have been used in the treatment of acquired PRCA in humans, but their use in veterinary medicine has not been reported.[51] Erythropoietin has been used in cases of canine and feline anemia associated with end-stage renal failure, but it has questionable benefits in patients with normal renal function.[53,65] In addition, the use of erythropoietin has been implicated in some cases of acquired PRCA in other species.[49,52] Although erythropoietin was administered to the ferret in the one published case report, it was not thought to be a factor in that ferret's remission. In other species, erythropoietin is effective only after administration for several weeks, and the ferret had a marked reticulocytosis within 5 days of initiating treatment with erythropoietin. The dosage of the ferret's cyclosporine had been increased at the same time and was thought to be the more likely cause of the regenerative response.[53]

Prognosis

In other species, prognosis depends on the inciting cause of PRCA. In people, cases of secondary PRCA due to medications are often transient and reversible when the medications are discontinued.[44] Most dogs (10 out of 13) responded well to immunosuppressive medications, although initial response to therapy had a median of 38 days (range 22–87 days) and complete remission had a median time of 118 days (range 58–187 days).[49] A rapid response (1.5–5 weeks) was noted in 6 of 7 cats; however, a relapse and/or refractoriness to treatment was noted if the cats were not treated promptly and aggressively with long-term immunosuppressive medication.[50] In addition, cats that develop PRCA after an infection with FeLV subgroup C do not respond to immunosuppressive therapy, and usually succumb to their anemia.[50]

The prognosis in ferrets is unknown because of the paucity of reports, but complete remission has been reported in one ferret treated with multiple blood transfusions and immunosuppressive therapy.[53] In the author's (S.C.) practice, 1 ferret (Case C) responded extremely well to prednisolone alone, had complete remission, and has not had a recurrence of its anemia 1 year later. A partial and short-term response was noted in 1 ferret (Case B), but the nonregenerative anemia returned while in the process of weaning off the prednisolone. It is unknown whether the ferret with concurrent insulinoma and hyperadrenocorticism (Case D) had a delay in the appearance of his PRCA because it was on long-term steroids, albeit not at an immunosuppressive dose. The case in the juvenile ferret (Case A) had no response to immunosuppressive therapy and multiple blood transfusions, which may have been due to suboptimal dosing of the prednisolone (see **Table 4**). Based on these cases, ferrets possibly respond in a similar manner to cats, for which prompt and aggressive long-term immunosuppressive therapy is required to prevent recurrence of erythroblast destruction and refractoriness to medication.

SUMMARY

There are several emerging diseases described in ferrets that occur with unknown frequency or may be overshadowed by those conditions that are more commonly seen. Based on current published data, it is unknown whether these emerging conditions occur sporadically or are increasing in incidence. Being cognizant of these diseases will allow for earlier detection and identification of affected ferrets. In turn, this can lead to more effective and successful treatment of affected patients in clinical practice. Diagnosis and reporting of cases is also crucial in expanding our understanding of these rarer diseases, and will facilitate elucidation of their incidence, etiology, and pathology.

REFERENCES

1. Hirsh D, Biberstein E. Yeast—cryptococcus, malassezia, and candida: veterinary microbiology. 2nd edition. Oxford (United Kingdom): Blackwell Publishing; 2004.
2. Sykes J, Malik R. Cryptococcosis. Infectious diseases of the dog and cat. 4th edition. Philadelphia: WB Saunders; 2011.
3. Franzot SP, Salkin IF, Casadevall A. *Cryptococcus neoformans* var. *grubii*: separate varietal status for *Cryptococcus neoformans* serotype A isolates. J Clin Microbiol 1999;37:838–40.
4. Duncan C, Schwantje H, Stephen C, et al. *Cryptococcus gattii* in wildlife of Vancouver Island, British Columbia, Canada. J Wildl Dis 2006;42:175–8.
5. Mitchell TG, Perfect JR. Cryptococcosis in the era of AIDS—100 years after the discovery of *Cryptococcus neoformans*. Clin Microbiol Rev 1995;8:515–48.
6. Skulski G, Symmers WS. Actinomycosis and torulosis in the ferret (*Mustela furo* L). J Comp Pathol 1954;64:306.
7. Malik R, Alderton B, Finlaison D, et al. Cryptococcosis in ferrets: a diverse spectrum of clinical disease. Aust Vet J 2002;80:749–55.
8. Lewington J. Isolation of *Cryptococcus neoformans* from a ferret. Aust Vet J 2008; 58:124.
9. Greenlee P, Stephens E. Meningeal cryptococcosis and congestive cardiomyopathy in a ferret. J Am Vet Med Assoc 1984;184:840.
10. Hanley CS, MacWilliams P, Giles S, et al. Diagnosis and successful treatment of *Cryptococcus neoformans* variety grubii in a domestic ferret. Can Vet J 2006;47: 1015.
11. Eshar D, Mayer J, Parry NM, et al. Disseminated, histologically confirmed *Cryptococcus* spp infection in a domestic ferret. J Am Vet Med Assoc 2010;236: 770–4.

12. Malik R, Martin P, McGill J, et al. Successful treatment of invasive nasal crypto-coccosis in a ferret. Aust Vet J 2000;78:158–9.
13. Morera N, Juan-Sallés C, Torres JM, et al. *Cryptococcus gattii* infection in a Spanish pet ferret (*Mustela putorius furo*) and asymptomatic carriage in ferrets and humans from its environment. Med Mycol 2011;49:779–84.
14. Ropstad EO, Leiva M, Peña T, et al. *Cryptococcus gattii* chorioretinitis in a ferret. Vet Ophthalmol 2011;14:262–6.
15. Lester SJ, Kowalewich NJ, Bartlett KH, et al. Clinicopathologic features of an unusual outbreak of cryptococcosis in dogs, cats, ferrets, and a bird: 38 cases (January to July 2003). J Am Vet Med Assoc 2004;225:1716–22.
16. Erdman SE, Moore FM, Rose R, et al. Malignant lymphoma in ferrets: clinical and pathological findings in 19 cases. J Comp Pathol 1992;106:37–47.
17. Malik R, McPetrie R, Wigney D, et al. A latex cryptococcal antigen agglutination test for diagnosis and monitoring of therapy for cryptococcosis. Aust Vet J 1996; 74:358–64.
18. Krockenberger M, Canfield P, Kozel T, et al. An immunohistochemical method that differentiates *Cryptococcus neoformans* varieties and serotypes in formalin-fixed paraffin-embedded tissues. Med Mycol 2001;39:523–33.
19. Plumb D. Amphotericin B desoxycholate/amphotericin B lipid-based. In: Plumb D, editor. Veterinary drug handbook. 7th edition. Ames (IA): Wiley-Black-well; 2011. p. 62–7.
20. Plumb D. Flucytosine. In: Plumb D, editor. Veterinary drug handbook. 7th edition. Ames (IA): Worldwide Print Distribution; 2011. p. 432–4.
21. Plumb D. Itraconazole. In: Plumb D, editor. Veterinary drug handbook. 7th edition. Ames (IA): Wiley-Blackwell; 2011. p. 558–61.
22. Plumb D. Fluconazole. In: Plumb D, editor. Veterinary drug handbook. 7th edition. Ames (IA): Wiley-Blackwell; 2011. p. 430–2.
23. CDC. Seasonal influenza: flu basics. Available at: http://www.cdc.gov/flu/about/disease/index.htm. Accessed January 3, 2013.
24. Huang SS, Banner D, Fang Y, et al. Comparative analyses of pandemic H1N1 and seasonal H1N1, H3N2, and influenza B infections depict distinct clinical pictures in ferrets. PLoS One 2011;6:e27512.
25. CDC. Influenza type A viruses and subtypes. In: CDC, editor. 2011. Available at: http://www.cdc.gov/flu/avianflu/influenza-a-virus-subtypes.htm. Accessed January 3, 2013.
26. CDC. 2009-2010 influenza (flu) season. Available at: http://www.cdc.gov/flu/pastseasons/0910season.htm. Accessed January 3, 2013.
27. Schrenzel MD, Tucker TA, Stalis IH, et al. Pandemic (H1N1) 2009 virus in 3 wildlife species, San Diego, California, USA. Emerg Infect Dis 2011;17:747.
28. Campagnolo E, Moll M, Tuhacek K, et al. Concurrent 2009 pandemic influenza A (H1N1) virus infection in ferrets and in a community in Pennsylvania. Zoonoses Public Health 2013;60:117–24.
29. Swenson SL, Koster LG, Jenkins-Moore M, et al. Natural cases of 2009 pandemic H1N1 influenza A virus in pet ferrets. J Vet Diagn Invest 2010;22:784–8.
30. Patterson AR, Cooper VL, Yoon KJ, et al. Naturally occurring influenza infection in a ferret (*Mustela putorius furo*) colony. J Vet Diagn Invest 2009;21: 527–30.
31. Smith W, Stuart-Harris C. Influenza infection of man from the ferret. Lancet 1936; 228:121–3.
32. Govorkova EA, Rehg JE, Krauss S, et al. Lethality to ferrets of H5N1 influenza viruses isolated from humans and poultry in 2004. J Virol 2005;79:2191–8.

33. Jackson S, Van Hoeven N, Chen LM, et al. Reassortment between avian H5N1 and human H3N2 influenza viruses in ferrets: a public health risk assessment. J Virol 2009;83:8131–40.

34. CDC. Influenza A (H3N2) variant virus. Available at: http://www.cdc.gov/flu/swineflu/h3n2v-cases.htm. Accessed January 3, 2013.

35. CDC. Information on avian influenza. Available at: http://www.cdc.gov/flu/avianflu/index.htm. Accessed January 3, 2013.

36. Govorkova EA, Ilyushina NA, Boltz DA, et al. Efficacy of oseltamivir therapy in ferrets inoculated with different clades of H5N1 influenza virus. Antimicrob Agents Chemother 2007;51:1414–24.

37. Pearson R, Gorham J. Viral disease models. In: Fox J, editor. Biology and diseases of the ferret. 2nd edition. Baltimore (MD): Lippincott Williams & Wilkins; 1998. p. 487–97.

38. Wagner R. Hypothyroidism in ferrets. Association of Exotic Mammal Veterinarians 11th Annual Conference. Oakland (CA), October 25, 2012. p. 29–31.

39. Scott-Moncrieff JC. Hypothyroidism. In: Ettinger SJ, editor. Textbook of Veterinary Internal Medicine. Elsevier; 2004. p. 1535–44.

40. Rand JS, Levine J, Best SJ, et al. Spontaneous adult-onset hypothyroidism in a cat. J Vet Intern Med 1993;7:272–6.

41. Heard D, Collins B, Chen D, et al. Thyroid and adrenal function tests in adult male ferrets. Am J Vet Res 1990;51:32–5.

42. Mayer J. Use of recombinant human TSH hormone for a thyrotropin stimulation test in euthyroid ferrets. Association of Exotic Mammal Veterinarians 11th Annual Conference. Oakland (CA), October 25, 2012.

43. Weiss DJ, Tvedten H. Erythrocyte disorders. In: Willard MD, Tvedten H, editors. Small animal clinical diagnosis by laboratory methods. 5th edition. St Louis (MO): Elsevier Saunders; 2012. p. 38–62.

44. Perkins SL. Pediatric red cell disorders and pure red cell aplasia. Am J Clin Pathol 2004;122:S70–86.

45. Ball S. Diamond Blackfan anemia. Hematology Am Soc Hematol Educ Program 2011;2011:487–91.

46. Moore A, Day M, Graham M. Congenital pure red blood cell aplasia (Diamond-Blackfan anaemia) in a dog. Vet Rec 1993;132:414.

47. Stokol T, Blue JT, French TW. Idiopathic pure red cell aplasia and nonregenerative immune-mediated anemia in dogs: 43 cases (1988-1999). J Am Vet Med Assoc 2000;216:1429–36.

48. Weiss DJ. Bone marrow pathology in dogs and cats with non-regenerative immune-mediated haemolytic anaemia and pure red cell aplasia. J Comp Pathol 2008;138:46–53.

49. Weiss DJ. Primary pure red cell aplasia in dogs: 13 cases (1996-2000). J Am Vet Med Assoc 2002;221:93–5.

50. Stokol T, Blue J. Pure red cell aplasia in cats: 9 cases (1989-1997). J Am Vet Med Assoc 1999;214:75.

51. Sawada K, Fujishima N, Hirokawa M. Acquired pure red cell aplasia: updated review of treatment. Br J Haematol 2008;142:505–14.

52. Randolph JE, Scarlett J, Stokol T, et al. Clinical efficacy and safety of recombinant canine erythropoietin in dogs with anemia of chronic renal failure and dogs with recombinant human erythropoietin-induced red cell aplasia. J Vet Intern Med 2004;18:81–91.

53. Malka S, Hawkins MG, Zabolotzky SM, et al. Immune-mediated pure red cell aplasia in a domestic ferret. J Am Vet Med Assoc 2010;237:695–700.

54. Morrisey JK, Kraus MS. Cardiovascular and other diseases. In: Quesenberry KE, Carpenter JW, editors. Ferrets, rabbits, and rodents: clinical medicine and surgery. 3rd edition. St Louis (MO): Elsevier Saunders; 2012. p. 62–77.

55. Chen S. Advanced diagnostic approaches and current medical management of insulinomas and adrenocortical disease in ferrets (*Mustela putorius furo*). Vet Clin North Am Exot Anim Pract 2010;13:439–52.

56. Grindem CB, Neel JA, Juopperi TA. Cytology of bone marrow. Vet Clin North Am Small Anim Pract 2002;32:1313–74.

57. Morrisey J, Ramer J. Ferrets. Clinical pathology and sample collection. Vet Clin North Am Exot Anim Pract 1999;2:553.

58. Williams BH. Disorders of rabbit and ferret bone marrow. In: Fudge AM, editor. Laboratory medicine - avian and exotic pets. Philadelphia: W.B. Saunders Company; 2000. p. 276–84.

59. Manning D, Bell J. Lack of detectable blood groups in domestic ferrets: implications for transfusion. J Am Vet Med Assoc 1990;197:84.

60. Plumb D. Diphenhydramine HCl. In: Plumb D, editor. Veterinary drug handbook. 7th edition. Ames (IA): Wiley-Blackwell; 2011. p. 338–40.

61. Marini R, Callahan R, Jackson L, et al. Distribution of technetium 99m-labeled red blood cells during isoflurane anesthesia in ferrets. Am J Vet Res 1997;58:781.

62. Lichtenberger M. Transfusion medicine in exotic pets. Clin Tech Small Anim Pract 2004;19:88–95.

63. Plumb D. Hemoglobin glutamer-200 (Bovine). In: Plumb D, editor. Veterinary drug handbook. 7th edition. Ames (IA): Wiley-Blackwell; 2005. p. 492–4.

64. Antinoff N, Williams BH. Neoplasia. In: Quesenberry KE, Carpenter JW, editors. Ferrets, rabbits, and rodents: clinical medicine and surgery. 3rd edition. St Louis (MO): Elsevier Saunders; 2012. p. 103–21.

65. Plumb D. Epoetin alfa, epoetin beta, erythropoietin, EPO, r-HuEPO. In: Plumb D, editor. Veterinary drug handbook. 7th edition. Ames (IA): Wiley-Blackwell; 2011. p. 384–6.

Index

Note: Page numbers of article titles are in **boldface** type.

Vet Clin Exot Anim 16 (2013) 495–521
http://dx.doi.org/10.1016/S1094-9194(13)00030-3
1094-9194/13/$ – see front matter © 2013 Elsevier Inc. All rights reserved.

Moving?

Make sure your subscription moves with you!

To notify us of your new address, find your **Clinics Account Number** (located on your mailing label above your name), and contact customer service at:

Email: journalscustomerservice-usa@elsevier.com

800-654-2452 (subscribers in the U.S. & Canada)
314-447-8871 (subscribers outside of the U.S. & Canada)

Fax number: 314-447-8029

Elsevier Health Sciences Division
Subscription Customer Service
3251 Riverport Lane
Maryland Heights, MO 63043

*To ensure uninterrupted delivery of your subscription, please notify us at least 4 weeks in advance of move.

Printed and bound by CPI Group (UK) Ltd, Croydon, CR0 4YY

13/10/2024

01773499-0002